Routledge Revivals

Midwives in History and Society

Originally published in 1986, this book examines the history of midwifery, concentrating on 19th and 20th Century Britain. It shows how the evolution of the midwife has been influenced by cultural waves which started in the Near East and Egypt in pre-classical times and slowly spread Northwards and Eastwards over Europe. The authors emphasize the effects of specialization and professionalization upon midwifery and also the influence of male authority and interest group politics. The evolution of the educated qualified midwife of the 20th Century is recorded, leading up to the ongoing debates about high technology birth vis-à-vis natural birth and home deliveries.

Midwives in History and Society

Jean Towler and Joan Bramall

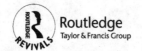
Routledge
Taylor & Francis Group

First published in Great Britain in 1986 by Croom Helm Ltd

This edition first published in 2023 by Routledge
4 Park Square, Milton Park, Abingdon, Oxon, OX14 4RN
and by Routledge
605 Third Avenue, New York, NY 10158

Routledge is an imprint of the Taylor & Francis Group, an informa business

© 1986 Jean Towler and Joan Bramall.

ISBN 13: 978-1-032-45658-4 (hbk)
ISBN 13: 978-1-003-37810-5 (ebk)
ISBN 13: 978-1-032-45663-8 (pbk)
Book DOI 10.4324/978100378105

Midwives in History and Society

Jean Towler, BA, SRN, SCM, MTD
and
Joan Bramall, BA, SRN, SCM

CROOM HELM
London   New York

First published in 1986 by
Croom Helm Ltd
11 New Fetter Lane, London EC4P 4EE
Pubished in the USA by
Croom Helm
29 West 35th Street, New York NY10001
Croom Helm Australia
44–50 Waterloo Road, North Ryde 2113,
New South Wales
Reprinted 1988

Printed in Great Britain by
Biddles Ltd, Guildford and King's Lynn

ISBN 0 7099 2453 4

British Library Cataloguing in Publication Data

Towler, Jean
    Midwives in history and society.
    1. Obstetrics—History
    I. Title   II. Bramall, Joan
    610.73′678′09   RG950

    ISBN 0–7099–2453–4

Library of Congress Cataloging in Publication Data

Towler, Jean
    Midwives in History and Society.
    Includes Index.
    1. Midwives — History. I. Bramall, Joan, 1922-
    II. Title (DNLM: 1. Midwifery — History. WQ 11.1 T742M)
    RG950.T69 1986   362.1′9820233   85-26508
    ISBN 0-7099-2453-4 (Pbk.)

CONTENTS

FOREWORD

The occupation of a midwife is one of the earliest specialised crafts to emerge in any society; it has affected all our lives and the lives of our ancestors. Yet apart from textbooks and technical publications, very little has been written about it and hardly anything at all by midwives themselves.

Miss Jean Towler, a distinguished midwife teacher and experienced practitioner of her profession, has devoted several years of patient research to this history. Miss Towler has been assisted in the writing by Miss Joan Bramall, whose experience includes 28 years' midwifery practice as well as a degree in English.

This book will be of great interest to midwives and other health professionals, and for the general reader will make a fascinating contribution to our social history. It is particularly appropriate that at this time of implementation of EEC Directives on midwives there should be a historical perspective to help in understanding the development of our midwifery service.

R.J. Fenney CBE
former Secretary,
Central Midwives Board

PREFACE

Midwifery ranks among the oldest professions in the world but it has also been one of the most maligned. The social and clinical status of Greek midwives *c.* 500 BC was high, but in the Dark Ages in Western Europe, midwives occupied a humble, often despised, position. This relegation could be attributed to the low status of women generally and to their exclusion from learning. Religious dogma of these times opposed both formal medicine and secular education; consequently there were few doctors, and these few, being men, were totally unconcerned with the biological events of pregnancy and birth. To aid women in childbirth, self-appointed midwives, often classed as witches and outlawed by the Church, experimented with herbal remedies and became the unofficial healers of the peasant subcultures.

By the fourteenth century, physicians, qualified at universities and reluctantly approved by the Church, systematically began to shake the faith of the people in the traditional 'old wives' and their remedies, and thus gradually assumed authority and power.

By the turn of the nineteenth century, the medical profession, now exclusively male, became highly organised and attempted to take over midwifery, thereby rendering obsolete the traditional female midwife. Some women, aware of the potential demise of the midwife, recognised that she too must become politically and professionally organised, and above all educated. Women fought a long battle to this end.

Twentieth-century medical science has provided diagnostic tools and monitoring equipment to aid those mothers with complicated pregnancies, but this technology has been indiscriminately applied. The physical needs of mothers may have been met but the psychological needs have not. The medical take-over of childbirth, with its emphasis on hospitalisation, pathology and unemotional science and technology, has resulted in the midwifery profession again being threatened with extinction.

Doctor-domination and male characteristics can significantly change the nature of childbirth, turning it into a mechanistic exercise. Midwifery rightly belongs to a woman's world where instinct, intuition and emotion as well as clinical competence and theoretical knowledge play their parts. In terms of everyday care, it remains the midwife who provides holistic care, which can transform pregnancy, labour and early post-partum days from a traumatic and negative experience to a positive and rewarding achievement. Midwives have an obligation to womankind to provide an ambience that facilitates a safe and satisfying birth experience.

Role changes creep into a profession and tend to go unnoticed by the individual rank-and-file midwife until a point of no return is reached. Some midwives have in fact opted out and are content to be doctor's assistants: in this respect the greatest threat to the future of the midwife may come from the midwife herself. It is up to midwives, both individually and collectively, to ensure that they do not lose the position won by the midwife pioneers of the past.

J.T.
J.B.

ACKNOWLEDGEMENTS

During the many years of research necessary for the compilation of this book we have encountered many helpful people. In particular we would like to thank Mr R.J. Fenney, former Secretary of the Central Midwives Board, for his support and encouragement. We are grateful to him and to Miss I. Ward and other Board Officers for allowing free access to CMB documents, reports and minute books, and for making available other relevant books and papers.

We are fortunate to have, within the University of Manchester John Rylands Library, the Radford Collection of historical midwifery and obstetric manuscripts and texts, and we would like to thank Mr D. Cook and Miss P. Cummings, Medical Librarians, for permission to read and extract from this invaluable collection of source material.

We are indebted to interested friends and colleagues for providing historical records, papers and photographs of some of the first Maternity Hospital and Midwifery Training Schools, for loaning original copies of old books, and for providing primary source material relating to some of our midwife predecessors. Among others we would like to thank: Margaret Adams, Queen Charlotte's Hospital, London; Margaret Aynsley, Newcastle General Hospital Maternity Unit; Beryl Davidson, The Jessop Hospital, Sheffield; Eileen Fisher, Princess Anne Maternity Unit, Bolton; Mary Waites, Fairfield Maternity Unit, Bury; and Janet Williams, Liverpool Maternity Hospital. Material relating to St. Mary's Hospital, Manchester, was collected by kind permission of Mrs Jean Fowler, Hospital Administrator.

Our thanks are extended to the following copyright holders for their courtesy in granting permission to reproduce pictures or quote extracts from texts:
Barbara Balch, Director of Professional Affairs, Royal College of Midwives, for a photograph of members of the Midwives Institute 1881; the Israel Department of Antiquities and Museums, Ministry of Education and Culture, Jerusalem, for Ashtoret (Astarte); Egyptian Museum, Ministry of Culture Antiquities Organisation, Cairo for Thoueris; Paul Popper, London, for the rock drawing of a woman giving birth from *Prehistoric Mythology, New Larousse Encyclopaedia of Mythology*; The Wellcome Institute Library, London, for photographs from the 1724 edition of *The Compleat Midwife's Companion* by Jane Sharp, and for

the reproduction of the *Mid-wives Just Petition*, also for the portraits of Agnodike and *Elizabeth Nihell*, from *Biographie des Sages-Femmes Célèbres, Anciennes, Modernes et Contemporaires*, P.A. Delacoux, Paris, 1834, for the title page from *The Byrth of Mankynd*, and for diagrams from Rueff's *Ein schön lustig Trostbuchle*; the Arts Library, University of Manchester, for the title page of *The Rosengarten*; Barry Feldman for a photograph of the birthing chair which he designed; Independent Photography Project, Woolwich, London for the photograph of Alice Gregory; the City of Manchester Cultural Services Department for the Certificate in Monthly Nursing, and the Kendal Records Office for permission to handle, extract from and reproduce a page from the anonymous midwife's diary. The picture of Birth EZ Birthing Chair is reproduced from the catalogue of the Century Manufacturing Company, Nebraska, USA. Oxford University Press gave permission to include the extract from *Lark Rise to Candleford* and The Open University granted permission for the inclusion of extracts from their publications. The Kawabata Press, Torpoint, Devon, authorised reproduction of the photograph of midwife Caroline Tarplee from *The Cropthorne Camera of Minnie Holland*. Leonardo da Vinci's 'fetus *in utero*' is reproduced by gracious permission of Her Majesty the Queen.

Mr Ron Murray and his staff of the Department of Medical Illustrations at the University Hospital of South Manchester have been particularly painstaking and unfailingly helpful, and we would like to record our thanks to him for photographs from books outside the copyright period, where not otherwise acknowledged.

Our special thanks go to our long-suffering friends and families, who have inevitably been somewhat neglected. We feel, however, that any personal deprivation has been more than compensated for by the pleasure we have derived from researching and recording the history of midwives and the midwifery profession, to which we are proud to belong. We trust that there is much more of the midwife's story still to be told.

1 IN THE BEGINNING . . .

Everyone is a miracle in miniature with a personal history linked with the history of men and women who lived, loved and gave birth to others since ever there were men and women.[1]

It seems fairly well established that the human species proper in the form of *Homo sapiens* emerged between 250 000 and 200 000 years ago, so that in terms of age man is a relative newcomer to the planet. In the preceding 2 million years his immediate predecessor *Homo erectus* was to be found primarily in Asia, but remains of this species have also been found in Africa and Europe.[2]

Paleolithic or early Stone Age man lived between 50 000 and 9 000 BC and has left some traces of his mode of life and physical characteristics. From cave murals and from fertility symbols of these times it is apparent that the women were of generous proportions, suggesting that they had adequate gynaecoid pelves (Figure 1).

Until about 9 000 BC *Homo sapiens* lived by hunting wild game such as deer and bison, by fishing, and by the gathering of fruit, nuts, seeds and honey. Early man experienced extremes of cold and heat, drought and flood,[2] but managed to adapt, survive and reproduce. It is perhaps reasonable to assume that in this nomadic cave-dwelling society the man spent frequent periods away from home in his pursuit of food whereas the woman did the foraging. With such hard environmental circumstances and spartan lifestyle to contend with, only those women capable of natural parturition could both successfully deliver a child and survive. At this time, pregnancy would be an accepted biological event of unknown duration and it seems quite likely that the woman delivered herself in the squatting position or with her buttocks or knees supported by boulders. She would separate herself from the baby by cutting the umbilical cord with a sharp flintstone, or by biting through it with her teeth, and she would instinctively suckle the baby. It is likely that she found some means of attaching the baby to her body (perhaps in a sling made from animal skin) for warmth and comfort, and by this means she could take the baby with her when she resumed her search for food. In some remote regions of the world there are still cave-dwellers today, and in some cultures and tribes (almost untouched by modern civilisation) there has been little change from the unsophisticated childbirth practices of very early times.

Figure 1: Rock Drawing of a Child's Birth with Sabaean Graffito

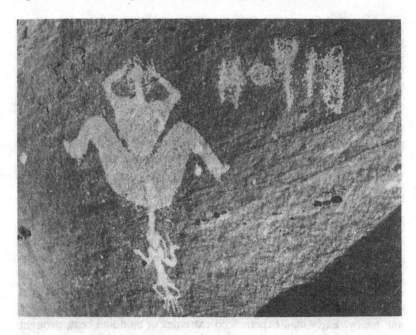

Source: Popperfoto, London.

Wives of the Kalahari Bushmen, the last surviving pygmies, still today give birth in a squatting position.[3]

Paleolithic nomadic hunting people would at times be compelled to go on very long journeys in pursuit of migrating prey. Shortage of food and the burden of carrying dependants meant that some babies and children would die or be abandoned or even killed *en route*. An excess of girls was regarded as a great misfortune, whereas boys, with their hunting potential, were preferred to females. It was essential for survival that babies should be breast fed for a considerable period of time, and long lactation contributed to some extent to population control. By 40 000 BC in favourable areas such as around the Mediterranean, bands of men, women and children were moving together in large groups. As man-and-woman units joined together to form more effective hunting teams, it is conceivable that the man remained with his wife and perhaps assisted with the birth.

A complete change in the way of life started towards the end of the last Ice Age (the Neolithic period). Some time between 10 000 and 8000 BC, favourable climatic conditions developed in certain areas that facilitated the evolution of an agricultural way of life. The most favoured area was the Fertile Crescent, the half-circle of plains and foothills bounded by the Zagros mountains to the East and by the ranges of the Taurus, Amanus and the Lebanon in the North and West. Within these boundaries now lie south-east Turkey and parts of Syria and Iraq. Gradually, by cultivation of the land, wanderers were able to settle. They made primitive dwellings in village compounds, and domesticated and bred animals to provide themselves with food and dairy produce. The animals were also used for farming as beasts of burden. It has been estimated that around the dawn of the agricultural era there were only between 2 and 10 million people on the whole of the Earth.[4] As agriculture developed and spread, and the strains and variety of crops improved, more people could be supported in one location. More babies and children survived, and as larger family groups were formed, so villages increased in number, size and complexity. Artefacts were produced, and local clay was used for brick making.[5] As man adapted to new environments, so towns and cities sprang up in many different locations. It is known that Catal Huyuk in Turkey was a flourishing city in 6000 BC, and remains of a clay statue from its ruins show a mother giving birth in a squatting position.[6] Jericho was already a large and thriving agricultural settlement.

During this period of increasing social organisation, elderly women, at first from within the family and then from within the community, replaced the men as attendants at birth. These 'experienced women' came to fulfil the role of midwife. Once they assumed the right to this office, they retained it, to the exclusion of men, for at least the next 10 000 years. In these pre-literate societies, empirical knowledge, such as there was, would be passed on by word of mouth, and practical skills would be acquired from observation and experience and in some cases from an inherent, instinctive aptitude.

Clay and terracotta figures found in the Fertile Crescent show women in the crouching and kneeling positions when giving birth, and similar figures have been found which date back into the Old Stone Age. In his 1882 study, *Labour among Primitive Peoples*[7] (of both pre-historic primitives and contemporary primitives), Englemann found that almost every conceivable position was used. It can therefore be assumed that women in the Neolithic period would give birth kneeling, squatting, sitting, standing or recumbent. The mode of giving birth in those times would to some extent limit the involvement of the 'midwife' to a *passive* role in the actual act of delivery but she would at least assist by receiving the baby. She would perhaps sever the umbilical cord by the use of a flint stone or by chewing through it with her own teeth. This latter practice has been observed among the Masai people of Kenya recently.[8] From very early times primitive men practised *couvade* (identification of the man with his pregnant mate), expressed by writhing with ostensible pain and moaning while the woman was in labour, and then taking upon himself the role of the lying-in mother just as though he had himself given birth.[9] Such a custom is practised today among the Basque people in Europe today.

As the ancient civilisations evolved through the centuries and society became more structured, so people began to develop trades and skills such as herding, carpentry, weaving, and building using bricks, stone and wood, and it is conceivable that the 'experienced woman' would come to care professionally for other women in disease and sickness as well as in childbirth.

Man's Instinct to Worship

It is not surprising that *Homo sapiens*, dependent as he was on nature, evolved deities to worship from natural forms and elemental forces. Because he did not understand the laws of the Universe, his world was full of magical influences and mysterious spirits which were mainly to be feared and propitiated. Gradually his imagination inspired him to create hundreds of gods to worship, each having a particular sphere of influence such as hunting or fertility, which were the most essential elements for survival.

References

1. Graham, H. *Eternal Eve* (Hutchinson, London, 1960).
2. Barraclough, G. (ed.) *The Times Atlas of World History* (Times Books, London, 1978).
3. van der Post, L. *Testament to the Bushmen* (Viking, New York, 1984).
4. Cipolla, C. *The Economic History of World Population* (Pelican, Harmondsworth, 1978).
5. Bronowski, J. *The Ascent of Man* (BBC Books, London, 1973).
6. Balaskas, A. and J. *New Life* (Sidgwick & Jackson, London, 1979).
7. Englemann, G.J. *Labour among Primitive Peoples* (J.H. Chambers, St. Louis, 1882).
8. MacLaine, S. *Don't Fall off the Mountain* (W.C. Norton, New York; Bantam edn, London, 1971).
9. Meltzer, D. *Birth. An Anthology of Ancient Texts, Songs, Prayers and Stories* (Northpoint Press, San Francisco, 1981).

Further Reading

Napier, J. *The Roots of Mankind. The Story of Man and His Ancestors* (Allen & Unwin, London, 1971)

2 MIDWIVES IN EARLY HISTORY

The Biblical Era

Peoples of the Biblical era included the Hittites, the Assyrians, the Babylonians and those who were later called Israelites. For all these peoples the bull symbolised male fertility and creativity, and was therefore revered and worshipped. The goddess of female fertility was Astarte (Ashtoret), a human form with hands symbolically placed under life-giving breasts (see Figure 2).

Such deities were forbidden to Israelites after the manifestation of Jehovah, but in fact polytheism, magic, witchcraft and superstition co-existed alongside the new monotheistic religion with its abstract God. There is evidence that, in times of doubt and stress, influenced by ancient habits, the Israelites reverted to overt idol worship, as when Aaron fashioned the golden calf.[1]

One of the first written references to midwives appears in the first book of the Old Testament within the story of the birth of Benjamin in approximately 1800 BC: 'and when they were some distance from Ephrath, the midwife said to her "Fear not, for now you will have another son" '. Presumably the midwife made a vaginal examination and was able to define the sex while discovering the breech presentation. 'And as her (Rachel's) soul was departing, for she died, she called his name Nenoni, but his father called him Benjamin.'[2] Perhaps this is the first recorded maternal death.

Midwives, recognised as skilful and valued professionals, appear in two more Biblical stories. The unusual case of the birth of Tamar's twins is one such story. This event took place approximately 1700 years BC

When the time for her delivery came, there were twins in her womb. And when she was in labour, one put out a hand; and the midwife took and bound on his hand a scarlet thread, saying 'this came out first'. But as he drew back his hand and behold his brother came out; and she said 'what a breach you have made for yourself'. Therefore his name was called Perez meaning 'come forth'. Afterwards his brother came out with the scarlet thread upon his hand and his name was called Zerah meaning 'to rise, shine or come forth'.[3]

It is evident from this passage that the midwife was present and active

6

Figure 2: Astarte (Ashoret)

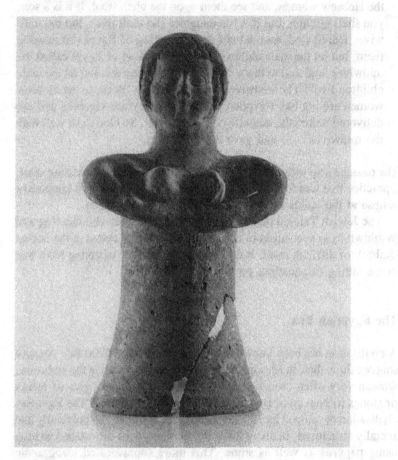

Source: Department of Antiquities and Museums, Ministry of Education and Culture, State of Israel.

during the labour and aware of the twin pregnancy, and was able to deal with a compound presentation. The survival of both the babies may indicate that competence of the midwife, in that she knew better than to pull on the prolapsed arm or to amputate it.

From the following passage it might be inferred that in this society (c. 1600 BC) midwives were not the old women of the tribe but women of childbearing years (unless, like Sarah, they conceived in old age):[4]

The King of Egypt said to the Hebrew midwives, one of whom was called Shiprah and the other Puah, 'when you serve as midwife to the Hebrew women, and see them upon the birth stool, if it is a son, you shall kill him, but if it is a daughter she shall live'. But the midwives feared God, and did not do as the King of Egypt commanded them, but let the male children live. So the King of Egypt called the midwives, and said to them 'Why have you done this and let the male children live?' The midwives said to Pharaoh 'Because the Hebrew women are not like Egyptian women; for they are vigorous and are delivered before the midwife comes to them'. So God dealt well with the midwives . . . and gave them families.[5]

The passage also includes the first reference to the use of a birthing stool, a practice that was to continue for some 3300 years, suffer a temporary eclipse at the hands of men and be revived in the 1980s.

The Jewish Talmud makes numerous references to childbearing and to midwives as specialists in normal birth who only called in the doctor (Rabbi) for difficult cases. It mentions that the mode of giving birth was in the sitting or squatting position.

The Egyptian Era

A civilisation has been known to exist in Egypt from 2700 BC. Ancient sources show that, in Mesopotamia and Egypt, and among the Hebrews, women very often crouched down in childbirth upon a pair of bricks or stones (o'*b*nayun of Exodus i 16) or on a birth stool.[6] The Egyptian civilisation developed into an advanced culture which was politically and socially structured. In about 2000 BC the Egyptians introduced writing using papyrus as well as stone. This more sophisticated ideographic writing superseded the earlier method of pictographic communication which had been expressed on stone. The Egyptian word *msi'*, 'to give birth', was often followed by the hieroglyph of a crouching woman in the act of birth, and in one late text the figure is actually shown crouching on two bricks or stones.[7]

The Egyptian people, even before the flowering of their civilisation, had invented the wheel, the plough and the sail. This elementary technology, together with their relative immunity from invasion because of their favoured geographical position, enabled them to advance their culture both artistically and academically. Medicine became a skill and profession with a basis of facts recorded on papyri. Despite the science and technology of this progressive society, religion and superstition remained as major forces, and a multiplicity of gods were invoked for help in daily living, which would of course include childbirth.

Among some ancient Egyptian papyri that are preserved in Leipzig University Library is the Ebers papyrus, which is dated not later than 1550 BC and possibly as early as 1900 BC.

Five columns of this papyrus deal with obstetrics and gynaecology. The obstetric rules and prescriptions relate to the acceleration of parturition . . . and to the birth prognosis of the newborn child, which depends upon the nature of its first cries and the way of holding its head.[8]

It is clear that in this culture midwifery was a recognised female occupation, with midwives attending normal deliveries including royal births. Bas reliefs in the royal birth rooms at Luxor and in other temples portray such events. One shows a queen in labour on an obstetric chair with four midwives in attendance, and another depicts a queen, assisted by five women, squatting to give birth. It is fortunate that some of the art of the Egyptians has survived since it serves to give insight into their way of life.

Even in the portrayals of Birth and the Lying-in Houses, which adorn the walls of the ancient Egyptian temples, it is interesting to note that the medical male gods (of which the Egyptians possessed many) are never included, whilst there are many representations of the goddess Isis, who was recognised as the goddess of birth.[8]

The Westcar papyrus, dated 1700 BC, includes instructions for calculating the expected date of confinement, and describes the use of both simple and sophisticated types of birth chairs.[8]

The Egyptians probably had considerable knowledge of drugs: 'for the fertile soil of Egypt is most rich in herbs, many of which are wholesome in solution'. Homer says that Helen of Troy was given a supply of many useful drugs, one of which was a powerful anodyne with which to assuage pain. An Egyptian lady, Polydamna, gave them to her.[9] Cleopatra is said to have been interested in drugs, both therapeutic and poisonous, and to have possessed great skill in their use.[10]

The early civilisations of the Middle East, India, Egypt and Persia gradually came to a realisation of the immense natural forces that governed their universe and controlled their way of life, and they consequently created gods and goddesses who represented the elements and became

Figure 3: Thoueris, an Egyptian Goddess of Fertility

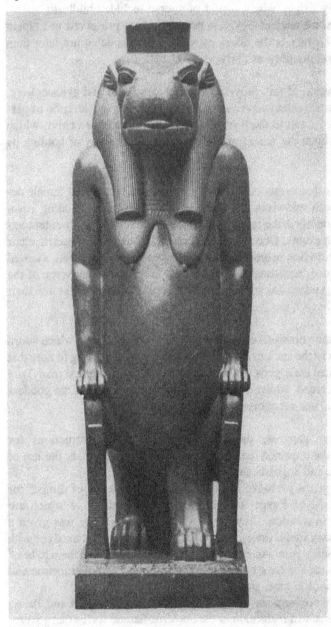

Source: Egyptian Museum, Ministry of Culture Antiquities Organisation, Egypt.

the major objects of their worship. The worship of minor deities, symbolised by idols of stone, gold and silver, continued, but slowly these creature idols came to take on some human characteristics of shape and form. These can be seen in Thoueris, an Egyptian goddess of fertility and safe childbearing, whose representation is part woman and part hippopotamus (Figure 3); and also in Hathor, an Egyptian goddess of love and childbirth depicted with human body but with a head bearing a pair of cow's horns. Other Egyptian goddesses of childbirth were Heket, a primitive frog-goddess who was thought to be one of the midwives who assisted every morning at the birth of the Sun, and Meskhent, who personified the two bricks on which some Egyptian mothers crouched for delivery. Sometimes Meskhent is portrayed in the form of one of these bricks, terminated by a human head. Midwives and labouring women would without doubt seek help from Thoueris, Hathor and Meskhent and other appropriate deities for safe deliverance.[11]

There is evidence of an Aryan Indian urban civilisation in the Indus Valley dating back to 2000 BC. It is known that prior to this time there was a village-based system of life and religion known as the Dravidian culture. It appears that these people had no understanding of the facts of human reproduction, not even of the connection between sexual intercourse and conception.[12] The Aryan polytheistic culture produced the *Vedas* or Sacred Books. A second group of Sacred Books, the *Upavedas*, included one written by Charaka who, it is thought, was the Court Physician to the King of Peshawar. Although written in the first century AD, it is accepted that this medical text probably reflects the obstetric practices of the earlier Aryan civilisation. It would appear that 'midwives' undertook *normal* deliveries and were instructed to call for the physician in the event of complications.[13]

Anahita (Anaitis) was the goddess of water, fecundity and procreation in the Persian civilisation of the ninth century BC. She is depicted as of entirely human form.[11]

The Greek Period

Greece became the centre of the first great European civilisation, and the influence of this advanced culture with its philosophers, scientists, lawyers, writers, artists, doctors and architects still pervades Europe and the Western world. By 800 BC an entirely anthropomorphic conception of gods was established, and the Greeks' representation of these gods was as magnificent human figures. Some gods, such as Neptune, personified the elements; others personified human qualities such as wisdom and love. All the gods were conceived to have supernatural powers while at the same time they behaved in an entirely human fashion, indulging in hate and jealousy as well as love. Greeks of this classical era were humanists, believing pre-eminently in man and in his unbounded ability in every dimension of life. They strived for physical perfection and for supreme qualities of the mind, and they sought to resolve fundamental issues about every aspect of life. Beauty was a passion and was enduringly demonstrated in Greek architecture and sculpture. The Greeks had an abundance of material goods such as marble, ivory, wood, precious metals and stones from which to create temples and artefacts of outstanding magnificence. Their philosophy of living and enjoying life to the full seemed to overshadow thoughts of death or life after death. They rather brought their enquiring minds to bear on social and political systems, and on the physique and physiology of the human body. The basic principles of Greek medicine and also of midwifery were derived from the Egyptian body of knowledge. However, even in this age in which the art of midwifery appeared highly developed, and midwives and doctors were clinically skilled practitioners, the Greeks made very little contribution to obstetrics.

Hippocrates, Aristotle and other philosophers wrote about pregnancy and its duration and about how to predict the sex of the unborn baby. Hippocrates believed that if the fetus were male, the mother's right eye would be brighter and her right breast would be bigger, and vice versa for a female.[14] He advised that malpresentations of the fetus be reduced to the 'natural' presentation and he regarded footling presentation as both unnatural and 'dangerous'. He also taught that the fetus had to fight its way out of the womb, breaking the membranes in its struggle. Consequently, difficult labour, he argued, was due to failure of the child to force its way out.[15] These writings were both speculative and unscientific, but at the time were regarded as authoritative.

In the time of Hippocrates and Socrates (*c.* 500 BC) midwives had social recognition and were an honoured class. Phainarete, the mother of Socrates, was herself a midwife. Under the Law of Athens it was a condition that a midwife be a mother and past the age of childbearing. Midwives at this time were divided into two grades, those of superior skill and experience, who were consulted in the case of abnormal and difficult labours, and those who assisted at normal births only. In addition the midwife on occasion called in either a male or a female doctor who would, when required, perform internal version followed by jaw flexion and shoulder traction to deliver the head in a breech presentation.[13]

Figure 4: Agnodike, 'the Midwife of Athens'

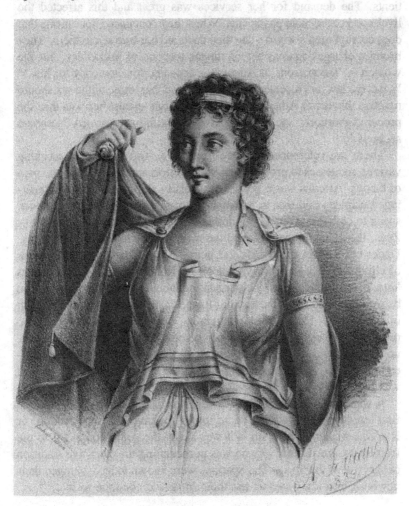

Source: The Wellcome Institute Library, London.

During the next two centuries it would appear that attitudes to women as healers and midwives changed radically, so much so that around 300 BC Agnodike (Figure 4), known as 'the Midwife of Athens', was put on trial for practising under false pretences. Agnodike, aware of women's modesty and their strong objection to being exposed 'to the hands of men', disguised herself as a man and studied midwifery under Herophilus, a famous physician and anatomist of Athens. She practised under the guise of a male although she revealed her identity to her patients. The demand for her services was great and this affected the livelihood of the male physicians. When they denounced her 'as one that does corrupt men's wives', she then declared her true sex to them. They brought charges against her of illegal practice of midwifery, but the women — 'the matrons of Athens' — appealed for clemency for her.[16] In fact the lawyers repealed the law and ruled that 'three of the sex should practise this art in Athens'.[17] Another charge against her was that she procured abortions. She is said to have successfully performed Caesarean sections.[18]

There are references to Greek midwives and mothers beseeching various goddesses to protect them in childbirth and help relieve the pain of labour. Artemis was a goddess especially associated with childbearing. Euripides said that in her capacity of midwife she would not even speak to childless women.[19] Another goddess was Hera, the consort of Zeus, the father of the gods and the major figure in Greek mythology. Under her Roman name of Juno Lucina she was known as the goddess of childbirth and was the symbol of the Roman matron. The cry was '*Juno Lucina, ser opem*' (help assist the labour).[16] Holding a newborn baby in one hand she is the familiar figure on the hat badge of the English midwife today. Hera had two daughters, both known as Ilithyias, who presided over birth: 'no child could be born unless they were present, no mother could find relief without them; the two Ilithyias finally merged as a single person. She is often depicted kneeling, a position which was believed to aid delivery . . .'[11]

It was the Greek custom for a father to inspect his child during the first ten days after its birth. If he found any physical imperfection, or if it was weakly, and often if it was a girl, he could commit it to die from exposure. In this way he was perpetuating the primitive tradition of survival of the fittest. The Spartans were known to have plunged their newborn into icy water to test their fitness to continue to live.[20]

The Roman Era

In about 500 BC the Greek civilisation reached its zenith, and during its decline the foundations of a Roman civilisation were being laid. As a result of traffic in trade and people, an enormous variety of goods and ideas were exchanged and as a result a Graeco-Roman style of life developed. The Romans also had their gods and goddesses, many of whom had a particular sphere and role. Egeria, one of Diana's water nymphs, discharged one of Diana's functions, that of succouring women in childbirth.

The Roman influence and power spread first throughout Italy and gradually throughout Europe, North Africa and the Near East, and lasted as an Empire until the fifth century AD. The regions colonised by the Romans benefited from their civil and military technology, in that the construction of roads, water systems, aqueducts and baths followed the invasion and occupation by Roman armies, as did the imposition of the Roman legal and monetary systems, which were to leave an enduring legacy.

Just as knowledge passed from the Egyptians to the Greeks, so in turn it passed from the Greeks to the Romans. Inevitably, midwifery practice would be inherited in the same way. Although little is known about Roman midwives, it can be assumed that by the Christian era midwifery was a well-established profession that required literate practitioners.

A Textbook for Midwives

The first notable physician of the Roman period was Soranus who lived at the beginning of the second century in the reign of the Emperors Trajan and Hadrian. He was a distinguished writer on obstetrics and gynaecology. One of his books, originally written in Greek but more familiarly known by the Latin title of *De Morbis Mulierium*, was the first textbook ever to be written for midwives. In it Soranus states that literacy is an important pre-requisite for a midwife, '. . . she must be literate in order to be able to comprehend the art through theory also'.[21] Two chapters of his book are devoted to the special qualities a midwife should possess. 'She must have a good memory; be industrious and patient, moral so as to inspire confidence; be endowed with a healthy mind, and have a strong constitution; and finally she must have long delicate fingers with nails cut short.'[8] He felt that the midwife must have theoretical as well as practical training, and be experienced in all branches of medicine so as to give dietetic as well as surgical and pharmacological prescriptions in order to draw correct conclusions from what she observed. She was to encourage the patient by cheerful talk, to help her sympathetically, and to be unflinching in any danger so as not to lose her head when giving advice. She must besides have given birth herself and must not be too young. Another chapter deals with female anatomy sufficiently accurately to indicate knowledge gained from postmortem dissection. Both normal and abnormal midwifery were within the province of the midwife, Soranus described at least ten positions that the fetus could adopt *in utero* (most of which would appear to be highly unlikely at term). One such presentation he described seems in these days quite extraordinary, and yet presumably were part of his experience. He instructed the midwives on how to extract the baby by arranging the legs together in the midline above the cervix and then to deliver as a double footling presentation.[15] The midwife was advised to support the perineum with a linen pad to prevent tearing during the second stage of labour.[13] Instructions on practical baby care were also given in this comprehensive book. These instructions describe how to tie off the umbilical cord and the subsequent care of the stump. Soranus also gave advice on the choice of a wet nurse,[15] the physical and moral qualities of whom have been the subject of pontification ever since. It has always been seen to be of importance because of the possibility of good and bad properties being transmitted via the milk to the innocent infant.

Although the original treatise was lost, the ideas and teachings of Soranus were the source on which other authors based their writings for the next millennium.

Britain from the Late Neolithic Period to the First Century AD

At the time when the Egyptian civilisation was flourishing, the population of Britain was probably not more than 20 000. Most of these people were still following a nomadic way of life, though there appears to have been domestication of animals, which might have allowed for a few small settlements. This type of society continued until at least the late Bronze Age (1000 to 500 BC) while in Europe at the same time the advanced Greek civilisation was dominant. It must be assumed that synchronous with the nomadic way of life was an equally unsophisticated way of birth. By the first century BC, the population may have risen to almost 250 000 as new tools for agriculture were both made and used. When the Belgae came, they brought still better implements for cultivating the land, so that by the time of the Roman conquest of Britain in the middle of the first century AD a population of about 400 000 could be supported.[22] It is probable that by this time the mother had an attendant when giving birth, although the nature of this self-selected 'midwife' is unknown. Nevertheless these 'midwives' — whoever they were — could be identified as the first British midwives.

Early Writers and Translators

The first translation into Latin of the textbook by Soranus was made by Moschion (or Moschio) in the sixth century AD. It is said to be a word-for-word copy.[23] (It was this Latin version that was translated by German, French and English writers in the sixteenth century, under various titles, the English title being *The Byrthe of Mankynde*. The first person to make a study of these manuscripts was Konrad Gesner (1516–65). He found a Greek manuscript in the library at Augsburg and compared it with the Latin text he had read at Basel and recognised that one was a translation of the other.[10] Since that time, other manuscripts, all derived from the work of Soranus, have been found in many European countries, including a copy in the Vatican Library and another, written in medieval English, among the Sloane manuscripts in the British Museum.[15] It is even conceivable that a Chinese translation was made, which found its way into Japan, where a book entitled *Tat Shang Pin* or *Midwifery Made Easy* first appeared in 1661. This book was concerned with midwives and their practice.[24] It is likely that during the process of multiple translations this book may have suffered many changes, partly as a result of the lack of understanding of this specialised subject by the scribes, and partly because of inevitable copying errors.)

Moschion is said to have lived in Rome, and is quoted as saying: 'in difficult births the parts are first of all to be relaxed with oil: if the passage of urine is obstructed . . . draw off the urine with a catheter; if the faeces are indurated a clyster [enema] should be given'.[25] Whether these practical 'tips' were original to Moschion, or simply copied from the instructions given by Soranus, is uncertain.

In addition to Soranus, other Roman physicians wrote on midwifery. These included Aurelius Cornelius Celsus, who lived in the first century AD. He described podalic version and breech extraction for fetal death in labour. In the second century AD, Galenus (Galen) wrote on diseases of women. Although he has gained and maintained a high reputation over the centuries for some of his anatomical observations, nevertheless the knowledge of female reproductive anatomy displayed in his writings was probably derived from animal studies.[13] The next and perhaps the last writer of the Roman period was Paulus Aeginetta (AD 630), whom Smellie describes as the first man-midwife. While acknowledging that head presentation was natural and preferable, Aeginetta taught that 'feet presentation' was also natural. He advocated that vaginal examination be performed to assess the degree of opening of the mouth of the womb and to determine whether a bag of forewaters was present.[25]

The Roman Empire was ended by the seventh century but the influence of both Greek and Roman medicine and midwifery had spread across the Arab world. After the Fall of Rome, medical teaching was mostly in the hands of the Islamic people who practised and preserved this inherited knowledge but made no significant contribution to its advance. There were, though, two outstanding Arab medical writers, who were knowledgeable in the theory and probably the practice of obstetrics. The first was Rhazes, who was born in 852 AD in Persia but practised as a physician/clinician in Bhagdad. His knowledge was derived from the teachings of Galen and Paulus Aeginetta. He is quoted as recommending 'piercing the membranes when they are too thick, or remain too long unbroke'.[14] He actually used a fillet to aid delivery, that is, a loop of woven material which was manipulated to encircle the head or a limb, so as to provide a hold for traction. Seclusion of Muslim women precluded men physicians from attending them, particularly in childbirth, and therefore care at this time was almost exclusively in the hands of midwives.

The other Arab writer was Avicenna, born in 980 AD in Bokhara, a city of Central Asia which had been conquered by the Arabs in the eighth century. He appears to have had an extensive knowledge of medicine, and he became famous for his medical treatises. He wrote on 'instrumental' deliveries, and it thus appears that obstetric forceps were available for extraction of the fetus in the case of obstructed labour.[25] In fact Aveling says it is beyond doubt that Arabian surgeons used 'obstetric' forceps.[26] The fillet, along with crude destructive instruments, remained in common use, but neither the forceps themselves, nor the concept of such potential live-saving instruments, survived beyond the Arabian period of influence. In fact forceps had to be reinvented in the seventeenth century.

The Byzantine Era

Between the fourth and sixth centuries Barbarians swept into Italy and destroyed Rome's ruling classes; but another Empire, the Byzantine, took over where the Roman Empire left off. It emerged in the fourth century and was to last until the fifteenth century during the so-called Dark Ages of Western Europe. Byzantium inherited and preserved the Roman traditions of Law and State Government, the Greek language, literature and culture, and Christianity. At its height the Byzantine Empire extended from its capital, Constantinople, to embrace parts of Italy and Sicily, east to the Caucasus mountains and parts of Russia, and north to include Yugoslavia and Bulgaria. The metropolis, a prosperous seaport, a centre of commerce and a showpiece walled city, was first called Byzas and later Constantinople after Constantine the Great who made it his city and capital. It displayed magnificent palaces, monasteries and churches in which were mosaics and frescoes; classical marble statuary adorned public buildings. It had shops, bazaars, public baths, aqueducts, piped water fountains, underground drains for the disposal of sewage and water, street lighting and fire brigades. There were Trade Guilds and there was a plentiful supply of materials with which craftsmen made artefacts of copper, gold, ivory, marble, leather and precious stones. Weapons, dyes and high-grade silks were also manufactured. There were several hospitals, and free medical care was provided by the Government and the Church for those who could not afford to pay. The records show that the construction of hospitals and homes for the aged and infirm was a frequent assignment for the architects and builders of Byzantium. The Hospital of the Monastery of St. Saviour Pantocrator, endowed by John II Commenus in the twelfth century, contained fifty beds divided into five wards, with separate wards for surgical cases, for medical cases and for women. It was attended by ten male doctors and one female doctor.[27] The birth of Imperial children took place in the porphyry (purple) chamber within the Imperial Gardens beside the Palace, and the title porphyrogenitus (born in the purple) was conferred on children of the ruling family.[27]

In such an advanced and highly organised society, influenced by Roman and Greek culture and medicine and by the Christian religion, it can be assumed that midwives had the same status and position as those of Greece and Rome. Constantinople was beseiged by Moslems twice in the seventh and eighth centuries, and finally fell to Muslim domination in 1453 AD.

References

1. Exodus 32:1–8.
2. Genesis 35:16.
3. Genesis 38:27–30.
4. Exodus 1:15 RSV.
5. Genesis 21:1–2.
6. *The New Bible Dictionary* (Inter-Varsity Fellowship, 1965).
7. Spiegelberg, W. *Aegyptologische Randglossen zum Alten Testament* (1904), pp. 19–25. (Quoted in ref. 6, under 'Midwives'.)

8. Dempsey, A.J. 'A Brief Survey of Early Midwifery Practice', *Ulster Medical Journal*, November 1949.

9. Homer. *The Odyssey*. Transl. E.V. Rieu (Penguin Books, Harmondsworth, 1946).

10. Rowland, B. *Medieval Women's Guide to Health* (Croom Helm, London, 1981).

11. *New Larousse Encyclopaedia of Mythology* (Hamlyn, London, 1979).

12. Ling, T. *The History of Religion East and West* (Macmillan Press, London, 1968).

13. Graham, H. *Eternal Eve* (Hutchinson, London, 1960).

14. Spence, D. *A System of Midwifery Theoretical and Practical* (1784).

15. Radcliffe, W. *Milestones in Midwifery* (John Wright & Sons, Bristol, 1967).

16. McMaster, G.T. 'Ancient Greece. The First Woman Practitioner (Agnodice) of Midwifery and the Care of Infants in Athens, 300 BC', *American Medicine, New Series B (4)*, 202–5, 1912.

17. *Archaeologia Graeca, vol. II*, pp. 324–5 (John Potter, London, 1764).

18. Chamberlain, M. *Old Wives' Tales. Their History, Remedies and Spells* (Virago, London, 1981).

19. Frazer, Sir J.G. *The Illustrated Golden Bough*, M. Douglas (ed.) (Doubleday, New York, 1978).

20. Bowra, C.M. *Classical Greece* (Time-Life Books, Amsterdam, 1965).

21. Benedek, T.G. 'The Changing Relationship between Midwives and Physicians during the Renaissance', *Bulletin of the History of Medicine, 51* (1977).

22. Hoskins, W.G. *The Making of the English Landscape* (Hodder & Stoughton, London, 1977).

23. Spencer, H.R. *The Renaissance of Midwifery* (Harrison, London, 1924) (quoting from *Codex Hafniensis*, Ingerslev, *Journal of Obstetrics and Gynaecology of the British Empire*, 1909).

24. Standlee, M. *The Great Pulse, Japanese Midwifery and Obstetrics through the Ages* (Charles E. Tuttle Co., Vermont, 1959).

25. Smellie, W. *A Treatise on the Theory and Practice of Midwifery*. Facsimile of First Edition (1752) (Bailliere Tindall, London, 1974).

26. Aveling, J.H. *The Chamberlens, and the Midwifery Forceps* (J. and A. Churchill, 1882).

27. Sherrard, P. *Byzantium* (Time-Life Books, Amsterdam, 1966).

Further Reading

The Israelites (Time-Life Books, Amsterdam, 1975)
Cook, S. *An Introduction to the Bible* (Penguin, Harmondsworth, 1945)
Smart, N. *The Religious Experience of Mankind* (Fount Paperbacks, London, 1971)
Winkleman, E. (ed.) *The Times Atlas of World History* (Time-Life Books, London, 1971)

3 CUSTOMS AND PRACTICES ASSOCIATED WITH CHILDBEARING IN THE DARK AGES AND MEDIEVAL PERIOD

The Dark Ages of Western Europe

As the civilisations and cultures of Greece and Rome died out, what unity and stability there was in Europe disappeared as various barbarian races struggled for supremacy. The next unifying force to emerge was Christianity, which eventually came to embrace the whole of Europe. But with the rise of Christianity came a preoccupation with the soul and the hereafter which resulted in a cessation of scientific investigation into physical and natural sciences. Consequently, little or no progress was made in medicine, partly because the human body was regarded as sacred and so its dissection was forbidden, and partly because religion and superstition took the place of rational thought.

The Islamic religion, which arose in the seventh century AD, spread rapidly throughout Asia, Asia Minor, North Africa and even parts of southern Europe, and its teaching also forbade human anatomical dissection.

While Europe stagnated, it is known that between the sixth and thirteenth centuries there was a highly developed industrial, commercial and agricultural Chinese civilisation to which immigrants from Japan, Turkey, Persia and India were attracted. The population in China increased spectacularly to reach 110 million by 1100 AD.[1] This population increase in such a highly organised cosmopolitan society argues for the existence of a similarly organised and skilled body of midwives.

A Japanese Empire can be dated at around 600 BC, but ancient Japan, in its 'mythological period', was — like China — dominated by legend, superstition and birth custom. In the Buddhist culture between 700 and 800 AD Buddhist nuns treated diseases with medicines and presumably acted as midwives. There were male physicians, but it is known that they were prohibited from treating ladies of the Court and so in 772 AD special training in midwifery was given to women who could neither read nor write. However, according to *History of Midwives and Midwifery in Japan* (Ministry of Public Health and Welfare, Tokyo, undated) these women were classified as 'occupational female doctors'.[2]

Very little was written in the truly Dark Ages of Europe between the end of the fifth century and the beginning of the eleventh century, and nothing at all is to be found about clinical midwifery practice. So the midwife of this time is a shadowy figure. However, it is almost certain that it would be this 'old wife' practitioner, and not the male physician, or even one of the very few female physicians, who would be in charge of confinements. Although these 'midwives' would certainly be uneducated, some would have empirical knowledge, skills and ability whereas others would be both ignorant and unskilled. It is not surprising, therefore, that, when midwives are next referred to by the writers of later centuries, they and their practices had fallen far below the standard deemed necessary by Soranus.

In Europe the focal point of society was the Church, and religion had a repressive influence on all other aspects of life because of its emphasis on the wrath and judgement of God and the enduring requirement of the sinner to repent. Only a small number of privileged men, and even fewer women, were educated in the Dark Ages, and in fact the only educational institutions in this period were monasteries, where monks, who made vows of poverty and chastity, isolated themselves for religious and charitable purposes. Scholarship was mainly theological, and mainly in Latin, and there was virtually no scientific enquiry and very little advance in technology. Even the arts were subjugated to the laws and needs of the Church. There were, of course, a few exceptions to the almost exclusive study of theology. One notable exception in England was the Venerable Bede, of Durham, who also studied medicine and astronomy. Writings in this period were, in the main, on religious and ecclesiastical matters, although the Anglo-Saxon Chronicle was a record of events of the day, and the Song of Beowulf was entirely pagan in its concept; both of these writings were in the vernacular.

In England the total population during the Dark Ages has been estimated to have ranged between one and one-and-a-half million. Population growth was minimal because both men and women were killed by invaders; life expectancy was short and a significant number were monks and nuns and therefore not free to raise families. It can therefore be deduced that the experience of those women practising midwifery, however few or many there were, was likely to have been limited.

Saxons invaded Britain between 400 and 600 AD and settled here. Saxons, Angles and Jutes brought with them a system of medical practice based on their wide knowledge of herbs and superstitious beliefs in incantations and charms.[3] The settlers cleared and cultivated large areas of the country and so produced more food to support an increased population. Christianity, which had been introduced into Britain early in the Roman occupation some time between the second and third centuries, almost vanished when the conquering Anglo-Saxons brought in their heathen gods. However, the Anglo-Saxons in turn were converted by Christian missionaries, and Christianity became the established religion of England despite successive waves of invasion by Vikings and Danes. The Church sought to establish rules about almost every facet of life including chastity in marriage, and declared that 'every religious woman should keep her chastity for three months before childbirth and for sixty nights and days after, whether the child be male or female'.[4]

Whole villages were burned and pillaged during invasions, and people fled for refuge to hilltops and forests. In these circumstances, where the need simply to survive was predominant, it is unlikely that much, if any, consideration was given to women's needs or to the mechanism or manner of birth.

The final invasion by the Normans in 1066 brought security to the land. With this security and with new customs a more structured and in fact highly organised society emerged and the life of the English people was gradually changed. In two decades a comprehensive survey of the entire kingdom, in the form of the Domesday Book, was produced. The Normans built castles, acquired great estates for themselves, and town and cities grew, but the mass of the native population worked as serfs ekeing out an existence during their short lifespan. They were subject to their masters, who could be Dukes, Lords or Barons. Life was spartan for these peasants at the best of times, but in the event of a bad harvest many died from starvation. Their homes were mud and wattle huts with bare earth forming the floor. These dwellings, which lacked both windows and chimneys, contained very little furniture or other creature comforts. Almost nothing is documented about the domestic life of this period and as the historians were men it is not surprising that childbirth seemed too unimportant to mention. Consequently not only are there no records of births, but there is also no indication of the number of children born into either aristocratic or peasant families.

In the face of continual local fights and skirmishes, the majority of women would become adept at treating wounds incurred in battles or in the course of everyday life, and also in nursing the sick, using inherited knowledge of herbal medicine in addition to their inherent feminine caring skills. In the Domesday Book, completed in 1086, groups of women are mentioned as 'living mostly near the place of pilgrimage and caring for the sick'.[3] Such a charitable act of nursing the sick, chronicled possibly for the first time in England, was obviously acceptable but attempts to cure were condemned by the Church.

Medieval Fatalism

In almost all religions, from the most primitive up to and including the
Christian religion, sickness and disease have been regarded as punishment for offences against God or gods, or as possession by demons.
Moreover, in the Christian faith, suffering and affliction were to be
regarded, even welcomed, as a test of faith and spiritual strength. Because
of this the official policy of the Christian Church in the Middle Ages
was totally opposed to both the practice of medicine and secular healing
because they were seen as reversions to pre-Christian practices or even
as collusion with devilish forces. 'On Sundays, after Mass, the sick came
in scores, crying for help, — and words were all they got. "You have
sinned and God is afflicting you. Thank him; you will suffer so much
the less torment in the life to come. Endure, suffer, die. Has not the
Church its prayers for the dead?'' '⁵ This attitude was perpetuated until
the Renaissance when it was challenged by creative and intellectual im-
pulses that initiated change towards a more scientific and humanistic approach to Man's life on Earth. However, even in medieval times the
official policy was inconsistently enforced, and although the Church at
times actively opposed the pursuit and application of medical knowledge,
it must also be credited with its preservation in the form of manuscripts
from previous ages, which were stored and studied in monastic libraries.
A few ecclesiastical dignitaries were in fact doctors of medicine, the most
illustrious being Pope John XXI in the middle of the thirteenth century.⁶
      Every monastery of size had an infirmary in which elderly and sick
monks were cared for by members of the religious order but

> the Lateran Treaty of 1125 forbade the attendance of monks and priests
> on the sick in any capacity other than as ministers of religion. This
> Decree was swiftly followed in 1131 by further restrictions prohibiting
> the study of medicine by monks and priests, and directed, interestingly,
> that they confine their role as physicians strictly to their own
> monasteries.⁷

This demonstrates the equivocal position in which the Church found itself.
In addition to monastic infirmaries, many other hospices and hospitals
were founded in an attempt to deal with the sick and infirm members
of the lay society. Whether or not these hospitals were attached to
monasteries or abbeys, the patients were nursed mainly, but not exclusively, by monks and nuns. One such hospital, St. John's, Winchester (built
in 1275), widened its scope in 1414 'to include assistance to women in

childbirth'.[8] Even before this time, St. Bartholomew's Hospital, London, which was founded in 1123, had included 'pregnant women' among its patients.[8]

The Middle Ages

The Dark Ages merged gradually into what is known as the Middle Ages, which could in England be roughly dated from the latter part of the eleventh century to the Renaissance and Reformation in the sixteenth century.

Europe in the Middle Ages experienced the violence and death that resulted from five major Crusades to the Holy Land and the Hundred Years War between England and France. England suffered, in addition, the Wars of the Roses. Armies returning from the Holy Land brought in their wake both venereal disease and the plague, which then became endemic throughout Europe. Major outbreaks of the plague brought such catastrophic loss of life that in England in the fourteenth century, the agriculture, trade and wealth of the entire country were seriously affected. The extent of this is seen in the fact that the population in England decreased from 3.7 millions in 1348 to 2.2 millions in 1377,[9] and from the latter date the population increase was only 1.5 million in the two centuries between 1400 and 1600.[10] It is impossible even to speculate on the amount of infant mortality and morbidity, in terms of skeletal and brain damage, that resulted from congenital syphilis.

Although throughout the Middle Ages people suffered the horrors of war, disease and poverty, at the same time the horizons of all Europeans were being widened. Trading increased and as people began to travel there was an intermingling of cultures which enriched life generally. People enjoyed the display of chivalry at colourful pageants and tournaments and also the entertainment provided by peripatetic troubadours and strolling players. Men and women travelled within England, mainly on horseback or on foot, to the many towns where fairs were by now a regular event, and in addition to buying and selling they 'made merry' by drinking and dancing. There was a development of secular activities in rural and urban communities, with people entertaining themselves by dancing round the maypole, by music-making and story-telling, and by playing games. In castles, manor houses and the homes of merchants and gentry, the women, who would have time on their hands, would be developing crafts such as fine sewing, tapestry and embroidery. An increase in the amount and variety of imports provided them with the necessary materials for these and other pursuits. Much of the making of everyday household essentials was by this time coming into the province of men. Drapers, silversmiths, goldsmiths, tinsmiths, tanners and shoemakers grouped together into trade guilds. The introduction of paper making, and of new writing and painting materials, forwarded these two arts, but especially allowed for literary expression and its wider dissemination. Mallory wrote on the romantic theme of King Arthur, and Chaucer wrote on a wide range of subjects and people (and despite the power of the Church, many of his tales have an anti-clerical flavour). In *Piers Plowman*, William Langland produced a great religious and social allegory. At the same time both Miracle and Morality plays were performed and were very popular. The first book was printed in Europe in 1445 and Caxton introduced the printing press into England in 1477.

The Emergence of Medical Study and Writing

In the eleventh century a Medical School was established in the Italian city of Salerno. As far as is known, this was the first School of Medicine founded in Christendom and must indicate some degree of tolerance by the Church towards medical learning. During the eleventh century a treatise on gynaecological and obstetric conditions was written in Salerno. This work is known under several titles: *De Passionibus mulierum curandarum, De aegritodinibus mulierum, De curis mulierum, Trotula major* or simply *Trotula*. Its authorship is generally ascribed to Trotula, but who Trotula was, and whether Trotula was a woman, is debatable. However, Trotula is a feminine name and so the writer may have been a woman doctor who graduated from the famous Medical School and who also practised midwifery; alternatively she may have been a midwife of Salerno. Trotula may, however, have been a male physician who assumed a female identity, because in that age it would have been offensive to women for men to interest themselves in such matters. Moreover it would have been regarded as beneath a man's professional dignity to do so.

The work was based on the original teachings of Soranus and other classical scholars. *Trotula* became the standard obstetric and gynaecological textbook of the medieval period. The very fact that such a treatise was written demonstrates a certain amount of concern for women. It appears that this Latin manuscript was translated into English in the early fifteenth century (some four centuries later). In this form it has been preserved as Sloane MS 2463, which has been examined in detail and rendered into Modern English by Beryl Rowland.[11] The majority of the chapters deal with a variety of gynaecological conditions, some of which are identifiable and some more abstruse such as 'suffocation of the uterus'. Only two chapters deal with obstetric conditions. These are entitled 'The Pain in Childbearing and the Terrible Suffering Women Have Before they are Delivered' and 'The Withholding of the Secundine and the Ache of the Uterus'. Natural labour and delivery are mentioned briefly but not discussed, and the text and drawings show a preoccupation with 'unnatural' labour and delivery. Sixteen malpresentations of the 'child' are described and illustrated. Some of the positions stretch the imagination and range from 'when the child extends both his hands with his two shoulders, with his hands one on one side and one on the other, and the head is turned back into a reversed position into the side' and 'when the child displays first one hand and one foot and covers his face with the other hand'. It is notable that the *doctors* are addressed regarding the gynaecological conditions but it is the *midwife* who is instructed on how to deal with all the obstetric complications and situations. Interestingly, if confronted with a retained placenta, she is advised to 'anoint her hands and with her nails pull out the secundine if she can; and if she cannot, bore holes in a stool and let the woman sit on it and make underneath a fumigation from goats' horns and the claws of their feet, so that the smoke stinks right up to her privy members'.[12]

It must be inferred that not only were the midwives the recognised practitioners of childbirth in the time of the original writer, Soranus, but that this was still so in the medieval period. Because the original text by Soranus has been copied, translated and edited into many languages and cultures, it is more than likely that the medieval Sloane MS 2463 was an inevitably distorted reflection of the primary teachings, but certainly some of his sound advice, such as the advisability of perineal suturing, remained unaltered. With the passage of time, cultural accretions appeared in the text. For example, the Arab doctor, Rhazes, born in the ninth century, is mentioned, but Soranus antedated him by eight centuries. Remedies, containing long lists of ingredients, were prescribed for many conditions; one even included the use of gunpowder together with one ounce of lupins and thirty other medicinal constituents.

Although Sloane MS 2463 was written in the vernacular, it was not circulated and so its practical 'instructions' would go unheeded by the great majority of midwives, who were unaware of its existence and unable to read it had they been aware. However, it is conceivable that a few midwives would be married to apothecaries, schoolmasters and guilded craftsmen, and may have been literate.

Medieval Midwives

In Scotland one reference to the existence of a midwife occurs as early as 1326.

> The Scottish Exchequer is recorded as paying 13s 4d to a man whose name was John. He lived in an age when many people did not have surnames, and it is significant that his distinguishing feature was not his place of origin, some aspect of his physical appearance, his father's name or even his own occupation. Instead his designation came from his relationship with someone who was obviously a well known figure in the locality — he features in the records as 'John, son of the Midwife of Tarbar'.[13]

There are also references to Royal midwives as early as the fifteenth century. Mention is made in the Royal Exchequer records of payment to a midwife by the name of Margery Cobbe. She is known to have delivered Queen Elizabeth Woodville of the future King Edward V on 1 November 1470 in the sanctuary of Westminster Abbey. It would appear that she was the Queen's midwife 'by appointment' because three years later the Rolls of Parliament decreed that her salary of £10 per annum be continued during her lifetime. Another Royal midwife was Alice Massy who received £10 per year for her attendance on Elizabeth of York. She received a pension of £5 per year after the Queen's death in 1503 which occurred during the puerperium after the birth of her seventh child which took place prematurely in the Tower of London.[14] A Scottish midwife named Margaret Asteane who attended Mary Queen of Scots in 1566 was presented with cloth and thread for a fine black wool gown trimmed with black velvet.[13]

Specific measures were taken to exclude men when Margaret of Anjou, Henry the Sixth's Queen, had her confinement in 1442. 'The order was that . . . in the second chamber must be a traverse which shall never but be drawn until she be purified. After that traverse there may not openly be no man officer or other come there nearer than the outer chamber. Instead of men officers must be gentlewomen.'[15] However, male astrologers were sometimes in attendance at births for the express purpose of casting the newborn baby's horoscope.[16]

Barber-surgeons' Guilds were set up during the thirteenth century. They regulated conditions for apprenticeship, admission to membership and standards of practice. Barber-surgeons were not doctors: they were 'tradesmen' who were adept in the use of instruments for a variety of purposes. Although in the main they were men, it appears that a few women apprentices were admitted to the Guild who later practised as barber-surgeons.[10] Alleviation of human suffering was undoubtedly one of their motives, and it is notable that this branch of healing performed by *men* was neither challenged by the Church nor persecuted by the State. In towns where barber-surgeons practised, they had exclusive rights and so midwives were debarred from using instruments, and were obliged, when faced with an obstructed labour, to call upon a barber-surgeon. His role was to remove the baby, which was usually dead, with the aid of surgical instruments; hooks and perforators were usually employed to deliver the baby piecemeal. Alternatively, a post-mortem Caesarean section was performed. In the event of a maternal death and where a barber-surgeon was not available, the midwife herself was required by the Church to perform an immediate Caesarean section in an attempt to secure a living child.[17]

During the thirteenth century, centres of learning distinct from monasteries had been set up in Oxford and Cambridge, and subjects other than divinity, such as law and medicine, came to be studied. In England, as distinct from other European countries, women were excluded from these universities. Hence the formalising of medicine as a subject to be learnt from written precepts of classical origin, and in which to be examined and professionally qualified, actually disqualified women, who previously, by custom and tradition, had been the informal practitioners of domestic medicine. Ironically, at this time, men physicians did not express any interest in women's conditions or in midwifery. This attitude to childbirth and to diseases peculiar to women no doubt stemmed from the doctrine of the Church with its misogynistic tendencies and its perpetuation of the Biblical teaching relating to God's punishment of women for the sin of Eve: 'I will greatly multiply your pain in childbearing, in pain you shall bring forth children. Yet your desire shall be for your husband, and he shall rule over you.'[18] Moreover, a woman's reproductive organs were regarded as 'forbidden territory' to any man other than her husband. As Harvey Graham puts it in *Eternal Eve*, 'midwivery was an unclean subject fit only for midwives and sow gelders'.[16]

Once medicine was taught in universities which were outside direct ecclesiastical jurisdiction, the Church had no alternative but to condone attempts to heal the sick, although even then 'the new University-trained physicians were not allowed to practice without first calling in a Priest to aid and advise them'.[19] In an attempt to keep control of the situation, the Church had already had to concede that 'in every community there be appointed ''at least one widow to assist women who are stricken with illness'' '.[19] However, this widow had to restrict herself to midwifery and related areas, and was accountable to the priest.[19] Because baptism was a prerequisite to salvation, the priest was often in attendance along with the midwife at the delivery in order to perform this sacrament and thereby save the child's soul should its bodily existence be in jeopardy.

It is highly likely that most women of childbearing age and in all classes of society would have a pregnancy every year except when the men were away at war. This would result in many women becoming grande multiparae who would present the 'mydwyf' with complications consequent upon this status. The mortality of mothers and babies would be great as a result of the inevitable high-risk factors such as malpresentations, ante-partum haemorrhage, prolapse of the umbilical cord, uterine inertia, post-partum haemorrhage or prematurity. The babies may have died from birth trauma or asphyxia. Even if safely born, they would be subject to the hazards associated with early arrival, to infections and to the hardship of a draughty, smoky, home environment.

Medieval Magic

Although ostensibly the Church exerted a powerful hold over every area of life, a reliance on ancient superstitions and magical rites and practices had never been relinquished by the common mass of people, despite the formulation of 'Punishments for Sorcery, Soothsayings, and Making Use of Potions':

> If any exercise divinations and soothsayings, or keep vigils at any spring, or at any other creature, except at the Church of God, let him fast for three years. A woman deserves the same if she cures her child by any sorcery or if she draws it over the ground to the cross roads.[4]

The event of birth and the beginning of new life has always engaged man's imagination, and its peril and secrecy have evoked wonder and superstition.

> Several aspects of the birth process at various times have acquired special meanings. Superstition surrounded the placenta, the umbilical cord and the caul . . . The caul was believed to confer eloquence and protection against drowning, to promote easy childbirth, and to bring various other pieces of good fortune.[20]

Midwives may have been tempted to appropriate the caul to sell, perhaps to a witch, as an ingredient for a potion.

One superstition which was important to pregnant women was chalcedony or a belief in the magical properties of certain precious and semi-precious stones. The use of chalcedony was an ancient and widespread custom which was believed to confer an occult power against evil and which would ensure continuation of pregnancy, a safe delivery and successful lactation. Precious or semi-precious stones, which included sapphire, jasper and agate, were worn as amulets or charms: 'being worne about a woman with chylde, it preserveth her from deliverance before her time'.[21] Other stones believed to prevent abortion and to facilitate birth were the aetites or eagle-stones, which have been known since the days of the Assyrians. Pliny described their use in the first century and Julius Solinus in the third century, and there are numerous other references to their use up to the 1800s.[22] Bartholomew (in 1539) and Rueff (in 1554) both write of the use of chalcedony in childbirth, as also did Trotula. 'It is also profitable to wear about them gemmes and precious stones, as the saphire, Iacint, Corall, the precious stone Corneola, Adamant, Thurchese.'[23] Because aetites contain stones within a stone, they were considered to be 'pregnant' stones and as such to exert sympathetic magic. These stones, sometimes discovered in eagles' nests, have been found in Persia, Hungary, China, South Africa and Scotland. It was also claimed that these haematite stones have 'powers of attraction' or magnetic properties. It is reported that in 1633, Richard Andrews, a London physician, wrote to the Countess of Newcastle on 10 May 1663 advising her that he had sent her 'an eagle-stone which in the time of labour being tied about the thigh will make labour easier'.[19] In 1658 a noblewoman who had worn an eagle-stone around her neck during pregnancy and early labour was slow to progress . . . 'wherefore taking off the eagle-stone from her neck and applying it to her thigh, upon the inward part, not far from her privvies, she had an easy and quick delivery'.[24]

Disapproval of the belief in the therapeutic virtues of aetites and chalcedony had been voiced by clerics, scholars and physicians throughout the Christian period. 'It is unlawful for clerics or laymen, to be sorcerors or enchanters, or to make amulets . . . If anyone makes amulets, which is detestable, he should do three years penance.'[4] The following clerical injunction was issued in County Clare in the seventh century: 'That no woman have amber round her neck . . . or have recourse to enchanters . . . . or to engravers of amulets.'[21]

Another device employed for protection against evil spirits was the practice of writing out a Biblical verse, often part of a psalm. In some cases the scriptural quotation was written on parchment and worn round the neck during pregnancy and labour. Often the ink was washed off the paper and the solution was then drunk. This practice was documented in *Brevarium Bartholomei*, which was compiled by a priest and scholar who was also a physician, John of Mirfield, in the late fourteenth century while practising at St. Bartholomew's Hospital.[19] He included the wording of a charm which was worn by parturient women but disclaims any personal belief in the use of scripture for magical purposes.

The most interesting and rather mysterious charm is the Sator 'magic' square, which may have Christian connotations but could be variously interpreted. The formula was inscribed on a medallion which was worn on the person or hung on the wall. Apparently the words were also written in butter, put on bread and eaten by the pregnant woman or by the sick for therapeutic purposes. Forbes states that 'sator' was an important charm for protection in pregnancy and childbirth.[24] Perhaps it was used in the same way as a *mantra* is used. The Latin words are:

S A T O R	'a sower of seed'
A R E P O	'I creep to'
T E N E T	'He holds . . . thread'
O P E R A	'works'
R O T A S	'wheel'

This has been loosely interpreted as 'Creative power holds the wheels by a thread'. Its use dates back to Roman times and it has been found in various sites on walls, pavements, doors and coins, and on various artefacts of stone, plaster, leather, paper and tiles in all parts of the Roman Empire. The most recent discovery of the text was on a broken amphora unearthed from a second-century rubbish pit in Deansgate, Manchester. Its exact meaning is uncertain, but another explanation is that the letters can be arranged as follows:

```
                        P
                        A
                        T
                        E
                        R
            P A T E R N O S T E R
                        O
                        S
                        T
                        E
                        R
```

The words of the cross thus formed mean 'Our Father'. The two Os and As of the formula not included may stand for Alpha and Omega, the Beginning and the End: fundamental elements of Christian belief. It is thought possible that when Christians were a persecuted minority in the Roman world they used these words as a cryptogram for identifying themselves to other Christians.

The Association between Witchcraft and Midwifery

In all religions and cultures since the emergence of man, people have believed in evil spirits and demons. Witches and witchcraft are mentioned and condemned in the Bible.

> Thou shalt not suffer a witch to live.[25]

> There shall not be found among you anyone who burns his son or his daughter as an offering, anyone who practises divination, a soothsayer, or an augur or a sorcerer, or a charmer or a medium or a wizard or a necromancer; for whoever does these things is an abomination to the Lord and because of these abominable practices the Lord your God is driving them out before you.[26]

> For rebellion is as the sin of witchcraft.[27]

> Now the works of the flesh are . . . idolatry, witchcraft . . .[28]

In the millennium between the fifth and fifteenth centuries, witchcraft was widely practised in Europe including England. In fact the secular laws of Cnut (King Canute, 1020–23) forbade heathen practices specifically including witchcraft.[4] Witchcraft was denounced by Pope Innocent VIII in his Papal Bull of 1484.[19] A witch was defined as 'a person who hath conference with the devil to consult him or to do some act' (Lord Coke, 1552–1634).[24] A 'witch-craze' in the late Middle Ages resulted in an orgy of witch-hunting and burning. Such witch-hunting was spearheaded by the Inquisition, which denounced witchcraft *per se* as a heresy. These hunts involved torture in order to extract a confession, and it is likely that some women died as a result. Although torture was used in England, witches were less persecuted than in Europe or Scotland, and although hunted by the church, it was the Civil Courts who meted out punishment appropriate to the crime, but burnt them only for murder.

In this period in history the devil was conceived of and feared not only as a supernatural evil force but also as possessing a physical form which could be summoned up by his agents, the witches. One such witch was Agnes Sampson, the midwife of Haddington, who in 1590 took part in a plot to destroy King James of Scotland by magic.

> James was present at the examination of the prisoners and listened very attentively to their confessions. At the end of it all he lost patience, and remarked that they 'were all extreme liars'. Then a very curious thing happened. Agnes Sampson suddenly declared that she would not wish the King to suppose her words were false, and thereupon, drawing him a little aside, she repeated to him the actual words that had passed between him and his bride on their wedding night in Norway. James was astounded, as well he might be, for there was no normal means by which she, or any other outsider, could possibly have known this. He acknowledged that her words were 'most true' and swore by the Living God that he believed all the devils in hell could not have discovered the same. Whatever the source of her mysterious knowledge may have been, it is clear that the King was deeply impressed by Agnes Sampson's account of what happened that night . . . What drove her into making so dangerous a statement no one knows. James' freely expressed incredulity must have seemed to offer her (and her fellow prisoners also) at least a hope of pardon and release; but this she deliberately rejected by going out of her way to admit knowledge that could only be explained by magic. She was, as far as is known, quite sane . . . She must have realised what the effect of such a declaration would be upon her own immediate fate, but nevertheless, she made it, without any sort of provocation or persuasion, and in due course she was executed in Edinburgh.[29]

In a society dominated by the Church, in which poor people had no influence or power, it is not surprising that some of them were tempted to tap a source of potential power such as witchcraft. The use of it by peasants, and particularly by peasant *women*, was a threat to the Church and State. Alongside these confessed witches, who were an organised force, were lay women who practised herbal medicine and who were the midwives, wise women, healers, therapists and in fact the general 'medical' practitioners of their communities. Unfortunately these women, whose motives were good and who were merely using inherited knowledge and inherent healing gifts, were also classified by the Church as witches, against their will. When it was recognised that so-called witches could be divided by their motives and activities into two categories, the term 'white witch' or 'blessing witch' was ascribed to the benevolent healers, and the term 'black witch' was given to the malevolent evil-doers. Most midwives would be categorised as white witches, but some would be black witches. It is possible that some white-witch midwives may occasionally have dabbled in witchcraft and black magic in an attempt to get help in desperate circumstances.

Women lay healers mainly, though not entirely, ministered to the poor, who were the most sorely afflicted by disease and deprivation. The rich could turn to qualified licensed physicians, who, by the fourteenth century, were beginning to be officially tolerated by the Church. However, the orthodox medicine practised by these physicians was relatively unsuccessful because of lack of progress in any of the sciences for many hundreds of years. In fact, on occasions, such physicians had to fall back upon the experiential knowledge of 'wise women'. 'In the 13th century, for instance, one Professor at Oxford rode forty miles to get a prescription from an old woman who cured jaundice with the cooked juice of plantain.'[18]

The Malleus Maleficarum or *The Hammer of Witches*,[29] the classical textbook on European witches first printed in 1486, the original text of which was a quarter of a million words, makes a number of extensive references to witch-midwives and their practices. Chapter 13 is entitled 'How Witch-midwives Commit Most Horrid Crimes when they either Kill Children or Offer them to Devils in Most Accursed Wise.' The authors claim that witch-midwives 'surpass all other witches in their crimes'. The following is an extract from this work.

Then follows an experience described by an honest God-fearing woman who lived in Zabern in the diocese of Strasbourg. 'I was, she says, pregnant by my lawful husband and as my time approached, a certain midwife importuned me to engage her to assist at the birth of my child. But I knew her bad reputation, and although I had decided to engage another woman, pretended with conciliatory words to agree to her request. But when the pains came upon me, and I had brought in another midwife, the first one was very angry and hardly a week later came into my room one night with two other women where I was lying. And when I tried to call my husband, who was sleeping in another room, all the use was taken from my limbs and tongue so that except for seeing and hearing I could not move a muscle. And the witch, standing between the other two, said 'See! this vile woman who would not take me for a midwife, shall not win through unpunished'. The other two standing by her pleaded for me saying 'she has never harmed any of us'. But the witch added 'Because she has offended me I am going to put something into her entrails, but, to please you, she shall not feel any pain for half a year, but after that she shall be tortured enough'. So she came up and touched my belly with her hands; and it seemed to me that she took out my entrails, and put in something which, however I could not see. And when she had gone away, and I had recovered my power of speech, I called my husband and told him what had happened. But he put it down to pregnancy, and said 'you pregnant women are always suffering from fancies and delusions'. And when he would by no means believe me, I replied 'I have been given six months grace, and if, after that time, no torment comes to me, I shall be leaving you.' She related this to her son, a cleric who was then Archdeacon of the District, and who came to visit her on the same day. And what happened? When exactly six months had passed, such a terrible pain came into her belly she could not help disturbing everybody with her cries day and night. And because she was most devout to the Blessed Virgin Mary, the Queen of Mercy, she fasted with bread and water every Saturday, so that she believed she was delivered by her intercession. For one day, when she wanted to perform an action of nature, all those unclean things fell from her body; and she called her husband and her son, and said 'Are these fancies? Did I not say that after half a year the truth would be known? For whoever saw me eat thorns, bones and even bits of wood?' For there were brambles as long as a palm as well as a quantity of other things.

Much of this tale seems in present times rather far-fetched but at the time of telling would, in almost every detail, be believed.

The book tells of another witch-midwife in the town of Dann in the Diocese of Basel who was burned after confessing that she had killed more than forty children by sticking a needle through the crown of their heads as they came out from the womb.

Another woman in the Diocese of Strasbourg confessed that she had killed more children than she could count. And she was caught in this way. She had been called from one town to another to act as midwife to a certain woman and, having performed her office, was going back home. But as she went out of the town gate, the arm of a newly born child fell out of the cloak she had wrapped around her, in whose folds the arm had been concealed. This was seen by those sitting in the gateway, and when she had gone, they picked up from the ground what they took to be a piece of meat, but when they looked more closely, and saw that it was not a piece of meat, but recognised it by its fingers as a child's arm, they reported it to the Magistrate, and it was found that the child had died before baptism, lacking an arm. So the witch was taken and questioned and confessed the crime, and that she had, as has been said, killed more children than she could count.

The text goes on to say:

Witches are taught by the devil to confect from the limbs of children an unguent which is very useful for their spells. Some children are blasphemously offered to the devil in this manner. As soon as the child is born, the midwife, if the mother herself is not a witch, carries it out of the room on the pretext of warming it, and raises it up, and offers it to the prince of devils, that is Lucifer, and to all the devils. And this is done by the kitchen fire. The reason given for this sacrilegious offering of babies was that the treachery of witches might increase, to the devil's own gain, when they have witches dedicated to them from their very cradles.

The charge that witch-midwives committed infanticide is seen repeatedly in the literature of the time, and not only in the condemnatory Church writings of the day. There is evidence that witches, having summoned up the devil and other evil spirits, indulged in incestuous orgies; and that they 'baked the ashes of the resulting babies, whom they killed eight days after birth, into a blasphemous communion bread'.[31] According to one writer's account of a trial of sorcerers and witches, the initiation ceremony involved drinking a potion the essential ingredient of which was the flesh of dead unbaptised babies.[32] If the witches were not midwives themselves, this practice would have required collusion (perhaps under threat) with the midwives who were the first to handle the newborn.

There take this unbaptised-brat,
boil it well: preserve the fat,
You know 'tis precious to transfer
our anointed flesh into the air . . .[33]

At one visitation in 1669, made by representatives of Elizabeth I, it was

asked 'whether you know anye that doe use charmes, sorcerye, enchaunt-
ments, invocations, circles, witchcrafts, soothsayings, or any lyke craftes
or ymaginations invented by the devyll and especallye in the tyme of
travayle'.[34]

As late at 1595 Hiltprand's *Textbook of Midwifery* states that 'many'
midwives were witches and offered infants to Satan after killing them
by thrusting a bodkin into their brains.[24] Written in 1575, Fromann's
Tractatus de Fascinatione says 'The devil arranges through the midwives
not only the abortive death of the fetuses lest they be brought to the holy
font of baptism, but also by the midwives aid he causes newborn babies
secretly to be consecrated to himself'.[35]

The extent to which midwives were actually associated with witchcraft
in Britain is not clear, but it would appear that it was to a lesser degree
than in other parts of Europe. In fact although severe penalties were meted
out to those convicted of witchcraft, there is no mention of midwives
in this or any other connection in the Statutes of the Realm from the
time of Magna Carta to the reign of Queen Anne, nor in any other legal
or ecclesiastical records.[24] Even so, the genuine wise-woman midwife
found herself in a peculiarly unenviable position in that if she did good
by participating in a successful birth in which the mother and the baby
were alive and well, she still fell foul of the Church by being labelled
as a witch. Should a midwife have the misfortune to participate in a
delivery with a bad outcome involving the death of either the mother
or baby, or the birth of a deformed child, then she would be classified
and condemned as a black witch by everyone concerned. Moreover her
position was precarious in the eyes of the civil authorities also. A
Witchcraft Act of 1542 specifically lists the good witch as being among
those whose activities were prohibited by law because she was an
unlicensed practitioner 'of medicine and other useful skills'[36] which
would include midwifery. Such wise-women midwives were valued by
the community because they were known and trusted, and therein lay
their challenge to the Church which hated both women themselves and
their power of healing. A famous English witch hunter wrote 'It were
a thousand times better for the land if all Witches, but especially the
blessing Witch might suffer death . . . these are the right hand of the
devill by which he taketh and destroyeth the soules of men.'[37] 'The white
witch was the servant of the sick individual. Just as the Priest considered
the white witch a theological charlatan, and persecuted her in the name
of the faithful, so the physician considered the unlicensed healer a medical
charlatan.'[36] The Church's condemnation of all 'witchcraft' was because
it 'involves an appeal to powers beyond those of God, a presumptuous

attempt to compel by human acts benefits which could be granted or denied only by the Divine Will'.[29] Moreover, the acquisition of power by peasant women posed a threat to the Church. In post-Renaissance, post-Reformation England, both God and the devil assumed less importance in man's thinking, and in the following ages of humanism and rationalism the witch came to be viewed merely as a malicious twisted old woman who seemed to possess certain magical powers. Because of her claims to cast spells as well as to heal, she became caricatured as a bent, aged crone with long crooked fingers and long crooked nose, who owned a black cat and a tall pointed black hat and who travelled on a broomstick. She stirred weird ingredients such as toads, bats, adders and blood in a steaming cauldron while at the same time she muttered incantations —

> Eye of newt and toe of frog . . .
> lizard's leg and howlet's wing . . .
> Root of hemlock digg'd i' the dark . . .
> Gall of goat and slips of yew . . .
> Finger of birth-strangl'd babe,
> Ditch-deliver'd by a drab.[38]

Thomas Shadwell writes of another and even more revolting concoction, of which the Pendle witch, Mother Demdike, boasted:

> To a mother's bed I softly crept
> and while th' unchristn'd brat yet slept,
> I suck't the breath and bloud of that,
> And stole another's flesh and fat,
> Which I will boyl before it stink;
> The thick for oyntment, thin for drink[39]

Also in Bale's *Comedy Concerning Three Laws* (1538) Idolatry boasts:

> Yea, but now I am she,
> And a good midwife, perde,
> Young children can I charm
> With whisperings and witchings,
> with crossings and kissings,
> With blastings and with blessings,
> That sprites do them no harm.

Figure 5: Leonardo's Study of the Human Embryo

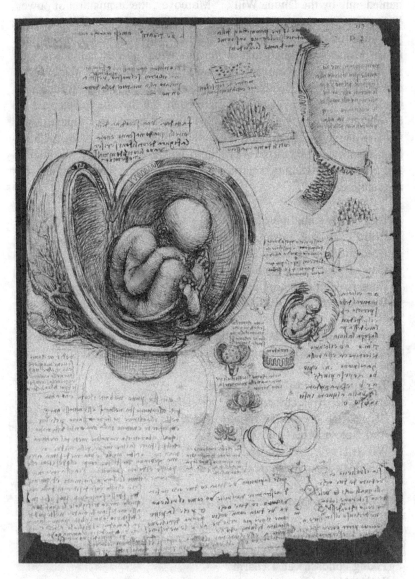

Source: Reproduced with permission of the Royal Library, Windsor Castle.

Progress through a Renaissance Artist

At the beginning of the sixteenth century, one man, who was both scientist and artist, kindled a light which has never been extinguished and which was to dispel the darkness of superstition and stagnation that had existed for many centuries. This man was Leonardo da Vinci, whose enquiring mind and pursuit of reality made him the first to practise human dissection in Renaissance Europe. He was a man of genius in many spheres and his artistic gift was used to further scientific progress. His famous drawing of the fetus *in utero* opened up a world of new knowledge in the obstetric field, although this was not fully appreciated or applied for several generations (Figure 5).

References

1. BBC TV History Documentary, 'China in Transition, 581–1279 AD', September 1980.

2. Standlee, M. *The Great Pulse. Japanese Midwifery and Obstetrics through the Ages* (Charles E. Tuttle, Vermont, 1959).

3. Gordon, E.J. 'Nurses and Nursing in Britain. 2. The Saxon Centuries', *Midwife and Health Visitor*, July 1970.

4. Scott, A.F. *The Saxon Age* (Croom Helm, London, 1979). (Quotation from *Penitential of Archbishop Ecgbert (735–66)*, B. Thorpe, 'Ancient Laws and Institutes of England').

5. Michelet, J. *Satanism and Witchcraft* (ARCO Publications, 1958).

6. Spencer, H.R. *The Renaissance of Midwifery* (Harrison, London, 1924).

7. Chamberlain, M. *Old Wives' Tales: Their History, Remedies and Spells* (Virago, London, 1981). (Quotation from *Harnack Medicinisches aus der Aeltesten Kirchen Geschichte*, Leipzig 1892, in *Old Time Makers of Medicine* (J. Walsh, New York, 1911)).

8. Gordon, E.J. 'Nurses and Nursing in Britain. The Medieval Monastic Tradition', *Midwife and Health Visitor*, August 1970.

9. McNeill, W.H. *Plagues and Peoples* (Blackwell, Oxford, 1976).

10. Donnison, J. *Midwives and Medical Men* (Heinemann, London, 1977).

11. Rowland, B. *Medieval Woman's Guide to Health* (Croom Helm, London, 1981).

12. Rowland, B. *Medieval Woman's Guide to Health* (Croom Helm, London, 1981, p. 147).

13. Marshall, R. 'Birth of a Profession', *Nursing Mirror*, 30 November 1983.

14. Dewhurst, J. 'Royal Midwives of Former Times', *Midwife, Health Visitor and Community Nurse*, October 1983.

15. Cunnington, P. and Lucas, C. 'Costumes for Births, Marriages and Deaths', in *The History of Childhood*, L. de Mause (ed.) (Souvenir Press, London, 1974).

16. Graham, H. *Eternal Eve* (Hutchinson, London, 1960).

17. Barker, G. *Early History of Surgery in Great Britain* (London, 1920).

18. Genesis, 3:16.

19. Chamberlain, M. *Old Wives' Tales. Their History, Remedies and Spells* (Virago, London, 1981).

20. Forbes, T.R. 'Midwifery and Witchcraft', *Journal of the History of Medicine, 17* (1962).

21. Forbes, T.R. *The Midwife and the Witch* (Yale University Press, New Haven,

1966, pp. 67).
22. Forbes, T.R. *The Midwife and the Witch*, 1966, pp. 65–6.
23. Rueff, J. *The Expert Midwife* (Griffin, London, 1637).
24. Forbes, T.R. *The Midwife and the Witch* (Yale University Press, New Haven, 1966).
25. Exodus 22:18 A.V.
26. Deuteronomy 18:10–12 R.S.V.
27. I Samuel 15:23 A.V.
28. Galatians 5:20 A.V.
29. Hole, C. *Witchcraft in England* (Batsford, London, 1977).
30. Sprenger, J. and Kramer, H. *Malleus Maleficarum*. Transl. M. Summers, 1928 (Loughborough Library copy).
31. McCall, A. *The Medieval Underworld* (Hamish Hamilton, London, 1979).
32. McCall, A. *The Medieval Underworld* (Hamish Hamilton, London, 1979, pp. 252–3).
33. Middleton, T. *The Witch*, Act I, Scene II (1610).
34. Pettigrew, T.J. *On Superstitions Connected with the History and Practice of Medicine and Surgery*, Barrington and Haswell (eds), (Philadelphia, 1844).
35. Forbes, T.R. *The Midwife and the Witch* (Yale University Press, New Haven, 1966, p. 127).
36. Szasz, T. *The Manufacture of Madness* (Routledge and Kegan Paul, London, 1971).
37. Hole, C. *Witchcraft in England* (Batsford, London, 1977). Quotation from Perkins, W. *A Discourse on the Damned Art of Witchcraft* (1608).
38. Shakespeare, W. *Macbeth*, Act IV, Scene I.
39. Shadwell, T. *The Lancashire Witches* (R. Clavell, London, 1691).

Further Reading

Eccles, A. 'The Early Use of English for Midwiferies. 1500–1700', *Neuphilologische Mitteilungen (Finland)*, 4, LXXVIII
Hughes, P. *Witchcraft* (Longmans Green, London, 1952)
Murray, M.A. *The Witch Cult in Western Europe* (Clarendon Press, Oxford, 1921)
Tuttle, E.F. 'The Trotula and Old Dame Trot: A Note on the Lady of Salerno', *Bulletin of the History of Medicine*, 50, 61–62 (1976)

THE EMERGENCE OF ENGLISH MIDWIVES AND EUROPEAN INFLUENCES ON MIDWIFERY PRACTICE

In England, the sixteenth century, which encompassed both the Renaissance and the Reformation, can be seen as a watershed between the medieval and the modern world. During the reign of Henry VIII, quite severe inflation had caused hardship to many people, particularly the peasants, large numbers of whom were dispossessed of their land by Enclosure Acts. However, as the century progressed, the economic situation gradually improved, and because many peasants had found themselves destitute, a social conscience developed which led ultimately to the passing of the Poor Law Act in 1601. The economic situation improved because the reign of Elizabeth I was an era of peace and stability and because trade and commerce expanded. Rich merchants founded hospitals, almshouses and schools, so that grammar-school education became available to all classes of boys.

England remained predominantly rural, with four-fifths of people living outside towns. The rich minority built themselves substantial houses but the poor majority still lived in 'gabled and thatched cottages of timber'.[1] It appears that the standard of living and nutrition, in terms of quantity and quality, was relatively good. It provoked a visiting Spaniard to remark, 'These English have their houses made of sticks and dirt but they fare commonly so well as the King.'[2] It is perhaps not surprising, therefore, that these people were fertile, and that despite high mortality and morbidity rates, the population of England rose from 2½ to 4 millions during the century. The greatest explosion was in London, where the number of people increased fourfold.[3]

As far as childbirth was concerned, the sixteenth century was to see the beginning of certain processes that were to lead ultimately to compulsory training and state recognition of the midwife, and to role conflict. It was also to see the entry of men into the sphere of childbirth — for better or for worse! In the early part of the century, however, there was little change in midwifery practice from that of previous centuries. The majority of midwives were still illiterate, and although they may have been skilled at normal delivery of healthy women, they had had no 'training' for the variety of obstetric and paediatric complications with which they had to deal, generally alone. There was no one to teach them, as male physicians, who were not acceptable to women giving birth, did not in any case concern themselves even with the theory let alone the practice of obstetrics. The midwife was in an unenviable position and her only source of help was from a limited number of barber-surgeons who were called in as a last resort. Even if she were the local midwife and knew the mother socially, she would have no knowledge whatsoever, prior to the labour, of what exactly presented itself beneath the mother's voluminous skirts. She may have been faced with a multiple pregnancy, or with a grande multiparous patient in premature labour with a malpresentation, uterine inertia, post-partum haemorrhage and an asphyxiated small baby; or with a woman convulsing and at the same time haemorrhaging from a placental abruption, and whose labour was obstructed due to a contracted pelvis; or with a permutation of any of these emergency situations. She was obliged in the interests of the mother to deliver the baby, alive or dead, whole or piecemeal. She was without analgesics, oxytocin or oxygen, she had no blood or other fluids for infusion, and there was no 'Flying Squad' to summon to her assistance. It is possible that she would carry herbal preparations in an attempt to deal with pain and bleeding, and her only recourse was to these remedies, which might have been efficacious in some instances. It is worth remembering also that the midwife would be without uniform and without equipment, and there would be very little of obstetric value for her to carry in her delivery bag. These were the days before the existence of thermometers, rubber gloves, syringes, needles and urine-testing equipment. Even such present-day useful items as cotton wool swabs and pads would be unknown to her. She may or may not have possessed a metal catheter, depending on whether she had any idea about how or when to use it. This untutored midwife had to make difficult clinical decisions, the result of which could have been death of the fetus, or the mother, or in some cases both.

There are no relevant official statistics for this time, but the maternal and perinatal mortality rates are known to be have been high. The physical pain and psychological anguish, suffering and morbidity some of the mothers endured are incalculable. Who could estimate the short- and long-term psychological trauma experienced by the midwife who was party to a disastrous end result to her handiwork but who had no means or knowledge to do anything else, or to improve the situation in the future?

It is not surprising that midwives lacked theoretical knowledge of even basic reproductive anatomy, physiology and pathology, given that women in general had no access to education of any kind. Although a forceful and highly educated Queen occupied the throne of England for four decades, the legal, social and educational subjection of women was not alleviated. Indeed the new learning available to certain *men* served not only to widen the gap between men and women but also to reinforce male supremacy. The deficiency in the knowledge of midwives was recognised in the mid-sixteenth century by at least one 'Doctour of physicke', Andrew Boorde, who wrote in *The Brevary of Helthe*:

> every midwife shulde be presented with honest women of great gravitee to the Byshoppe, and that they should testify for her that they do present: she shulde be a sadde woman, wyse and discrete, havynge experience and worthy to have office of mydwyf. Then the Byshoppe with the consent of a doctor of physicke ought to examine her and to instructe her in that thynge that she is ignorant, and thus proved and admitted in a laudable thynge, for and if this were used in Englande, there should not be halfe so many women myscarry, nor so many children perish in every place in Englande as there be. The Byshoppe ought to look into this matter.[4]

It is interesting to speculate about who Boorde thought would be able to instruct the midwife. Perhaps the physician could have taught her some basic anatomy, physiology and pathology, but it is very unlikely that he knew anything of the physiology of pregnancy, labour or the puerperium. He almost certainly would not even have witnessed a normal delivery, and would therefore have no experience at all of abnormal presentation or complications. Physicians' skills were primarily diagnostic and not curative, so although they were quite likely to be interested in conception and the diagnosis of pregnancy, they considered the actual birth process to be both outside and beneath their professional province. Lacking normal delivery experience it would have been impossible for them to undertake the manoeuvres required for the delivery of malpresentations, obstructed labour, prolapsed limbs or cords, or to deal with any third-stage complications, whereas the midwives' practical skills would be gained by observation and personal experience.

The first glimmer of light in these dark ages for the midwife came in the middle of the sixteenth century with the publication of a book in English called *The Byrth of Mankynd*, made possible by the revival of classical thought and learning and the advent of printing (Figure 6). Its appearance was perhaps to meet a demand from the educated upper classes and the emerging 'middling' class who were beginning to recognise the deficiencies of their midwives. This book was a modern

Figure 6: Title Page of *The Byrth of Mankynd*, by E. Roesslin. Translated by T. Raynald, London, 1552

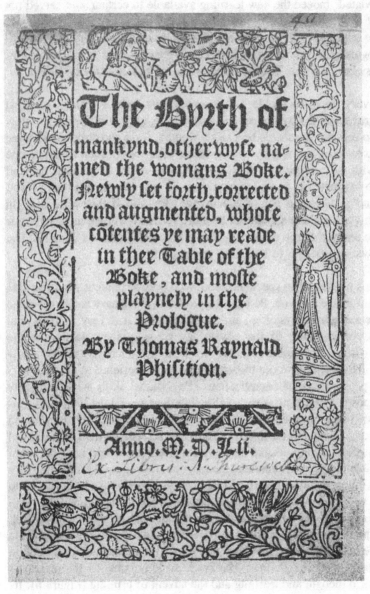

Source: Wellcome Institute Library, London, with permission.

and translated version of the text first written by Soranus 1400 years before, entitled *Instructions for Midwives*, which was later revised by Moschion (Moschio). A translation made by Eucharius Roesslin of *Instructions for Midwives* appeared in German in 1513. Roesslin entitled his book *Der Swangern Frauwen unt Mebammen Roszgarten*, generally abbreviated to *The Rosengarten* (Figure 7). Roesslin's son is believed to have translated this work into Latin, giving it the title *De Partu Hominis*. At the same time he latinised his father's name to Eucharius Rhodion. (Roesslin was the City Physician of Frankfurt and one of his duties was to supervise the work of the official city midwives. Was such a Medical Supervisor of Midwives the forerunner of the Medical Officer of Health in England in the twentieth century?)

De Partu Hominis was translated into English in 1540 by Richard Jonas, a studious and diligent clerk, under the title *The Byrth of Mankynd*.[5] A second amended and amplified English translation was made by Thomas Raynald, Physician, in 1545; he also used the Latin edition by Roesslin the younger.[6] Later editions appeared in 1552, 1564, 1565, 1598, 1604, 1626, 1634 and 1654, and these editions were variously illustrated; they all appeared under Jonas's title. In his prologue to the new edition, Raynald describes how:

> gentlewomen have been in the habit of visiting confinements 'carienge with them this booke in theyr handes, and causynge such part of it as doth chiefly concerne the same pourpose, to be red before the mydwife, and the rest of the wemen then beyng present' with such good effect that despite the criticism of prudes, right-minded women were glad 'to have the booke red by sum other, or els (such as could) to read it themselves'.[7]

Though it was acceptable for subject matter relating to reproduction and childbirth to be circulated among and between women, it was offensive to the modesty of women and respectable men that such intimate and feminine matters should be written in plain English so that 'every boy and knave had of these books, readyng them as openly as the tales of Roben hood'.[8]

A comprehensive study of *The Byrth of Mankynd* has been written by Dr J.W. Ballantyne. The English work is divided into the following parts:

Figure 7: Title-page of the 1524 Edition of *The Rosengarten* showing the midwife bathing the infant with her bare legs in the bath: from G. Klein's reprint of *The Rosengarten* (1910)

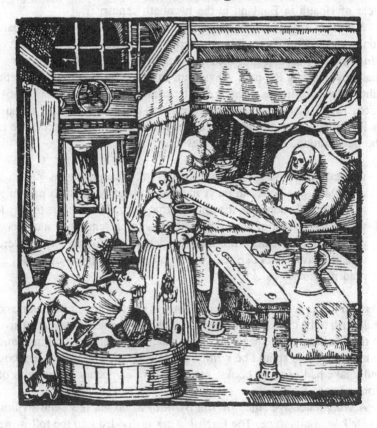

Source: Arts Library, University of Manchester, UK.

I. Anatomy or 'Inward Partes of Women' including 'coates, fleshye or Skin; . . . muskles and peritoneum; matrix; mother-port or cervix; bladder, woman's stones or ovaries'

II. This is concerned with 'howe a woman with childe shal use her selfe, and what remedies be for them that have harde labour'

III. This considers the choices of a wet-nurse

IV. 'Conception and the Overcoming of Sterility'

The chapter on labour and birth instructs midwives on the management of the labouring women. It starts with the following definition: 'Naturall byrth is when the chylde is borne both in due season and also in due fashion. The due season is most commonly after the ninth month, or about fortie weeks after the conception'.

Various ointments and baths were recommended before labour. 'Annointmentes wherewith ye may sople the privie place, be these. Hennes grese, Duckes grese, Goose grese, also oyle olife, Linsede oyl, or oyl of Fenegreke, or the viscositie of holyoke'. The mother was to bathe in water 'in which have been seethed malowes, Holyoke, Camomel, Mercury, Maiden haire, Lyneseede, Fenegreke seede, and such other thynges which have vertue to mollifie and sople'. She was also to 'exercyse the bodye in doing some thinge, styring, moving, goynge or standinge, more than otherwise she was wont to doe'. Hints are given as to what she must do once labour pains have commenced: '. . . it shall be verye profytable for her, for the space of an houre to syt styll, then (rysynge agayne) to goe up and downe a payre of stayres, crying or reaching so loude as she can, so to styre her self'. The midwives were advised that when the birth was imminent 'then shall it be mete for her to sit downe leaninge backwards in manner upright'. When using the birth stool 'the mydwyfe herselfe shal syt before the labourynge women, and shall dilligentlye observe and wayte, how much, and after what meanes the chylde styreth it selfe, also shall with her handes, fyrste annoynted with the oyle of almondes. . . . rule and dyrect every thynge as shall seme beste'. Also the mydwife was to 'enstructe and comfort the partie, not only refreshing her with good meate and drink, but also with swete wordes gevinge her good hope of a spedefull delyveraunce'. To assist the delivery, the midwife was told she should gently stroke the upper part of the abdomen, and if the membranes were still intact, 'it shal be the mydwyfes part and office, with her nayles easely and gentellye to break and rent it, or yf that may not conveniently be done, then rayse up betwene your fyngers a peece of it, and cut it with a payre of shieres, or a sharpe kynfe, but so that ye hurt not the byrth with the cut'.[5] Standing and walking during labour, and sitting for delivery were evidently standard practices at this time as they probably were when the original Greek text was written.

Midwives were given specific instruction on the care of the neonate. The cord was to be severed 'three fingers breadth from the belly and so knit up'. After the cord stump had separated, the midwife was advised to 'apply powder of burnt calves ashes or of snails shells, or the powder of lead, called red lead tempered with wine'.[9] This last preparation would create a raised level of lead in the blood, the consequences of which the author would be blissfully ignorant.

Midwives and their helpers who were present at the birth were 'dressed in their everyday clothes with the possible addition of an apron'. A late sixteenth-century list of the midwife's necessities is found in Thomas Delaney's *The Gentle Craft*. These include soap and candles, beds, shirts, biggins, waistcoats, headbands, swaddlebands, crosscloths, bibs, tailclouts, mantles, hose, shoes, coats, petticoats, cradle and crickets. 'Soap to cleanse mother and child; an assortment of clothes for the baby including the tailclout, his diaper and bigginbonnet; a crosscloth to tie about the mother's forehead to prevent wrinkles; and the cricket-low stool for the attendant midwife.'[10]

Babies born in the sixteenth century were given popular saints' names such as John, Thomas, Anne, Margaret and Catherine, or Royal names such as Edward and Elizabeth. Sometimes they were given such holy names as Pentecost and Baptist.

Stimulus from European Practitioners of Midwifery

In post-Renaissance Europe, men who were educated at secular universities were beginning to enquire, research, investigate, reason, observe and change the existing thinking and understanding in many subjects. Some of these 'scientists' turned their attention to the study of female anatomy and to the practice of 'abnormal' midwifery.

Some physicians in Germany, Holland, Switzerland, and France interested themselves in midwifery as early as the fifteenth century and began to organise and regulate the practice of midwives. In 1452, what is thought to be the first municipal system of midwife regulation in Europe was set up in Regensburg, Bavaria. Gradually other cities followed its example, and by the sixteenth century these municipal authorities were paying more attention to the technical competence of the midwife than to her moral character.[11] In country areas of Germany, however, the scene was so vastly different as to require a law to be passed in 1580 forbidding shepherds and swineherds to attend women in labour.[12] In parts of Bavaria the status of the midwife was so low that midwives were even 'despised by the barber, the knacker and the executioner and the midwife's son might be excluded from a Trade Guild because of his mother's occupation'.[13]

In the sixteenth century an Ordinance was enacted in Paris. Its regulations were detailed, and the midwives were told:

if they realise that the child presents other than head first . . . and before the woman is in extremity, they must call for advice either from physicians, or from official Master Surgeons of the Palace in Paris, or from senior Mistresses and expert Matrons of Paris, and not persons who are ignorant in this matter.[14]

They were also instructed to take off their rings and wash their hands before attending to the mother.[15] It would appear that in this century France was particularly advanced and progressive in the fields of medicine, surgery and obstetrics, and the Hotel Dieu in Paris was the most renowned establishment in Europe for lying-in mothers. This hospital was originally run by the Chapter of Notre Dame, but in 1505 it was transferred to a Board of Lay Governors appointed by the Paris Parlement. A famous obstetrician-surgeon at this hospital for a large part of the sixteenth century was Ambroise Paré, who, although a Protestant, was appointed surgeon to no less than four French kings. Halfway through the century, Paré wrote two obstetric treatises in colloquial French in which he clearly describes his technique for the delivery of the child by the feet, originally described by Soranus, but which he appears to have revived. His work, called *De la generation de l'homme* (1573), contains 'the anatomical and other figures, including the birth chair copied from Roesslin and Rueff'.[6] Not only did he, like Mercurio (a contemporary Italian obstetrician), define and categorise natural and unnatural labour, but he also allocated the normal cases to midwives and the abnormal cases to doctors. He realised that midwives were unable to deal satisfactorily with complicated cases, and that this could cause great suffering and often the death of both baby and mother. His concern led him to equip himself to provide skilled obstetric care and to instruct some of the Parisian midwives, and he therefore established at the Hotel Dieu what was probably the first School for Midwives in modern Europe. Admission to the midwifery course was conditional on being a married or widowed French national.[16] With Paré came the innovation of delivering a woman on a bed should she require assistance with the birth, but he did, however, advocate the continued use of the squatting position and stool for normal deliveries. He pioneered and taught suturing of torn perineums and he described the movements of the fetus *in utero* which could be felt on palpation, and also endorsed the view of Hippocrates that the life of the baby born at eight months is 'brief or null'.[6]

One of Paré's student midwives was Louise Bourgeois (the wife of an army surgeon), who practised at the Hotel Dieu and became famous throughout Europe. She also worked with and was influenced by Jacques Guillemeau, who had studied under and worked alongside Paré. Bourgeois was an educated woman who became an outstandingly skilful midwife, and her clientele included members of the French court and royal family. According to Harvey Graham, she was 'a much superior type to the bedraggled midwives who had previously trundled their obstetric chairs from house to house'.[17] French midwives in general, though, were classed as peasants because their income was so small that they were pitiably poor.[18]

Jacques Guillemeau wrote a book for midwives entitled *Childbirth or the Happy Deliverie of Women*, which was translated and available in English in 1612. In this work he enumerated the qualities a midwife should possess. She was to be, he said, beyond the age of childbearing, but neither too young nor too old. She was to be healthy and have no diseases nor be deformed in any part. She was to be neat in her dress and in her person. Her hands were to be small, and with nails pared, very clean and even. She was not to wear rings when she was about her business. She was to have a pleasant and merry disposition and be accustomed to hard work so that if necessary she could stay awake two or three nights. She was not to be gossipy, nor to repeat anything she might hear or see in the privacy of the childbirth room.[19] It is interesting to note that right through the ages very similar moral, physical and psychological attributes have been required of the ideal midwife. It seems that it was recognised early that her very disposition could provide emotional support to the mother in her inevitably painful and often long labour.

The first Italian to write a book for midwives was an obstetrician called Scipione Mercurio who published *La Comere o Riccoglitrice* in 1596. (The translation of *La Comere* is midwife or 'with woman'.) On visits to France, Mercurio had learnt about the Caesarean-section operation on living women and he introduced this into Italy.

The text of Mercurio's book is divided into three parts. One deals with pregnancy, natural labour, and care and feeding of the newborn child. The second part considers preternatural labour and teaches 'how the midwife should deal with these difficult and dangerous cases'.[6] Abnormalities of mother and baby in the puerperium are covered in the third part. His advice that women should reduce their dietary intake by one-third in the last three months of pregnancy may be unsound, but seemed wise to him; indeed it is likely from his description of the position in which very fat women should be placed for delivery that grossly overweight women were not uncommon.

In the middle of the sixteenth century a Swiss doctor, Jacobus Rueff, who was responsible for the instruction and examination of midwives in Zurich, wrote a *Guide for Midwives, Pregnant Women and Women in Childbed*. He persuaded the Burgomaster to supply free copies to all the midwives and nurses in the Canton. This book was published in 1554 in the German vernacular under the title of *A Very Cheerful Booklet of Encouragement Concerning the Conception and Birth of Man and its Frequent Accidents and Hindrances etc.*; this rather long title was often shortened and Latinised to *De Conceptu et Generatione Hominis* (Figure 8). This book was the set text for the examination of the Zurich midwives who were obliged to have the appropriate section read aloud by an educated woman, if possible, during the first stage of labour at any confinement they attended.

Baptism, Oaths and Licences

In 1277 the Trier Synod stipulated that priests were to instruct lay women in the words of emergency baptism.[20] However, Aveling says that there is evidence in *Monumenta Ecclesiastica* that midwives were called upon by the Archbishop of Canterbury as early as the seventh century to perform this sacrament. In *Liber Penitentialis* of Theodore, Archbishop of Canterbury, it says 'Mulier baptizare nonpralesumat nisi cognenti necessitate maxima': in other words, a woman should only baptise an infant in a grave emergency.[21] In 1303, Robert Mannyng declared that midwives must understand thoroughly the procedure relating to baptism. He recounted how one midwife who failed to use the correct words 'loste a chylde both soule and lyfe'.[22] Because baptism was a necessary prerequisite to the salvation of the soul, midwives were under an obligation to ensure that the ultimate destiny of a baby unlikely to survive was the Kingdom of God and not the Kingdom of the Devil. To this end an English manual for parish priests of 1540 specifies the midwife's

Figure 8: Title page of Jabocus Rueff's *De Conceptu et Generatione Hominis* (1580), showing the midwife drinking

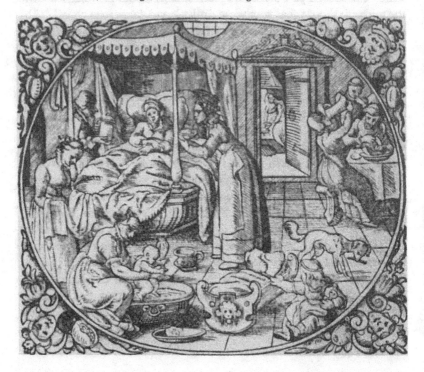

Source: *The Renaissance of Midwifery*, H.R. Spencer, 1924 (Lloyd Roberts Lecture delivered under the Conjoint Scheme of the Royal College of Physicians, the Medical Society of London, and the Royal Society of Medicine).

ecclesiastical and professional duties in an obstetric emergency. These duties are beautifully spelt out in verse:

> And teche the mydwyfe never the latere
> Then heo have redy clene watere,
> Then bydde hyre spare for no schame,
> to folowe [baptise] the chylde there at hame,
> and thoghe the chylde bote half be bore,
> Hed and necke and no more,
> Bydde hyre spare never the later
> to crystene hyt and caste on water;
> And but sche mowe se the hed,

Loke sche folowe hyt for no red;
And ef the wommon thenne dye
Teche the mydwyf that sche hye [hasten]
for to undo hyre with a knyf,
And hye that hyt christened be,
For that ys a ded of charyte.[23]

Records exist of emergency baptisms by midwives. In an East Sussex parish register is the following entry: '1579. Was baptised Joan Birmingham, the daughter of John Birmingham and Joan his wife, by the midwife at home, and it was buried on the 20th day . . .'[13] At Lichfield on 12 October 1591, we find Margaret, 'dr. of Walter Henningham de Pypehall, baptised by the mydwyfe, and, as yet not brought to the Churche to be there examined and testified by them that were present'.[21]

In one case it appears that perhaps the midwife made a mistake. The parish register of Hanwell, Middlesex, records: 'Thomas, son of Thomas Messenger, and Elizabeth his wife, was born and baptised October 24, 1731, by the midwife at the font called a boy and named by the godfather, Thomas, but proved a girl.'[22]

Licences

Whereas in Europe ecclesiastical licensing of midwives was being superseded by municipal licensing, in England episcopal licensing only began in the 1500s and was not officially replaced until the twentieth century.

In 1512, in the reign of Henry VIII, an Act permitted the Church to grant licences for the practice of medicine and surgery, and the licensing of 'qualified' midwives by Bishops began soon afterwards.[24] Forbes also states that, from records he has seen, licensing of midwives by Bishops was taking place in England during the first half of the sixteenth century.[22] It is certain that Bishop Bonner was issuing licences in London by the middle of the century. This continued until the eighteenth century with the exception of the time when, as a result of the victory of the Parliamentarians and Puritans in the Civil War, the Established Church with its Bishops collapsed. With the restoration of the monarchy in 1660 came the re-establishment of the Church of England and so the practice of granting ecclesiastical licences was resumed. However, it appears not to have been as widespread as before and to vary from diocese to diocese. Bishops' licences, whether granted to physicians, surgeons, apothecaries or midwives, were doubtless very useful in enabling the

poorly educated people of those days to choose between 'licensed' practitioners and pretentious charlatans. Possession of a licence guaranteed
both an accepted standard of behaviour and certain virtues, but it was
not proof of knowledge or clinical competence.

It seems that a secular form of licensing was instituted between 1642
and 1662. This took place at Chirurgions' Hall in London after the midwives had satisfied 'six skilful midwives and as many chirurgions, expert in the art of midwifery' in three examinations. In 1688 Elizabeth
Cellier, a famous London midwife, writing the above in a 'letter concerning midwives', expressed her preference for a professional authority granting licences to practice *by examination*, as against the granting
of licences to practice following the production of character references,
the taking of an oath and the payment of a fee. Her reasoning was that
during the years of lay licensing the London mortality figures dropped
markedly.[24] This alternative method of licensing could only have applied to midwives in London, as those in other parts of the country would
have found it almost impossible to journey to London, especially during
the period of the Civil War. On the other hand it has been claimed in
retrospect that, with the fading out of episcopal licensure, standards of
midwifery practice dropped.[25] The implication is that midwives *en masse*
were neither competent nor morally or ethically reliable.

One of the earliest preserved oaths made by a midwife prior to her
receiving a licence is the one made by Eleanor Pead who was licensed
on 26 August 1567. Not only was she questioned about her knowledge
of midwifery by the Archbishop of Canterbury and eight women
(presumably experienced and respected midwives) but she was also expected to carry out, irreproachably, the office of midwife in regard to
many ethical issues. She had to swear as follows:

> I, Eleanor Pead, admitted to the office and occupation of a midwife,
> will faithfully and diligently exercise the said office according to such
> cunning and knowledge as God has given me; and that I will be ready
> to help and aid as well poor as rich women being in labour and travail
> of child, and will always be ready both to poor and rich, in exercis-
> ing and executing of my said office.
> *Also* I will not permit or suffer that women being in labour or travail
>   shall name any other to be the father of her child, than only
>   he who is the right and true father thereof; and that I will not
>   suffer any other body's child to be set, brought or laid before
>   any woman delivered of child in the place of her natural child,
>   so far forth as I can know and understand.

Also I will not use any kind of sorcery or incantation in the time of travail of any woman; and I will not destroy the child born of any woman, nor cut, nor pull off the head thereof, or otherwise dismember or hurt the same, or suffer it to be so hurt or dismembered, by any manner of ways or means.

Also that in the administration of the sacrament of baptism in the time of necessity I will use apt and accustomed words of the same sacrament, that is to say, these words following, or the like in effect; I christen thee in the name of the Father, the Son and the Holy Ghost, and none other profane words. And that in such time of necessity, in baptising any infant born, and pouring water upon the head of the same infant, I will use pure and clean water, and not any rose or damask water, or water made of any confection or mixture; and that I will certify the curate of the parish church of every such baptising.[26]

In 1551–52 the clergy of the diocese of Gloucester and Worcester were asked by their Bishops 'whether the midwives at the labour and birth of any child . . . do use salt, herbs, water, wax, cloths, girdles, or relics or any other such like thing or superstitious means contrary to the word of God and the laws of the realm'.[27] One of the injunctions at the visitation of Bishop Bonner (1554) was the following: 'A mydwyfe shall not use or exercise any witchcrafte, charmes, sorcerie, invocations, or praiers, other than suche as be allowable and may stand with the lawes and ordinances of the Catholike Churche'.[21] A Directive of the Bishop of Chester (1584) specified that in their Oath midwives should state that they do not use 'any witchcraft, charms, relics, or invocation of any Saint in time of travail'.[28]

In Scotland during this century, under the direct influence of the European Reformation, the church required midwives to notify them of all births. This requirement stemmed from an attempt to eliminate immorality and illegitimacy by persuading the mother to divulge the name of the father and if possible to legitimise the birth.[29] This procedure originated in Edinburgh in 1564 so that the 'Kirk session' could immediately investigate any suspicious circumstances surrounding the birth.

Almost a century after the Oath made by Eleanor Pead, a Book of Oaths[30] issued in 1649 includes the wording of an oath which makes even greater professional, ethical and moral demands on the midwife and in effect catalogues a list of abuses in which midwives had been known to be involved. The practices she had to forswear exceeded those made by Eleanor Pead in that midwives in the seventeenth century were also required to swear that they:

1. *Would* call upon the aid of other midwives if they were in doubt about the outcome of a difficult labour.

> So often as you shall perceive any perill or jeopardie, either in the woman or the childe, in any such wise, as you shall bee in doubt what shall chance thereof, you shall thenceforth in due time send for other midwifes and expert women in that facultie, and use their advice and counsell in the behalfe.

2. *Would not* use 'medicines' to abort the fetus or to facilitate premature labour. (Induction was performed by midwives who seemed to have reasoned that if the baby was small the greater would be the chance of a normal vaginal delivery.)

> You shall not give any counsell, or minister any herbs, medicine or potion, or any other thing, to any woman being with childe, whereby she should destroy or cast out that she goeth withal before her time.

3. *Would not* extort extra fees.

> You shall not enforce any woman being with childe by any paine, or by any ungodly wayes or means, to give you any more for your paines or labour in bringing her to bed, than they would otherwise do.

4. *Would not* collude with the woman to hide anything under cover of darkness.

> You shall not consent, agree, give or keep counsell, that any woman be delivered secretly of that which she goeth with, but in the presence of two or three lights readie.

5. *Would* keep the secrets of the woman.

> You shall be secret, and not open any matter appertaining to your office in the presence of any man, unless necessity or great urgent cause do constraine you so to do.

6. *Would* treat with dignity the body of a stillborn baby, and ensure its safe burial to prevent retrieval for unlawful purpose.

> If any childe bee dead-born, you yourselfe shall see it buried in such secret place as neither hogg nor dogg, nor any other beast may come into it, and in such sort done, as it may not be found or perceived, as much as you may; And that you shall not suffer any such childe to be cast into the Jaques or any other inconvenient place.

7. *Would* report any midwife guilty of disobedience to these edicts and any woman known to be practising as an unlicensed midwife.

> If you shall know any midwife using or doing anything contrary to any of these premises, or in any other wise than shall be seemly or convenient, you shall forthwith detect open to show the same to me [the Bishop] or my Chancellor, all such women as you shall know from time to time to occupie and exercise the roome [rank] of a midwife within my foresaid Diocese and Jurisdiction without my Licence and admission.

8. *Would* deal fairly with their sister-midwife colleagues.

> You shall use yourselfe in honest behaviour unto the woman being lawfully admitted to the room [rank] and office of a midwife in all things accordingly.

9. *Would not* employ an 'unqualified' deputy.

> You shall not make or assigne any Deputie or Deputies to exercise or occupie under you in your absence the office or room of a midwife, but such as you shall perfectly knowe to be of right honest and discreet behaviour, as also apt, able and having sufficient knowledge and experience to exercise the said roome and office.

10. *Would not* allow baptism except into and by the laws of the Church of England.

> You shall not be bee privie, or consent, that any Priest, or other Partie, shall in your absence, or in your companie, or of your

knowledge or sufferance, Baptise any childe, by any masse, Latine
service, or Prayers, than such as are appointed by the Lawes of
the Church of Englande; neither shall you consent, that any childe,
born by any woman, who shall be delivered by you, shall be carried away without being Baptised in the Parish by the Ordinarie
Minister, where the said childe is borne, unless it be in the case
of necessitie Baptisted privately, according to the Booke of Common Prayer; but you shall forthwith upon understanding thereof,
either give knowledge to me the said Bishop, or my Chancellor
for the time being.

It is rather strange that this Book of oaths should appear in the year
in which the Church of England became disestablished. All midwives
were not members of the Church of England: some would be Papist midwives and others would be adherents of one of the many non-conformist
sects that had come into being by this time, but many of them may have
been prepared to pay lip service to Anglican regulations and conform
to Article 10.

Whether the midwives were charged for licences to practice from the
beginning is uncertain but records show that they paid 18s 6d in 1662,
8 guineas in 1714, and £10 in 1738.[31] These licence fees seem extor-
tionate, and except for those few who attended wealthy patients, midwives generally would have difficulty in raising such a sum of money.
Evidence of gifts given to midwives at christening feasts in the sixteenth
century is found in the Privy Purse expenses of Henry VIII. '1530. To
the Nurse and Mydwif of my Ladye of Worcestre, by way of reward
£4 . . . 1532. To the Nurse and Mydwif of Sir Nicholas Harvy cheilde
£3 6s 8d.' Entries concerning gifts of the Princess Mary to midwives
are numerous, the sums ranging from 5 to 15 shillings according to the
rank of the parents.[32]

According to Burn[33] midwives practising without a licence or otherwise violating professional regulations (as in articles of oath) could be
brought before an Ecclesiastical Court and fined or otherwise punished.
It appears that midwives were allowed a period of practice (perhaps as
apprentices) before presenting themselves to be licensed. This is apparent
from the following extract from evidence presented in 1661 on behalf
of Judith Newman of the Parish of All Hallows the Less in London.

shee is in our judgements able and sufficient for the office and ffunction of a midwife which shee hath many years past been exercised
in, and therefore we Recommend her unto yr honor for the exercise

of such an office and ffunction.

Signed by Curate, two Churchwardens and two common Counsellmen, one midwife and the mark of another.

A licence written in Latin on parchment was granted.[22]

Licences were certainly issued in the Diocese of Chester in the seventeenth and early eighteenth centuries, and in the thirteen years between 1667 and 1680 records state that 41 women were 'licensed to the office of midwife'. The Bishop of Chester, on visitations to the various parishes, granted these licences or 'faculty to practice within the Diocese of Chester' and midwives are named in the parishes of Chorley, Leyland, Tarvin, City of Chester, Duddon and Whalley. In 1705 four 'obstetrices' were licensed in the city of Chester, and in 1712 on an episcopal visit to the parish of Bowden, Altrincham, three were granted licence to practice. In the same year four other 'obstetrices' in the parishes of Frodsham, Grappenhall and Knutsford were licensed. The details of these women show that they were married and that the common Christian names of the time were Biblical: Mary or Maria, Sarah, Elizabeth, Anne or Anna.[21]

Another enduring record of a licence granted to a midwife can be found on a tombstone in Charlestown, USA, which reads:

Here lyes interred the body of Mrs Elizabeth Phillips, wife of Mr John Phillips, who was born in Westminster, in Great Britain, and commissioned by John, Lord Bishop of London, in the year 1718, to the office of midwife, and came to this country in the year 1719, and, by the blessing of God, has brought into the world above three thousand children. Died 1761, aged 76 years.[21]

There are also records of ecclesiastical licences granted in Norwich to 30 midwives between 1770 and 1786 when the practice appeared to cease in that diocese.[35]

One eighteenth-century midwife's licence was worded as follows:

Joseph, by Divine Permission, Bishop of Rochester, to our well-beloved in Christ ELIZABETH CHAPMAN of the parish of St. Warburg, otherwise Hoo, in the county of Kent, and our Diocese of Rochester, send greetings in our Lord everlasting: Whereas we understand by good testimony and credible certificates that you the said Elizabeth Chapman are apt and able, cunning and expert, to use and exercise the office, business and function of a Midwife. We therefore, by virtue of Our Power Ordinary and Episcopal, do admit and give you power to use and exercise the office, business and function of a Midwife in and through our Diocese and Jurisdiction of Rochester with the best care and diligence you may or can in this behalf, indifferently both to poor and rich, as also to perform and accomplish all things about the same, according to your oath thereupon given you upon the Holy Evangelists, as far as God will give you Grace and enable you. In witness thereof we have caused the Seal of our Chancellor to be affixed to these presents this Twenty-first day of July in the year of our Lord, One thousand seven hundred and thirty-eight, and in the seventh year of our Translation.[21]

The general oath that the midwife had to swear varied little from the seventeenth-century oath.

By the end of the sixteenth century, books had been written in the vernacular for midwives in most European countries and certainly in England, France, Italy, Switzerland and Germany. On the whole all these books were based on the original obstetric text of Soranus, but new scholarship added new knowledge, and new techniques were evolved from experience. With the exception of Louise Bourgeois, it was the sixteenth-century physicians and surgeons who were becoming interested in pregnancy and childbirth (in spite of public opinion), and who compiled these books for the enlightenment of both midwives and mothers. It is regrettable that the vast majority of women remained unhelped, as neither they nor their midwives had been taught to read.

References

1. Trevelyan, G.M. *English Social History* (Longmans Green, London, 1944).
2. Harrison, W. 'Description of England in Shakespeare's Youth', 1588, in reference 1, p. 159.
3. Hurstfield, J. and Smith, A. *Elizabethan People, State and Society* (E. Arnold, London, 1972).
4. Boorde, A. *The Brevary of Helthe* (London, 1547).
5. Ballantyne, J.W. 'The Byrth of Mankynd (its Authors and Editions)', bound reprint from *Journal of Obstetrics and Gynaecology of the British Empire* (Sherratt & Hughes, London and Manchester, October 1906).
6. Spencer, H.R. *The Renaissance of Midwifery* (Harrison and Sons Ltd, London, 1924).
7. Eccles, A. 'The Early Use of English for Midwiferies. 1500–1700', *Neuphilologische Mitteilungen, 4*, LXXVIII (1977), quoting Raynalde, *The Byrthe of Mankynde*.

8. Eccles, A. 'The Early Use of English for Midwiferies. 1500-1700', *Neuphilologische Mitteilungen*, *4*, LXXVIII (1977).

9. Mause, de Lloyd. *The History of Childhood* (Souvenir Press, London, 1976). (Quoting from the translation of E. Rösslin's *The Byrthe of Mankynd*.)

10. Mause, de Lloyd. *The History of Childhood* (Souvenir Press, London, 1976). (Quoting from *Costumes for Births, Marriages and Deaths*, P. Cunnington and C. Lucas (eds), (London, 1972)).

11. Donnison, J. *Midwives and Medical Men* (Heinemann, London, 1977).

12. Radcliffe, W. *The Secret Instrument* (Heinemann, London, 1947).

13. Forbes, T.R. 'Midwifery and Witchcraft', *Journal of the History of Medicine*, *17* (1962).

14. Benedek, T.G. 'The Changing Relationship between Midwives and Physicians during the Renaissance', *Bulletin of the History of Medicine* (1977). (Quoting from R.C. Petrelli, 'The Regulation of French Midwives during the *Ancien Regime*', *Journal of the History of Medicine*, *26*, 276-91 (1971).

15. Benedek, T.G. 'The Changing Relationship between Midwives and Physicians during the Renaissance', *Bulletin of the History of Medicine* (1977).

16. Donnison, J. *Midwives and Medical Men* quoting E. Coyecque, *L'Hotel Dieu de Paris, 1889-91, Vol. I*.

17. Graham, H. *Eternal Eve* (Hutchinson, London, 1960).

18. Forbes, T.R. 'Midwifery and Witchcraft', *Journal of the History of Medicine*, *17* (1962). (Quotation from P. Gosset, 'Les sages-femmes du Pays Remois au XVIIe et au XVIIIe siecle', *Un. Med. Scient. Nord-Est, 33* (1909)).

19. Guillemeau, J. *Childbirth or the Happy Deliverie of Women* (1612).

20. Shorter, E. (ed.) *A History of Women's Bodies* (Allen Lane, London, 1982).

21. Aveling, J.H. *English Midwives: their History and Prospects* (Hugh K. Elliott, London, 1967).

22. Forbes, T.R. *The Midwife and the Witch* (Yale University Press, Newhaven, 1966).

23. Merc, Canon J. *Instructions for Parish Priests* (1450).

24. Atkinson, S.B. *The Office of Midwife (in England and Wales) under The Midwives Act 1902*.

25. Aveling, J.H. 'On the Instruction, Examination and Regulation of English Midwives', *British Medical Journal, 1*, 308-9 (1873).

26. Forbes, T.R. 'Midwifery and Witchcraft', *Journal of the History of Medicine*, *17* (April 1962). (Quoting J. Strype, *Annals of the Reformation and Establishment of Religion* (Clarendon Press, Oxford, 1822)).

27. Forbes, T.R. 'Midwifery and Witchcraft', *Journal of the History of Medicine*, *17*, 278 (April 1962). (Quoting W.H. Frere and W.M. Kennedy, *Visitation Articles and Injunctions of the Period of the Reformation* (Longmans, London, 1910)).

28. Raines, F.R. *The Derby Household Books* (Chetham Society, 1853). Remains Historical Literature.

29. Marshall, R. 'Birth of a Profession', *Nursing Mirror* (30 November 1983).

30. Forbes, T.R. *The Midwife and the Witch* (Yale University Press, Newhaven, 1966). Quoting from a *Book of Oaths and the Severall Forms Thereof both Ancient and Modern* (1649). (Surveyed by W. Lee, M. Walbancke, D. Pateman and G. Bedle, London, 1895).

31. Forbes, T.R. *The Midwife and the Witch* (Yale University Press, Newhaven, 1966).

32. Aveling, J.H. *English Midwives: Their History and Prospects* (Hugh K. Elliott, London, 1967, p. 20).

33. Burn, R. *Ecclesiastical Law* (A. Strahan, London, 1797).

34. Chester Records Office, Licences and certificates, Box 3 EBX.

35. Barnes, H. 'On the Bishop's Licence', *Transactions of the Cumberland and Westmorland Antiquarian and Archeological Society*, 1903, 3.

5 THE DEVELOPMENT OF MIDWIFERY AS A SCIENCE AND THE BEGINNING OF OBSTETRICS IN ENGLAND

Mydwif Monopoly Challenged

Seventeenth century society continued to be patriarchal. There was intense social, political and religious activity and upheaval, which, together with educational and scientific developments, changed the cultural life of the country. It was a century in which the plague returned and in which smallpox was common; in which the first democratic political party was born; in which the established Anglican Church collapsed, giving way to a multiplicity of religious sects; and in which there was economic crisis, mass unemployment, inflation, exceptionally severe winters, bad harvests and near starvation. There was revolution, civil war, regicide and then restoration of the monarchy, and re-establishment of the Church.

In spite of all these cataclysmic events and disruptive influences, tremendous strides were made in all the fields of science, by men such as Newton, Bacon and Harvey. There was a change in the style and content of poetry, epitomised by John Milton and John Dryden; and drama, after its total eclipse in the Commonwealth years, changed its character completely to social comedy and satire. Many diarists emerged, and so everyday events were described in detail from the pens of men of such diverse occupations, backgrounds and interests as Samuel Pepys, a Government official, Ralph Josselin, a country parson and farmer, and John Evelyn, a cultivated gentleman and traveller. Suppression of the established Church provoked the creation of a variety of extremist sects who often presented very unorthodox beliefs. There was expansion in education, and consequently schooling was available for greater numbers of boys than previously. On the whole, though, only prosperous families could afford to send their children to school, and two-thirds of adult men and even more women were illiterate throughout their lives.[1] A number of books on women and for women were, however, written during this century. An example of one such work was *The Sick Woman's Private Looking Glass* by J. Sadler.[2]

The belief which had been accepted down the ages that sickness and misfortune were the punishments for sin survived the seventeenth century revolutions and was perpetuated by Puritan doctrine. This emphasised that nothing happened by chance and that everything was expressly ordained by the providence and will of God. In writing on providence, Keith Thomas says

physical disorders in the heavens were believed to presage or reflect moral and social disorders upon earth. They also permeated the science of embryology. Moralists had always taught that incest, adultery and other forms of sexual immorality were punished by ill-health and monstrous births; this belief was taken over by doctors and midwives, who as late as the 18th century held that deformed children might well result from indecent sexual relations.[3]

There is some agreement, based on evidence such as inventories of possessions, preserved dwellings, contemporary writings and Gregory King's calculations (from the Hearth Tax 1688)[4] that at least 90 per cent of the population were in the lower socio-economic group, and that a large proportion of those lived at or below subsistence level. On the lowest rung of the social scale were a million people who were dependent on alms. (This figure represents close on one-fifth of the estimated 5½ million total population.)[5]

A considerable number of people lived as vagrants in forests, and dwelt in flimsy insubstantial self-constructed shelters or hovels; some had been driven to this way of life as a result of Enclosure Acts. Obviously life for many was a grim struggle for survival. Some attempt had been made by legislation to deal with the legitimate poor, and the Poor Law Act of 1601 required each parish to levy a poor rate. Some farm labourers lived in outbuildings which were purpose-built combined dwellings for man and animals with a shared middle dividing wall but separate entrances.[6] Some agricultural workers had smallholdings, and urban industrial labourers, along with small traders and craftsmen, lived in a variety of homes ranging from stone cottages, to tenement dwellings (often one room only) to small timber, stone and in a few cases brick houses. It is quite likely that the floor in many homes was still of bare earth and that the walls were plain and uncovered. Creature comforts were minimal; furniture was very basic and there is evidence that many people had few possessions and that what they had was often broken or old.[7] Artisans and traders, who included the stonemason, saddler, blacksmith, cooper, joiner, baker, glover and draper, lived in substantial small houses, often attached to their work premises. Certain women who were relatives of men from the artisan class are known to have practised as midwives, for example Elizabeth Collins, daughter of a glazier, who was licensed in 1662, and Elizabeth Hunt, who was the wife of an instrument maker.[8] A butcher's wife, Elizabeth Walthur, is also mentioned as a midwife in the writings of Dr Percival Willoughby.[9]

The emerging urban 'middling' class — the lawyers, bankers, merchants, clergymen and teachers — lived in slightly larger stone or brick houses, which possibly had chimneys and windows. The type and quality of housing varied from region to region, and because the South and East were the 'rich' regions, the people were materially and educationally advantaged whereas those in the poorest counties in the North and West of England were deprived.

The rich dwelt in mansions, halls or spacious country or prodigy houses.[10] This upper social group consisted of earls, barons, courtiers, noblemen, dukes, knights, landed gentry and bishops. Their dwellings contained elaborate furniture and cultural artefacts such as paintings, sculptures, stained-glass windows, silk hangings and tapestries, and very often housed a library also.[11] Undoubtedly they would have a bed with coverings and drapes. In contrast, 'pillows were thought meet only for women in childbed. As for servants, if they had any sheet above them, it was well, for seldom had they any under their bodies to keep them from the pricking straws that ran oft through the canvas of the pallet and razed their hardened hides.'[12] It is not therefore too difficult to visualise the homes and conditions into which our midwife predecessors went to deliver their mothers and care for the newborn. Only a little imagination is required to 'accompany' a midwife knocked up in the night by relatives of a woman in labour. In towns she would travel on foot through dark and dirty streets, possibly carrying her birth chair, and both examine and later deliver the mother in a room, which in some cases would be cold, possibly damp, and none too clean, by the light of tallow candles. Sometimes, where the population was sparse, the midwife had to travel long distances to confinements. One such lengthy journey, which took place in June 1610, is documented in the *House and Farm Accounts of Gawthorp Hall, Padiham, Lancashire.* The debit column reads:

> spente by Will'm Woode and Cooke, Wiffe and twoe horses, when they wente for the midwiffe of Wigan, being a day and a night away. 111js [4 shillings]
> Spente by Richard Stones, when he brought the Wigan (mid)wiffe home and a night away. xx1jd [22 old pence]
> To the midwiffe. x1jd [12 old pence]

An interesting entry appears in the same accounts for January 1612:

. . . given to midwiffe which helpe a cowe that could not calve. 1js vjd. [2s 6d][13]

The relative values of wife and child and cow and calf are illustrated here.

Sometimes, as in the case of a rapid labour, the midwife would not get to the delivery. A delivery in the absence of the midwife is mentioned in the famous diary, which covers the years 1645–60, of the Reverend Ralph Josselin, whose parish was Earls Colne in Essex. He records that his wife Jane had ten live births and five miscarriages in twenty years. His entry for 5 May 1649 reads:

> My dear wife had been very ill for three weeks; now towards night pains come fast on her and she was delivered before nine of the clock of her fifth child and third son. My wife was alone a great while with our good friends Mrs Mary Church and her mother; some few women were with her *but the midwife not*, but when God commands deliverance there is nothing hinders it [our italics].[14]

On 29 May 1661 Samuel Pepys recorded in his diary that he went to Walthamstow for the christening of his godson. He took gifts of a silver porringer and six spoons but in the event, because the baby was not named after him, he withheld the gifts. He did, however, give a generous tip of ten shillings to the midwife and five shillings to the nurse.

In contrast to the rather small sum paid to the midwife at Gawthorp Hall, the Royal midwives were handsomely recompensed. Alice Dennis, who attended Anne of Denmark (wife of James I), received £100 when she delivered Princess Mary in 1605 and Princess Sophia in 1606. An even larger sum was paid to Mrs Judith Wilkes, midwife to the queen of James II, who received 500 guineas in 1688.[15] Margaret Mercer was sent with an entourage to Heidelberg in 1616 to deliver the baby of Elizabeth of Bohemia, the daughter of James I. For her services she received a total of £84.[16] However, a small sum was the usual payment.

> a shilling or two was the normal fee at the beginning of the 17th century; whereas towards the end of it the anonymous business diary of a midwife shows a prosperous trade with some form of sliding scale. In 1696 this midwife recorded about two deliveries a month with payments varying from five shillings to ten shillings. On 24th August 1698 Mrs Rowell paid her 12s 6d for the delivery of a daughter at the awkward time of seven o'clock on a Sunday morning — but since the midwife was also able to record that she 'laid Mrs Clarke next

door' in the course of the same visit, she only charged the 2s 6d. By 1719, this midwife was attending approximately three confinements a month and charging an average of £1 a visit; all of which amounted to a handsome income. The midwife had a large practice in the Old Bailey area of the City of London, but a connection with the Barnardiston family — she attended a number of their confinements — took her as far as Cornwall where she 'laid Madam Barnardiston'. All the same the midwife was also aware of her social duty: when she 'laid a woman in the market' no payment was recorded, presumably because the mother was of the poor.[17]

In 1636 John Hayne, a dealer in serges, woollen goods and cotton paid the midwife the sum of £1 10s when she delivered his wife. He bought a cradle for the new baby for 11s.[18] In *Of Domestical Duties* William Gouge showed that some men could not afford the fees of certain midwives and had to look for one who charged less: 'when the time cometh, if their wife be desirous of a Midwife that requireth somewhat more charges than she that is next, she shall have none if she will not have next'.[19]

The seventeenth century experienced what has been called 'The Great Age of Puritanism'. Puritans consisted of men, many of whom were Calvinists and merchants of the 'middling' class, who wanted to purify the existing church of its rites and ceremonies, sacraments and liturgy and return to the simplicity of the primitive church. The Puritan way of life was characterised by morality, discipline, hard work, high ideals and service to the community, and was responsible for the spread of elementary education because of its emphasis on the reading of the word of God. They taught a doctrine of spiritual equality of all believers, which was a revolutionary concept.

The breeding, bearing and bringing up of children was such a serious matter for Puritans that one of their ministers, Thomas Gataker, who lost two of his four wives as a result of complicated childbirths, warned unmarried women, in his book *A Wife Indeed*, to recognise the requirements and consequences of being a wife and mother. William Gouge, a famous Puritan clergyman, also gave advice about childbearing. His own wife gave birth to thirteen children but died during the birth of the last one in 1624 as a result of complications. He charged the *mother* with the major responsibility for *prenatal* care. The first age of a child was its infancy, he wrote, and the first part of the infancy was while the child was in the mother's womb, so he encouraged a mother to take special care of herself throughout her pregnancy so that the child would go to full term. Gouge's advice on care during the antenatal period was generally sound, and what he advocated is still the basis of today's parentcraft classes. He advised on diet, exercise, clothing and the role of the father.

The *diet* was to be substantial but minus spicy and salty foods. It was to include bread made of good wheat well baked; meat consisting of chicken, capon, young pigeons, turtle, pheasant, veal, mutton; any kind of fruit. Starchy foods such as peas and beans were to be avoided. *Exercise* was to be moderate and the woman was to avoid running, leaping and dancing and riding long distances. Her *dress* was to be light and comfortable and she was to avoid lacing herself tightly to match the fashions. Husbands were advised to treat their wives kindly and tenderly during pregnancy and to do their utmost to ease their pain and discomfort with sweet loving words.[19]

Puritans, however, accepted that pain during labour was justifiable, being the curse put on women through the sin of Eve. Such teaching was in fact traditional, and an Elizabethan poet William Hunnis incorporated it into his poem *A Meditation to be Said of Women with Child.*

The time draws nigh
of bitter painful throes,
How long I shall
the same endure, God knows.
Oh Lord my God,
I humbly ask of Thee,
Make haste, sweet Christ,
and safe deliver me.
Although by sin
deserved I have right well
Such pain as this,
yea, more than tongue can tell;
Yet ah, my God
turn not away thy face,
Nor me forsake
in this so sharp a case.
This womb and fruit
that springeth in the same,
Hast thou create
to glory of thy Name.

Oppressed with pain,
Oh Lord when I shall be,
make less the same,
so much as pleaseth Thee:
And grant, good God
thy creature may proceed
Safely on live,
with mercy at my need;
In Christ his name,
I will my travail show;
Now Holy Ghost
come comfort me in woe.
Come father dear,
and let thy power descend:
Oh Jesu Christ,
thy mercies great extend.
Ah God behold
my dolour and my smart;
Sweet Holy Ghost,
my comforter thou art,
Take part with me,
and hear my woeful cry:
Exaudi me,
miserere mei.

(Seven Sobs of a Sorrowful Soul, 1583)[20]

The midwife and a few neighbours were usually present during the labour and delivery to support and aid the mother. It was customary for several women to be present in order to witness and verify the birth and also to learn what to do in case they were called to a birth in an emergency. Babies were born with the mother in the squatting, lying or sitting position. The Puritans did not offer any scriptural evidence in favour of any particular position. Writing on *English Puritans and Childbirth*, R.V. Schnucker gives a detailed description of the birth stool as set down in the *Expert Midwife* by Jacobus Rueff.

The birth stool was similar to a very sturdy chair with a strong back and most of the seat cut away so that the remaining part was in the form of a new moon. Around the bottom was draped black cloth and the seat covered with cloths so that the woman would not be bruised and neither the child as the two of them moved about in the process of labour.[21]

The Puritan attitude towards breast feeding was based on scripture. It was felt that God expressly commanded it through the example of women in both the Old and New Testaments. They recognised both physical and psychological advantages to the baby of being fed by its own mother rather than by a wet-nurse. Schnucker includes the view of a mother and writer, Elisabeth Clinton (the Countess of Lincoln), who wrote that she was convinced that those of her children whom she had personally fed were physically healthier than those given to wet-nurses. The Puritans believed that certain 'qualities' were transmitted through the milk from the mother that would determine the child's future characteristics. A husband who hindered or forbade his wife's nursing, or complained about the inconvenience of it, or refused to buy what she needed to nurse the infant better, or who did not actively encourage her and suggested a wet-nurse, was warned that he was an accessory to sin. The husband was not to forget that he was for the most part responsible for his wife's pregnancy and certainly she could not abuse his child by denying it its mother's milk. 'If husbands would only take a positive attitude towards nursing where one mother now nurseth her child, twenty would do it.'[22] Despite the fact that the Puritans taught that it was an offence against God not to breast-feed, nevertheless many women offered the same sort of reasons or excuses for not doing so as are still commonly heard today. These included poor lactation, sore nipples, inconvenience, disturbing the sleep of both parents at night, that it was messy and spoiled the clothes, dislike of exposure of the breasts to the public, or fear that the breasts would sag and so age the mother.

The Emergence of Doctors on the Childbearing Scene

During the seventeenth century, certain English midwives and doctors distinguished themselves in midwifery. Men who became directly involved originally called themselves 'men-midwives' but gradually other titles came to be used. These include andro-boethygynist (man helper of women), accoucheur (one who brings to childbed) and finally obstetrician, from the Latin *obstetrix* (to-stand before).

The Father of English Midwifery

The great medical scientist of the Age and to whom directly or indirectly doctors in many fields are indebted was William Harvey. His fame rests primarily on his achievements in physiology, particularly in his discovery of the circulation of the blood. He wrote the first original English work on midwifery in 1651. The book was written in Latin under the title of *De Generatione Animalium* and was translated into English in 1653. This was based on his own scientific knowledge and observations as well as on considerable practical experience. The book includes chapters on the development of the embryo and fetus and on practical management of labour and delivery. Harvey's main precept was to wait on nature and only intervene when it was absolutely necessary, and his method of intervention, for certain difficult cases, was podalic version and breech extraction. William Harvey has been rightly termed 'The Father of English Midwifery' because, as a result of his study of reproductive anatomy, physiology and parturition, *obstetrics* was for the first time placed on a scientific basis.

Percival Willoughby, Man-midwife

Another influential figure was Percival Willoughby, who was born in 1596. Following his apprenticeship to a barber-surgeon he developed an interest in midwifery. He attributed his theoretical knowledge to William Harvey, and by combining this theory with his technical skills he became one of the foremost practitioners of midwifery of his time. He practised in Derby, Stafford and London, and returned to Derby in 1659. He wrote a text that included 150 case histories, and although intended for the edification of midwives, and of physicians who were called to assist in difficult cases, it remained in manuscript form until a printed edition of one-hundred copies appeared in 1863. One of these is in the Radford Collection in the Medical Library of the University of Manchester.[23] It seems a tragedy that a text so full of excellent and sound practical experience and advice was to remain unprinted and unpublished for over 200 years. Willoughby left for us a very clear picture of the obstetric scene in the seventeenth century, mentioning cases of convulsions, white leg, puerperal sepsis, maternal death with fetus undelivered, and cephalo-pelvic disproportion. Prolapsed limbs, especially the arms, were a common occurrence, and dismemberment and decapitation not uncommon. This was a grim picture which needed remedying, and Willoughby's remedy was education of the midwives: 'A woman is not born a midwife; it is education, with practise that teacheth her experience. And midwives have need of good memories to help their judgements in all their undertakings.' He also expressed contempt for some 'doctors' who were ignorant practitioners, claiming that male practice at its worst was without doubt as bad as that of the most ignorant midwife. It seems likely that because he taught midwives he gained their confidence, and they called him in when they were in doubt or difficulty. His daughter was a midwife who apparently often called for his assistance, which he had to render surreptitiously. As men were not welcome in the birth chamber, he was obliged to crawl into the room on hands and knees and perform his life-saving work under cover of a sheet.

He records a confinement to which he was summoned by his daughter.

In Middlesex anno 1658 my daughter, with my assistance, delivered Sir Tennebs Evanks lady of a living daughter. All the morning my daughter was much troubled, and she told me shee feared that ye birth would come by ye buttocks. About 7 o'clock that night labour approached. At my daughter's request, unknown to the lady, I crept into the chamber on my hands and knees, and returned and it was not perceived by the lady. I said that it was ye head, but shee affirmed the contrary; however if it should prove ye buttocks then shee should know how to deliver her. She could not be quieted until I crept privately again the second time into ye chamber, and found her words true. I willed her to bring down a foot, the which shee soon did, and being much disquieted with fear of ensuing danger shee prayed mee to carry on with the rest of the work.

Another case Willoughby mentions is of the delivery of twins by a midwife who, having put his teaching to the test, let him know of its success.

Margaret Cliffe, the wife of Thomas, a weaver dwelling at Newton in Staffordshire, Jan the 7th 1671 was delivered of twins, the first was a boy, the second came enclosed in a secondine, and was a female; and the midwife laid this birth in her lap, and opened the secondines and took forth the child. Life was scarce perceived in it, but by laying the afterbirth on hot coales, and stroking the navel-string toward the belly, the child recovered and liveth. This was certified to mee by Margaret Kempe, a midwife at Abbots Bramley, that laid her of these two twins.

Willoughby's Pleas for Non-interference by Midwives. It seems from his writing that it was common practice at that time for midwives to induce labour by tearing the membranes with their nails or with scissors early. How early is not stated, nor is any reason given, but it appears that it was before term and before engagement of the presenting part because Willoughby comments upon the frequent occurrence of prolapsed limbs and the high incidence of 'dry labours'. It is interesting to speculate on the shape and length of scissors or instruments used to perform this quite difficult operation, which would of course be unsterile. It is also interesting to ponder on the reasoning behind such inductions. Was it to avoid obstructed labour in the belief that the smaller the baby the easier would be its passage? Or was it because the period of gestation was often in doubt and either the mother or the midwife became impatient? Their meddling was deplored by Dr Willoughby, and he entreated them to adopt his own policy of non-intervention. He begged midwives not to pull on prolapsed arms, nor to push on the fundament, nor to hasten birth by stretching the passages with fingers and hands. Willoughby strongly advocated natural childbirth, and he begged midwives to leave cases of natural labour to the safe conduct of 'the invisible midwife, Dame Nature'. He advised the midwives to give an enema and to persuade the mother to 'make water', explaining that otherwise a full bowel and bladder could impede descent and contribute to uterine inertia. He also realised that the enema could be used to 'stir up the expulsive faculty'. He was distressed that a midwife's endeavours to secure delivery of the baby often resulted in severe or fatal injuries to the mother or baby or both, but his criticism of these untrained midwives was constructive.

The 'Handy Operation'. Willoughby believed that the answer to all obstetric difficulties was *version* of the fetus and extraction by the feet, which he termed the 'handy operation', and he taught midwives how to perform this manoeuvre. 'And this way of practice *in all difficult births* to deliver women by the child's feet, *I shall wish all midwives to follow*' [our italics]. It seems unclear as to how this manoeuvre could have helped if the labour was 'difficult' because of pelvic inadequacy. He records that in 1654 he was

> brought to Bromidgham, Staffordshire to a woman in labour, and her midwife could not deliver her, though the child came in a natural birth. I found the child alive, I speedily altered the posture of the birth. As she *kneeled* on a bolster, I turned back the head, and I brought down the feet. By them I soon delivered her of a living sonne, and the mother and child lived. I saw them both afterward in May 1656 [our italics].

Willoughby's Philosophy. His aim seemed to be to help midwives improve the lot of women.

> My endeavours shall bee to very little meddle with diseases, physick or medicines, but to show the handy operation to midwives, how to

produce the fetus, when perfectly formed, and how to help poor suffering women in distresses, and chiefly to direct the young country midwives, giving them several examples, and caveats, with persuasions, intreating them not be too busie afore fitting time. So their women will be more easily, and better helped in their sufferings, and their own repute advanced in the practice of midwifery, by observing what hath been by mee performed at severall times in diverse places.

Care in Labour. It is interesting to learn from Willoughby that the obstetric cream of the day with which they anointed 'the places concerned with travail' consisted of fresh butter, goose grease, capon's or hen's fat. Another concoction to counteract the 'dryness of the privvies' was a mixture of oil of sweet almonds and lilies and a beaten egg. The case studies show that a few women were delivered lying on a bed, whereas others knelt, stood, or sat on the midwife's stool. It is obvious that at this time the mother delivered in the position of her own choice, and Willoughby's discourse on the environment for labour and the posture for and manner of delivery could be read as a blueprint for some of the present-day progressive natural- and active-birth units.

> And, for the labouring woman's chamber, let it bee made dark, having a glimmering light, or candle-light placed partly behind the woman or on one side, and a moderate warming force in it, and let it not bee filled with much company, or many women; five or six women assisting will be sufficient. [No mention is made of the husband.] And having her body annointed with Balsamum Hystericum, let her now and then (if shee please) walk gently in her chamber, or to lie quietly on her bed, untill Dame Nature shall will her to lie on her bed or come to her knees, for her more quick and easy delivery . . . And I would have no medicines given to force throwes, unless nature faint, and that towards the end of her travaile. If the woman bee weak, a pallet bed may bee thought the most convenient place. But, if shee bee strong, and of an able body, and the child lively, I then know no cause contradicting, why shee may not bee as well, or rather better kneeling on a bolster (than lying on a pallet-bed) when that her body is fitted for the birth . . . I have advised some women, that have formerly suffered much bitterness and pain by their hasty midwives' proceedings, not to bee too forward to thrust themselves into their midwives' hands, and not to let the midwife force them to sit on her stoole, or woman's lap, or to come to their knees, nor to touch them,

more than to anoint their bodies, untill the waters should flow of themselves, without any enforcement from the midwife . . . assuring them that it was no part of the midwife's office to force the birth, her part and duty was only to receive the child.

Posture for Giving Birth. Willoughby clearly favoured the kneeling position for delivery.

> In a natural birth the labouring woman, *kneeling* at a convenient and fitting time, in a bending posture, holding her hands about another woman's neck, that sitteth afore her, having a pillow laid on her lap, on which the labouring woman rests her belly, will have more command of herself and of her belly, *in this bending position*, and more than if shee did sit on a woman's lap, or on the midwife's stoole, for that the birth will be pressed somewhat forward by the pillow, and her own thighes, and through this bending posture, shee will bee the speedier delivered, leaving the midwife nothing more to do, than to receive the child [our italics].

Willoughby expressed his dislike of the midwife's stoole.

> Several midwives (chiefly about London) use Midwives Stools; many in the country make use of a bolster, stuffed with hay or straw. Others, in several places make use of both. For a woman to lie on her back, on her bed, is an unnatural birth, or to use a midwife's stool is not so convenient, as to kneel on a bolster . . . the placing of a woman in a fitting posture doth much facilitate the birth. A Midwife's stool is good for little, or, rather for nothing, yet severall women do highly commend them.

Delivery of the Placenta and Membranes. Willoughby claimed that the 'after-burden' was more easily delivered if the woman *knelt*, and he felt that it was troublesome to deliver if the woman lay on her back. He taught that the placenta usually descended into the vagina with the birth of the baby, but if not, he encouraged the midwife to deliver it actively by moving the 'navel-string' from side to side, or if necessary by inserting her hand into the uterus and gathering the afterbirth into her hand, and then withdrawing it with the aid of the mother who would be asked to cough, boken (retch) or sneeze. In an attempt to arrest 'flooding' (post-partum haemorrhage), strained hog's dung with sugar and nutmeg was given orally!

Willoughby's recommended management of birth asphyxia was to place the placenta on hot coals and with the baby's feet towards the fire to stroke the cord towards its body.

Apparently the usual lying-in period was three days but Dr Willoughby advocated that this should be extended to five days.

The Chamberlens and their Forceps

Dr William Chamberlen and his wife fled to England from France as Huguenot refugees in the 1560s. Two of their sons were called Peter and both of them were doctors. The second Peter also called one of his sons by the name of Peter. He also practised as a doctor, and three of his sons were doctors, and Hugh the eldest held a licence, issued by the Bishop of London, to practice midwifery within six miles of the city of London. Another son, Paul, was also a doctor, and as there were three called Peter and one called Paul, who all signed themselves 'P.C.', this has led to some confusion over the years.

The Chamberlens practised in England during the last decades of the sixteenth century, for the whole of the seventeenth century, and into the next. This family of medical men has had a profound and lasting influence on the practice of both midwifery and obstetrics in England and in other European countries. The Chamberlens gained such a reputation, almost certainly as a result of their intense interest and skill in midwifery, that they gained favour with Stuart royalty. Dr Peter III attended Queen Henrietta Maria in childbirth and is reputed to have attended the birth of Prince Charles who became King Charles II.

Effective metal obstetric forceps were invented within this family, but it is difficult to determine which one of them in particular can be credited with the achievement. Although some instruments were used before, 'the weight of evidence points to the invention of short straight-handled forceps by some member of the Chamberlen family, probably Peter the Elder'.[24] It is fascinating to speculate who actually made the original forceps, which were fashioned from iron and were short with curved blades to accommodate the fetal head. Because they only had the cephalic curve, their use was limited to outlet extractions. Both Peter I and Peter II practised contemporaneously in London, and they, as well as Peter III and Hugh (senior and junior) and Paul, all used forceps in their practice. Doctors Peter I and II were members of the Barber-Surgeons Company but were debarred from membership of the College of Physicians as neither of them had been educated at Oxford or Cambridge. There are reports of animosity between the Doctors Peter and the Barber-Surgeons Company, and on more than one occasion the doctors were fined for not attending meetings or because their dress was regarded as frivolous and flamboyant. They were summoned before the College of Physicians for repeatedly prescribing medicine contrary to the rules of the College.

The news of the Chamberlens' 'secret instrument' spread rapidly when it was realised that its use could shorten the agony of labour by overcoming obstruction, and that a living baby was more frequently being extracted from a living mother where previously one or both may have been sacrificed. It appears that the Chamberlens went to almost farcical lengths to conceal the nature of the invention. Apparently the forceps were transported to the confinement in a large box covered with gilt which was carried by two men. The impression given was that the box contained some large, complicated machine. Before the forceps were taken out of the box, the mother was blindfolded and the midwife locked out of the room, and during the forceps extraction sound-effects such as ringing of bells and slapping of sticks were employed in an effort to disguise the chinking of the metal blades.[25]

These pioneer instrumentarians soon became vocal on the social and political aspects of their calling. Because of their unique ability to facilitate vaginal delivery, they were made acutely aware of the limitations of the midwife's practice and of her lack of knowledge. At this time many midwives themselves began to be concerned about their lack of theoretical knowledge and conceded that even the most skilled among them needed to be yet more skilled. They felt the need to organise themselves to form a society, as other 'medical' professionals had already done. In 1616, midwives of the City of London petitioned King James I for permission to form a society. It would appear that the midwives' petition was not entirely of their own initiative and was supported, if not prompted, by both Doctors Peter Chamberlen I and II, who also proposed to the King 'that some order may be settled by the State for the instruction and civil government of midwives'. This petition was referred by the King and his Privy Council to the College of Physicians for their consideration, but after deliberation they decided that it was not necessary for midwives to form a self-governing corporation. They did, however, admit the need for improvement of the practice of midwives, and proposed that prior to being granted a Bishop's licence, midwives could first be examined and approved by the College of Physicians and any deficiency in their knowledge remedied by attendance at lectures and dissections: this proposal was not implemented. It appears that despite the outcóme of the 1616 Petition, Dr Peter Chamberlen II still attempted to teach the London midwives unofficially. This attempt was evidently resisted by some midwives who resented being threatened that Dr Chamberlen would not attend their patients in an emergency unless they had attended his lectures. Dr Peter III also attempted to gain the support of midwives; he wined and dined some of them as a bribe to this end. In an endeavour to make his teaching mandatory, Dr Peter III petitioned the King in 1633 for permission to establish a Corporation of Midwives with himself as Governor. Peter Chamberlen III had an immense practice. 'The burthen of all the midwives in and about London, lay only upon my shoulders', he said, and lamented:

ignorant women, whom either extreme poverty hath necessitated, or hard heartedness presumed, or the game of Venus intruded into the calling of midwifery (to have the issue of life and death of two or three at one time in their hands, besides the consequences of health and strength of the whole nation) should neither be *sufficiently instructed in doing good nor restrained from doing evil* [our italics].[26]

The London midwives, almost *en masse*, counter-petitioned the King because they were understandably suspicious of his motives, which seemed to threaten their independence. A month later, the midwives, led by Mrs Whipp and Mrs Hester Shawe, presented a petition to the College of Physicians which in effect was a strong protest about the unauthorised control Dr Chamberlen was attempting to exert over them. The College believed the complaint of the midwives to be a just grievance, and so their petition was referred to the bishops and an enquiry was held in the Palace of Lambeth in October 1634 in the presence of the Archbishop of Canterbury and the Bishop of London. The matter was referred to the ecclesiastical hierarchy because this was the official licensing authority and any proposed changes in procedure had to be considered by them. This was the first public confrontation between midwives and doctors. At this enquiry the midwives claimed that their 'business' was being interfered with by Dr Chamberlen, and that he was in no position to teach them the 'art' of midwifery because, they claimed, he had no experience of the normal birth process. In fact they went so far as to say:

Dr. Chamberlen's work and the work belonging to midwives are contrary one to the other for he delivers none without the use of instruments by extraordinary violence in desperate occasions, which women never practised nor desyred for they have neither parts nor hands for that art.[27]

The motives of both parties were questionable. Each contained a strong element of self-interest but also equally an element of concern for their patients. Dr Chamberlen's case rested on the fact that he could claim that medical intervention and forceps extraction were life-saving. The Bishops supported the midwives' case and did not grant Dr Chamberlen authority to instruct them. Indeed they proposed that Dr Chamberlen should apply for a licence to practise midwifery. In the succeeding years, Dr Peter III continued to express concern about the deficiencies in the practice of midwives, and in 1647 he published an autobiographical pamphlet called *The Crie of Women and Children* in which he called midwives 'the uncontrolled female arbiters of life and death'. It appears that he was still smarting from his failure to establish a Corporation for the education of midwives, which he claimed would be to their advantage and above all to the advantage of many women and their unborn babies. Dr Chamberlen was not alone in his criticism of the untrained midwife practitioners; Dr Willoughby, one of his contemporaries, was also lamenting: 'I could heartily wish yt some public good order might be made for ye better educating of all, especially ye younger midwives, for ye healing and saving of mothers.'[23]

This aspiration was not confined to England. In 1668 Mauriceau in his *Traité des maladies des femmes grosses* stressed that it was vital for midwives to recognise the limits of their practice and the need to send for help so that 'many women and children may be preserved, that now perish for want of seasonable help'. Sympathetic to this aim, Dr Hugh Chamberlen translated this book into English in 1672 for the benefit of midwives.

The Chamberlens kept their new 'instruments of delivery' a secret within the family for generations and they were found only accidentally in 1813 by a Mrs Kemball at Woodham Mortimer Hall, Malden, Essex. In an upper room at the front of the house she noticed loose plugs of wood on the dusty floor. When the floorboards were taken up, 'curious instruments' were found, which included some about a foot long and shaped like coal tongs. They were recognised as early midwifery instruments and, in fact, as the Chamberlen forceps. Three sets were found, belonging to Peter III, his father Peter II and his uncle Peter I. These forceps were presented to the Medical and Chirurgical Society, London, where they are now preserved.[27] Coins found at the same time serve to place roughly the date when the articles were hidden as being during the reign of Charles II.[28] How different things might have been if the Chamberlens had been willing to reveal their invention, and if, rather than antagonising the London midwives, they had gained their goodwill and co-operation. This might have led to the acceptance of their offer of education, the midwives having already perceived that they lacked certain theoretical knowledge which would be to the benefit of themselves and therefore of the mothers they served.

Literary and Pictorial Revelations

As the century progressed, midwives could have gained some useful knowledge from the spate of books that came on to the market. Whether original or copy, of value or worthless, much about pregnancy and childbirth was committed to paper by men during this century. These works, translated into English from Latin or other European languages, or originally written in English, made subject matter concerning conception, the female body and the act of birth available to the public. Detailed descriptions of the female genitalia, sometimes with illustrations, were included. That such words were written in English was regarded as 'shocking', but the use of Latin was contraindicated, being counterproductive to the educational objectives of the authors. There was obviously still the connotation of shame and modesty attached to mention of such 'private' parts.

One very useful book, actually written in the sixteenth century (see Chapter 4 and Figure 9) but translated into English in the 1700s was *The Expert Midwife*.[29] This was a comprehensive book originally entitled *De Conceptu et Generatione Hominis*. The translator's preface reads:

> Some say it is unfit that such matters as these should bee published in a vulgar tongue, for young heads to prie into. True, but the danger being great and manifold, whether it is better that millions should perish for want of helpe or knowledge, or that such means, which though lawful in themselves, may yet by some be abused, should be had and used. — But young and raw heads, idle serving men, profane fiddlers, scoffers, jesters, rogues; avaunt pack hence! — I neither meant it for you, neither is it fit for you.

This book covered the reproductive anatomy and physiology relating to conception, embedding, embryology, uterine and fetal growth and development, pregnancy, labour, birth and the newborn baby. According to the frontispiece it was 'compiled in Latin by the industry of Jacobus Rueff, a learned and expert chirurgion and translated into English for the general good and well being of this Nation'. It was addressed to 'all grave and modest Matrons, especially to such as have to do with women in that great danger of childbirth, as also to all young practitioners in Physick and Chirurgery'.

Herbal remedies were prescribed for swooning and other minor disorders of pregnancy and the 'treatment' for vomiting was syrup of pomegranates, musk, lignum, aloes, cinnamon and sorrel in water. For the management of premature labour the midwife was advised to use 'suffumigation of frankincense upon the coales', to strengthen the matrix and infant. Suffumigation was a traditional remedy and consisted of allowing pungent fumes to be directed towards the uterus by way of the vaginal passage. 'After let her bathe her outward parts with allome, galls, comfrey decocted and sodden in raine water, wine and vinegar.' During the labour Rueff advised the midwife to exhort women to pour forth devout prayers to God and 'after, let her bring the labouring woman to the stool which ought to be prepared in this fashion' (Figure 19).

Birth, Seventeenth Century Style

The stool was to be used as follows:

> The midwife shall place one woman behind her back which may gently hold the labouring woman, taking her by both the armes, and if need be, the paines waxing grievous, and the woman labouring, may stroke and press down the womb and may somewhat drive and depress the infant downward. But let her place other two by her sides which may both with good words encourage and comfort the labouring woman. Let the midwife herself sit stooping forward before the labouring woman and let her anoint her hands with the oile of lillies and of sweet almonds and the grease of a hen mingled and tempered together. Let the midwife instruct and encourage the party to her labour, to abide her paines with patience and then gently apply her hands to the works as she ought by feeling and searching with her fingers how the child lieth, and by relaxing and opening the way and passage conveniently for him, while his mother is in paine and also where there is needs by enlarging and stretching out the neck of the matrix warily. Let her conveniently receive the infant and let her presently cut the navell string, about the length of four fingers being left, and let her bind it hard with a double thread as near to the belly of the child as may be. The navell must be sprinkled with powder of Bole Armeniacke, Sanguis Draconis and Myrrh and to be pressed down with a double cloth laid upon it. Let her have care of the secundine or after-birth. Let her move and stirre it. If the birthe be hindered by driness or straightness of the neck of the wombe a little quantity of sneezing powder and pepper is to be blowne into the nostrile of the woman

Figure 9: Rueff's Chair and Fetuses *in Utero*

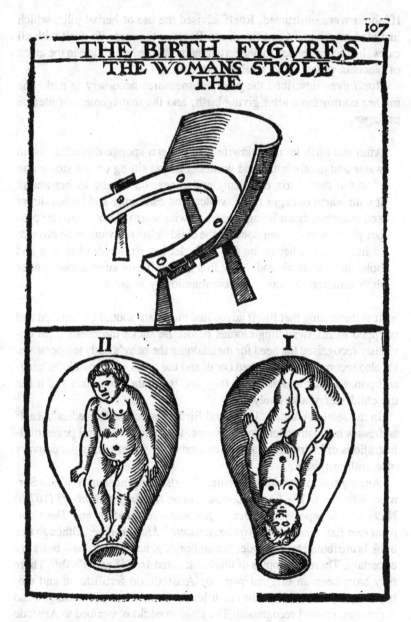

Source: J. Rueff, *Ein schön lustig Trostbuchle*, Zurich 1554, fol. bb4ᵛ.
Courtesy of the Wellcome Institute Library, London.

with a quill, and sneezing provoked.

If labour were obstructed, Rueff advised the use of herbal pills, which included myrrh and Gum Bdellium. Because the midwife dealt with all cases, he recommended to her certain herbal remedies for use in the event of placenta praevia and retained placenta.

Rueff even described the practical measures necessary to make the mother comfortable after giving birth, and the management of uterine prolapse.

> After the birth let the midwife take a clean sponge dipped in warm water and gently bathe and wash her as yet sitting on her stoole and if any of the matrix doth hang and appear outwardly let her anoint it with warm oiles, or roses, violets and camomile and let her direct and reduce it again being cherished with warm clothes into her proper place, which being done let the child-delivered woman be brought to her bed. Let her lie on her back, let her stretch out her legs and hold them wide abroad — by this means if any superfluous matter doth remaine, it may more commodiously passe away.

It is interesting that Rueff advocated the infant should be 'washed and wrapped in his swaddling clothes before he sucke the brests'. He obviously recognised the need for maintaining the baby's body temperature. He also recommended that 'red corall and the seeds of the pionie be hanged upon his neck and arms for they doe strengthen, comfort and make the child merry and lively'.

In the section entitled 'Unnatural Birth, Cures and Remedies', Rueff addresses his instructions to midwives. He includes several pages of illustrations of instruments for use by midwives for effecting the delivery of a stillborn fetus.

Among the most widely circulated texts were those of William Sermon, who wrote *The Ladies Companion* or *The English Midwife* (1671), Nicholas Culpeper's *A Directory for Midwives* (1650), and *The Compleat and Experienc'd Midwife or Aristotle's Masterpiece*. Although this book is attributed to Aristotle, the authorship, authenticity and basis are uncertain. There are copies of this book dated 1690[30] and 1700.[31] There may have been an original work by Aristotle on fertilisation and embryology, but throughout the centuries the content has been changed and augmented beyond recognition. The English editions ascribed to Aristotle have been numerous and seem to have been updated to conform to the knowledge and practices of the particular era. It seems likely that this book was very useful and in demand. There appear to have been several editions, and many undated copies (of a nineteenth-century edition) are in circulation at the present time. This edition (and presumably previous ones) has a large section headed 'The Midwife', with a subsection 'A Guide to Child-bearing Women'. The pseudonymous Aristotle who wrote or edited this section was obviously very observant and experienced in the minutiae of labour, birth and care of the newborn. The writer's understanding of the psychological needs of the mother and his/her conviction of the efficacy of herbal and other remedies, including the use of the aetites stone, make for absorbing reading.

Charitable Lay Midwifery

It seems that during the seventeenth century the Lady of the Manor or Mistress of the Household accounted it part of her function to attend her servants and neighbours in childbirth.

> Lady Margaret Hoby was the pattern of the great lady ordering her servants and her estates, although unusual in that she kept a diary, half personal, half spiritual, between 1599 and 1605 (the first known British woman's diary). Of one particular Wednesday she wrote: 'In the morning at six o'clock I prayed privately: that done, I went to a wife in travail of child, about whom I was busy until one o'clock, about which time, she being delivered and I having praised God, returned home and betook myself to private prayer.' There are numerous other references to her attendance at the labours of local women; delivery being a basic female skill it was not considered relevant that Lady Margaret was herself childless.[32]

Mrs Pepys also had no children but she was summoned to the bedside of Betty Mitchell in July 1668 'when she began to cry out; she helped to deliver the child, and when it proved to be a girl, acted as her godmother'.[33]

The Quaker movement was founded and became influential during the seventeenth century. It was progressive in its view of women and their active participation in society. Quakers provided schools for women and approved of them speaking at their meetings. Some of these educated, self-disciplined and caring women became midwives.

> The fame of a Quaker midwife in Reading, Frances Kent, was sufficient for the Verney family, after the Restoration, to consider employing her despite her awkward beliefs (they were assured that Mrs Kent

never discussed religious matters with her patients) and her price: she could command as much as £25. In 1684, however, when Sarah Fell was about to be delivered of her first child at the age of forty-two, Frances Kent's Quakerism was of course an added bonus: 'She is a fine woman', wrote Sarah, following her successful *accouchement*. 'It was the Lord sent her to me. It was the Lord's mercy that I had her, who is a very skilful and tender woman for that employment.'[34]

Causes of Concern to 'Professional' Midwives

Although the majority of women continued to be delivered by female midwives, a certain number in London and its environs favoured men midwives, whose numbers seemed to be growing, probably as a result of the influence and success of the Chamberlens. The threat from this incursion into a previously wholly female preserve was a cause of considerable concern to London midwives in particular. Another cause of concern arose from the great disruption of life in England created by the Civil War which was fought between the years 1642 and 1646. Large numbers of men had to leave their families for the four-year duration of the war and there was considerable loss of life in many great battles. This obviously affected the birth rate and consequently the livelihood of midwives, and their anxiety was expressed by a group of apparently educated, literate midwives, who, in 1643, presented a Petition to Parliament called the *Mid-wives Just Petition*, part of which reads as follows:

> We were formerly well paid and respected in our parishes for our great skill and midnight industry; but now our art doth fail us, and little gettings have we in this age, barren of all natural joyes, and only fruitful in bloudy calamities. We desire, therefore, for the better propagation of our owne benefit, and the general good of all women, wives may no longer spare their husbands to be devoured by the sword.

They then enumerate the battles which had resulted in the deaths of many thousands of potential husbands and fathers (Figure 10).

It seems that their loss of earnings was to the midwives more important than the fact that the country was impoverished and in a state of anarchy and revolution. The petition thus exhibits both political naivety and an extraordinary degree of self-interest.

Figure 10: Title Page of the Mid-wives Just Petition, London, 1643

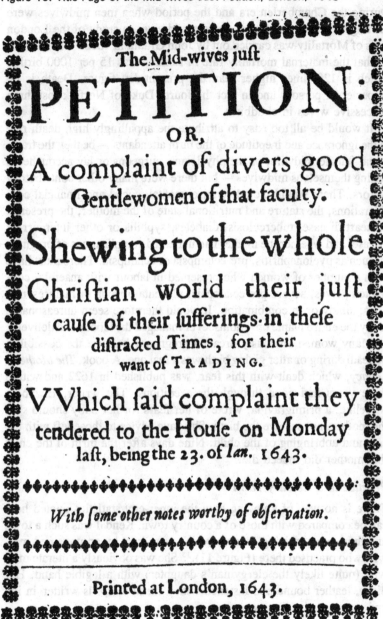

The Mid-wives juſt

PETITION:

OR,

A complaint of divers good
Gentlewomen of that faculty.

Shewing to the whole

Chriſtian world their juſt
cauſe of their ſufferings·in theſe
diſtracted Times, for their
want of TRADING.

VVhich ſaid complaint they
tendered to the Houſe on Monday
laſt, being the 23. of *Ian.* 1643.

With ſome other notes worthy of obſervation.

Printed at London, 1643.

Maternal Mortality Statistics: Contributory Factors

During the Chamberlen era and the period when men midwives were starting to practice alongside female midwives, a study of the London Bills of Mortality was carried out by John Graunt in 1662.[8] This revealed that the maternal mortality rate in London was 15 per 1000 births, which is 120 times higher than the present-day figure. Death is no respecter of persons and in fact the fourth Duke of Norfolk lost three successive wives in childbirth.[6]

It would be all too easy to attribute the appallingly high death rate to the ignorance and ineptitude of the birth attendants — be they the traditional female midwife, or the physicians, surgeons or lay accoucheurs calling themselves midwives — but there were many other contributory factors. These would include environmental, social and financial considerations, the stature and nutritional state of the mother, the presence of heart disease, tuberculosis, diabetes, syphilis or other intercurrent disease, and whether the mother had untreated complications of pregnancy such as pyelonephritis, pre-eclampsia or eclampsia. There must have been a number of women who presented in labour with anaemia, contracted pelves, severe pre-eclampsia, placenta praevia or malpresentations, singly or in combination. It would therefore seem unreasonable to lay the entire blame on whomsoever managed the labour and delivery.

Many women obviously dreaded pregnancy because the possibility of death during or after giving birth was a real one. A book, *The Mother's Legacy*, which dealt with this fear, was published in 1622 and within three years had gone through three editions. The writer, Elizabeth Josceline, a primigravida, wrote of her fears for her baby should she, the mother, not survive the birth. She gave advice to those left with the care and upbringing of the child. Nine days after the birth of the child this mother did indeed die.[17]

Practice in a Country Town

There is no way of knowing how the inner-city statistics quoted here can be compared with those of a country town. Kendal was such a town and there are surviving records which were kept by an unnamed midwife who practised there (Figure 11).[35] She was obviously a literate midwife (quite likely the clergyman's daughter) with a legible hand. Her diary, leather bound and fastened with a metal clasp, is written in ink and states on the first page:

Figure 11: Page from Diary of a Country Midwife

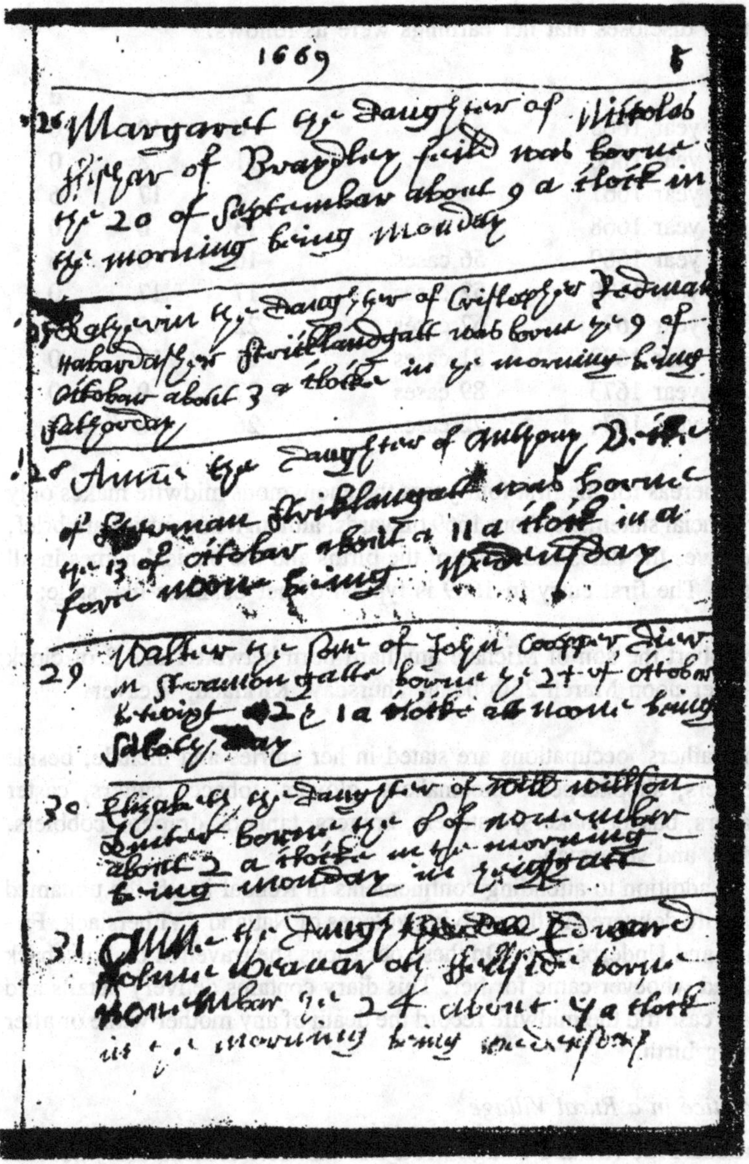

Source: Kendal Records Office, Kendal.

'The accounts of what mony I ever had given as a midwife.'

It then discloses that her earnings were as follows:

		£	s	d
the year 1665		0	19	0
the year 1666		11	8	0
the year 1667		3	17	6
the year 1668		13	6	0
the year 1669	56 cases	16	6	6
the year 1670	52 cases	17	17	0
the year 1671	62 cases	22	15	0
the year 1672	81 cases	24	10	0
the year 1673	89 cases	27	9	0
the year 1674	72 cases	26	18	2

Whereas for the first four years the anonymous midwife makes only a financial statement, from 1669 onwards, although her entries are brief, she gives the dates and times of the births and the babies' names in all cases. The first entry in 1669 is typical of her business-like style:

Robert the son of Michael Studhard born betwixt 1 and 2 of clock after noon March 25th being Thursday, Kirkland. Weaver.

The fathers' occupations are stated in her entries and include, beside weavers, shopkeepers, shoemakers, glovers, tobacco cutters, caster makers, basket makers, butchers, knitters, tanners, drapers, cobblers, dyers, and shearmen.

In addition to attending confinements in Kendal itself, the unnamed midwife delivered in the outlying villages of Natland, Witherslack, Firbank and Underbarrow. On these occasions she travelled on horseback behind whoever came for her. This diary contains delivery details and in no case did the midwife record the death of any mother while or after giving birth.

Practice in a Rural Village

Around 1700 Richard Gough wrote a remarkable contemporary account of the lives of all the people who lived in the Parish of Myddle. The village of Myddle was the centre of this remote rural parish in Shropshire which consisted of several small settlements or hamlets. Gough paints a vivid picture of the social and domestic scene by describing in detail family and village life including births, marriages, deaths, trades and professions. The following extract is his account of one woman's birth experience.

> This [Richard] Clarke had several children by his first wife, all which dyed while hee was a quaker and were buried by him in the oarchyard [orchard]. When his second wife Anne was in travail of a child, the midwife told him that the child was dead in the womb, and unless it was drawne from the woman, shee would dye also; and thereupon Clarke made iron hooks in his lytle smith's forge, according to the midwife's direction, and therewith shee eased the woman of her burthen and the woman recovered. But when she was with child agen, and the woman was in the same condition, hee would not suffer the midwife to do the like, soe the woman dyed . . .[36]

Myddle did not have its own doctor and it would appear that the nearest lived in Shrewsbury; consequently the midwife had no professional help on which to call and would have to make diagnoses and undertake any necessary measures to secure delivery. In this case she had obviously diagnosed fetal death *in utero* during labour, which may have been obstructed. That she had to wait for Richard Clarke, who was a blacksmith, actually to forge the instruments she used suggests that she did not possess such tools. Had she seen hooks used for this purpose during her 'apprenticeship', or was she just an ingenious midwife at her wit's end? Having saved this woman's life it must have been a tragedy for her to lose the mother during her next labour.

Famous Midwives of the Century

Jane Sharp

A midwife who lived in the seventeenth century and practised during the period of the Civil War, the Interregnum and the Restoration of the Monarchy was Mrs Jane Sharp of London. Not a lot is known about this woman. However, she was certainly capable of reading, learning and reasoning, and her background must have been such that she had access to books. After thirty years' practice as a midwife, she wrote a book which she entitled *The Midwives Book or the Whole Art of Midwifery Discovered*.[37] By so doing she became the first English midwife to write a 'textbook'. This book appeared in several editions, the third of which was called *The Compleat Midwife's Companion*.

Jane Sharp addresses her book 'to the Midwives of England':

Sisters

I have often sate down sad in the consideration of the many miseries women endure in the Hands of unskilful Midwives; many professing the Art (without any skill in Anatomy, which is the principal part essentially necessary for a Midwife) meerly for lucre's sake. I have been at Great Cost in Translations of all books, either French, Dutch or Italian of this kind, all which I offer with my own experience.

By Mrs Jane Sharp. Practitioner in the Art of Midwifery above 30 years.

She quotes in her introduction the story of the midwives of Israel, and goes on to remind her readers that Holy Scripture has recorded midwifery as being to the perpetual honour of the female sex 'there being not so much as one word concerning men midwives mentioned there that we can find'. The inference is that her feminine instinct recognised the need for women to defend their profession against the incursion of men. She seems to have combined considerable practical experience with common sense and knowledge, acquired from her reading of 'obstetric material' from a variety of sources, particularly European. She devised her own table which she used to calculate the 'time of birth'. Even in these comparatively recent times it seems that a factual physiological basis for estimating the expected date of confinement was lacking. It was obviously extremely difficult to arrive at anything approaching an accurate EDC (expected date of confinement), given the limited knowledge of the physiological process which would, in those days, be complicated by possible lengthy amenorrhoea due to anaemia or malnutrition, or prolonged breast feeding of a previous child. Jane Sharp recognised that it was important for the midwife to have some knowledge of female anatomy, perceiving that a midwife required 'theory as well as practice, art as well as science' (Figures 12 and 13).

Advice for Labour and Delivery. Jane Sharp tells midwives:

When the Patient feels the Throws coming, she should walk easily in her Chamber and then again lie down, keep her self warm, rest her self and then stir again, till she feels the Waters coming down and the Womb to open, let her not lie long a Bed, yet she may lie

Figure 12: From Jane Sharp's *The Compleat Midwife's Companion*, 3rd edn (J. Marshall, London, 1724)

Book IV.   *The Compleat* MIDWIFE.   115

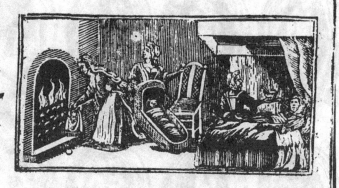

BOOK IV.

CHAP. I.

Rules for Women that are come to their Labour.

ALL Women, Midwives especially should be well provided against this time of necessity, with all things that may cause them to be easily delivered, and Childbed Linnen at hand, having first invoked the Divine Assistance by whom we live and move and have our being.

When the Patient feels her Throws coming, she should walk easily in her Chamber, and then again lie down, keep her self warm, rest her self and then stir again, till she feels the Waters coming down and the Womb to open ; let her not lie long a Bed, yet she may lie sometimes and sleep to strengthen her, and to abate pain, the Child will be the stronger.

Sometimes

Source: Courtesy of the Wellcome Institute Library, London.

Figure 13: Fetal Positions, from Jane Sharp's *The Compleat Midwife's Companion*, 3rd edn, engraving numbered 'pa. 199' (J. Marshall, London, 1724)

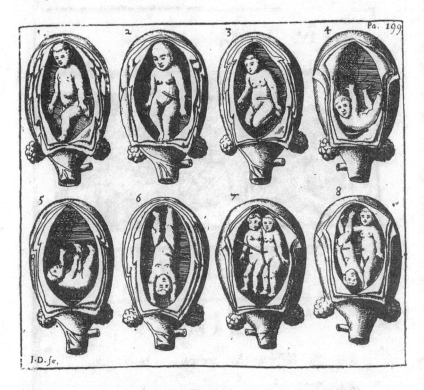

Source: Courtesy of the Wellcome Institute Library, London.

sometimes and sleep to strengthen her, and to abate pain.

If 'travail be long', the midwife was to

> refresh her with some chicken's broth or the yolk of a poached egg with a little bread or some wine or 'strong water' but modestly taken — and withal to cheer her up with good words, and stroaking down her belly above her navel with her hand, for that makes the child move downwards.

'When the waters run forth the birth is near', she declared, '. . . for when those skins are broken the infant can no longer stay there than a naked man in a heap of snow'. She says that the midwives 'do ill to rend these skins open with their nails to make way for the waters to come forth . . . but if the water breaks away long before the birth it is safe to give medical means to drive the birth after the water'. For this she adviced 'Featherfew or Mugwort boyled in white wine or dram of the powder of cinnamon in wine or the distilled water of mugwort, betony, dittander, penniroyal or featherfew'. Sharp exhorted the midwives to 'take notice that all women do not keep the same posture in their delivery; some lye in their beds, being very weak, some sit in a stool or chair, or rest upon the side of the bed, held by other women that come to the labour'. Before performing internal examinations or manipulations, she advised the midwife to 'anoint her hands with oyl of lilies and oyl of almonds and so with her hands handle and unloose the parts and observe how the child lyeth, and stirreth, and so help as time and occasion direct, but', she warned, 'above all take heed you force not the birth till the time be come . . .'. The midwife was to stroke down the birth from above the navel easily with her hand, she said. She claimed that *'particular helps* to delivery are to lay the woman first all along on her back, her head a little raised with a pillow, and a pillow under her back and another pillow larger than the other to raise her buttocks and rump . . . with her legs backwards and upwards' (!). This unnatural position would seem more unhelpful than helpful for the descent of the fetus. She advised that the mother should 'hold in her breath as much as she can, for that will cause much force to bring out the child'. It is only in this century and decade that such advice has been recognised as being undesirable because of its adverse effect on placental perfusion.

No actual delivery technique is included; Jane Sharp describes the mother as being active in *giving* birth, the midwife passive in *receiving* the baby as it is born. She emphasises the need for cleanliness during the delivery — and this was long before Semmelweiss! She mentions that to aid the delivery of a dead fetus some commended the use of the eagle-stone held near the 'privvy parts', but that she herself 'never saw it tried'.

Sharp's Advice for Delivery of Placenta and Membranes. 'The smoke of mary-gold flowers taken in by a tunnel at the "secrets" will easily bring forth the secundine though the midwife have let go her hold. Mugwort boil'd soft in water and applied like a poultice to the navel, brings birth and after-birth away'.

Jane Sharp was perceptive enough to warn that women were in great danger if membranes were left behind or incomplete. 'Midwives' long nails may do mischief . . . for if it be retained till it corrupt, it will cause

Feavers, Imposthumes, Convulsions'. To aid expulsion she recommended 'snuff to sneeze, herb vervain boyled in wine, syrup of tansie, featherfew and mugwort'.

Jane Sharp was a dedicated woman who conveyed her sense of the 'high calling' of a midwife, telling her readers that 'the art of midwifery is doubtless one of the most useful and necessary of all arts for the being and well-being of mankind.'

Elizabeth Cellier

On to the midwifery scene in the late seventeenth century came Elizabeth Cellier. She 'set up and practised the craft of midwifery in the city of London'.[16] Cellier was energetic in the political life of London and was one of the main participants behind the Catholic Meal Tub plot, for which she was tried but acquitted of treason on her own defence. After this unsuccessful plot she turned her attention to the politics of midwifery by reviving the agitation for instruction of midwives through a self-governing corporation or college. In a grandiose scheme, addressed to King James II, she laid down plans for a large Royal Foundling Hospital to be governed and funded by midwives, and for twelve other houses in which poor women would be delivered and maintained by the Charity during the puerperium. She claimed that the King had promised to unite the midwives into a Corporation by Royal Charter, but that, because of the King's exile in the following year, this promise was not fulfilled.

Mrs Cellier drew up detailed rules and regulations for the proposed charity hospitals and saw herself as the governess with a man-midwife as the principal clinician. Her rules required that this man should be a surgeon or physician who would lecture to the midwives on a regular basis. She proposed that surgeons and physicians who intended practising midwifery should attend the lectures along with the midwives.

Elizabeth Cellier should perhaps be given credit for her idea of in-service training for practising midwives, but her plan to enlist a thousand midwives, who would each pay £5 annually, seems unrealistic. Such an 'establishment' was in any case too high for the workload as records show that the number of births per annum in London at that time was under 15 000. When it was recognised that her scheme was unworkable and unacceptable to the doctors, her attitude towards these self-appointed men-midwives changed completely. In response to the queries of one doctor she wrote:

> We desire you not to concern yourselves until we desire your company, which we will certainly do as often as we have occasion for

your advice in anything we do not understand, or which doth not appertain to our practice. I hope doctor these considerations will deter any of you from pretending to teach us midwifery, which ought to be kept a secret amongst women as much as possible.[38]

Elizabeth Cellier was obviously a clever woman midwife with a forceful personality, and she was acknowledged to be 'of great ability'.[39] She had a concept which had the potential to influence, for good, the standard of midwifery practice in this country, but other interests and self-interest prevented the realisation of her aims.

The midwife was a key figure in society in the seventeenth century, when pregnancy and childbirth dominated the life of every woman 'so that in this period the midwife, not the prostitute, was the true "priestess of humanity" in Lecky's classic phrase'.[17]

The importance of the midwife to mankind is summed up by the Swiss doctor, Jacobus Rueff, as follows:

It is observable that in all the ages of the world, and throughout all countries in the world, the help of grave and modest women, (with us termed midwives) hath ever been useful for release and succour of all the daughters of Evah, whom God hath appointed to bear children into this world.[29]

References

1. Hill, C. *et al*. 'Education in England to 1660', Block 4, Course A203, *17th Century England* (Open University Press, Milton Keynes, 1980).

2. Eccles, A. *Obstetrics and Gynaecology in Tudor and Stuart England* (Croom Helm, London, 1982).

3. Thomas, K. 'Providence: The Doctrine and its Use', in *Seventeenth Century England. A Changing Culture*, *Vol. 2*, W.R. Owens (ed.) (Ward Lock Educational, London, 1980).

4. Trevelyan, G.M. *English Social History* (Longmans Green, London, 1942).

5. Trevelyan, G.M. *English Social History* (reference 4), p. 276.

6. Hill, C. *The Century of Revolution*, 2nd edn (Nelson, Surrey, 1980).

7. Steer, F.W. 'Farm and Cottage Inventories of Mid-Essex 1635–1749', in *Seventeenth Century England. A Changing Culture*, Vol. 1, A. Hughes (ed.) (Ward Lock Educational, London, 1980).

8. Donnison, J. *Midwives and Medical Men* (Heinemann, London, 1977).

9. See Chapter 3.

10. Benton, T. and Rowling, N. 'Architecture and Society in a Changing Culture', Block 2, Course A203, *17th-century England* (Open University Press, Milton Keynes, 1980).

11. Harrison, W. 'The Manner of Building and Furniture in our Houses, 1587', in

Seventeenth-century England. A Changing Culture, Vol. 1, A. Hughes (ed.) (Ward Lock Educational, London, 1980).

12. Harrison, W. 'The Manner of Building and Furniture in our Houses' (reference 11), p. 10.

13. *Shuttleworth Accounts*, House and Farm Accounts of Gawthorpe Hall, Padiham, Lancashire (Chetham's Library, Manchester).

14. Josselin, R. *Diary for 1616–1683*, A. Macfarlane (ed.) (Oxford University Press for the British Academy: Records of Social and Economic History, 1976).

15. Dewhurst, J. 'Royal Midwives of Former Times', *Midwife, Health Visitor and Community Nurse*, October 1983.

16. Aveling, J.H. *English Midwives. Their History and Prospects* (Hugh K. Elliott, London, 1967).

17. Fraser, A. *The Weaker Vessel. Woman's Lot in 17th-century England* (Weidenfeld and Nicolson, London, 1984).

18. Burton, E. *Jacobeans at Home* (Secker and Warburg, London, 1962).

19. Gouge, W. *Of Domestical Duties* (John Haviland, London, 1622, pp. 401–2).

20. Hunnis, W. 'A Meditation to be Said of Woman with Child', in *Penguin Book of Elizabethan Verse*, E. Lucie-Smith (ed.) (Penguin Books, London, 1965).

21. Schnucker, R.V. 'The English Puritans and Pregnancy, Delivery and Breast Feeding'. *History of Childhood Quarterly, 1* (4), 1974.

22. Gouge, W. *Of Domestical Duties* (John Haviland, London, 1622).

23. Willoughby, P. *Observations on Midwifery. A Country Midwife's Opusculum*. Ed. from original manuscript by Henry Blenkinsop. John Rylands Library, University of Manchester Radford Collection.

24. Cutter, I.S. and Veits, H.R. *A Short History of Midwifery* (W.B. Saunders, Philadelphia, 1964).

25. Simpson, M. *Simpson the Obstetrician* (Gollancz, London, 1972).

26. Aveling, J.H. *English Midwives. Their History and Prospects* (Hugh K. Elliott, London, 1967, p. 24).

27. Aveling, J.H. *The Chamberlens, and the Midwifery Forceps* (J. and A. Churchill, 1882).

28. Radcliffe, W. *The Secret Instrument. The Birth of the Midwifery Forceps* (Heinemann, London, 1947).

29. Rueff, J. *The Expert Midwife* (E. Griffin, London, 1637).

30. Rowlands, B. *Medieval Woman's Guide to Health* (Croom Helm, London, 1981).

31. Eccles, A. 'The Early Use of English for Midwiferies, 1500–1700', *Neuphilologische Mitteilungen, 4*, LXXVIII, 1977.

32. Fraser, A. *The Weaker Vessel. Woman's Lot in 17th-century England*. (Quoting Lady Margaret Hoby, The Hoby Diary) (Weidenfeld and Nicolson, London, 1984).

33. Pepys, S. Diary, July 1668.

34. Fraser, A. *The Weaker Vessel. Woman's Lot in 17th-century England*. (Quoting Verney Memoirs) (Weidenfeld and Nicolson, London, 1984).

35. An unnamed midwife's diary (Kendal 1669), Kendal Records Office.

36. Gough, R. *The History of Myddle*, D. Hey (ed.) (Penguin Books, London, 1981).

37. Sharp, J. *The Midwives Book* (London, 1671).

38. Aveling, J.H. *English Midwives. Their History and Prospects* (Hugh K. Elliott, London, 1967, p. 83).

39. Spencer, H.R. *History of British Midwifery, 1650–1800. The Fitzpatrick Lecture for 1927* (John Bale, Sons and Danielsson Ltd, London, 1927).

6 HE-MIDWIFE OR SHE-MIDWIFE? EIGHTEENTH-CENTURY MIDWIVES AND THEIR BATTLE FOR SURVIVAL

Social Growth and Development

The population of England and Wales at the beginning of the century numbered approximately 5½ million. The ports of Bristol, Norwich, Newcastle and Liverpool were already populous towns but were in no way comparable in size and prosperity to London. The middle of the century saw the invention of industrial machinery which was to revolutionise English, and later British, society. The ports grew and new cities emerged as industry expanded. Many large villages and towns were un-affected initially, but industrial growth created a shift in population from the country to manufacturing towns such as Manchester, Birmingham and Sheffield.[1] In these new industrialised areas, people were marrying younger and having larger families.[2,3] The latter half of the century experienced 'tumultous industrial change and a runaway population rise'.[4] In consequence, in the century preceding 1801, the population of Lancashire rose from 160 000 to 695 000;[1] by 1760 the population of England had risen to approximately 6 million and by 1801 to approximately 9 million.[5] This was despite the fact that both maternal and infant mortality rates were very high.[6]

In general the standard of living was better than in previous centuries for all but the wretchedly poor. The rich lived in luxury in town mansions and country houses; shopkeepers, small employers and artisans lived in well-built dwellings in some degree of comfort; villagers now dwelt in cottages of brick and stone. Much 'industry' especially spinning and weaving, was carried on in these cottages, some of which resembled miniature factories with the father, mother *and* children of the family being both skilled operators and 'factory hands'.

Daniel Defoe formulated seven social groupings which he defined by wealth and consumption. His classification[7] was:

1. The great, who live profusely.
2. The rich, who live plentifully.
3. The middle sort, who live well.
4. The working trades, who labour hard but feel no want.
5. The country people, farmers, etc. who fare indifferently.

6. The poor, who fare hard.
7. The miserable, that really pinch and suffer want.

Child deaths were common to rich and poor alike. It was not uncommon for women to have a pregnancy every year. Queen Anne herself
had 17 pregnancies in 17 years and all her 6 liveborn children died before
the age of twelve.[8] A Bishop of Norwich appointed in 1792, when only
36 years of age, had a family of 11 children.[9] Lady Bristol suffered 18
pregnancies in as many years, and although 16 babies were liveborn,
few survived beyond early childhood. Edward Gibbon, the historian,
was the only one of his parents' seven children to survive infancy.[10]
The mother of the famous Wesley brothers married when aged 19 and
subsequently had 19 children of whom only 10 survived infancy.[11]
One in five babies died in their first year but the death toll among
the children of the poor was even higher. 'In the 1740s in certain London
parishes about 3 in 4 children died before the age of six.'[6]
The eighteenth century saw a huge expansion in the number of school
places. One or two of the fifteenth-century grammar schools had become
fee-paying public schools and by the end of the century at least six of
such institutions existed, namely Westminster, Eton, Harrow, Rugby,
Charterhouse and Winchester. Every town had some sort of endowed
school, many of which had a religious foundation, and others were
initiated by a local benefactor. These charitable schools were intended
for the education of the poor, but it was the better-off who actually took
advantage of the opportunities provided. In the villages it was generally
the parson who provided education, although many of the poor children
went only to Dame's schools, where they received a rather inferior
education. However, because schooling was not compulsory, a large
number of children, particulary the girls, received little or none. Interestingly, though, the ten Wesley children were all taught at home by
their mother, the three boys later going on to public school.[11] There
is some evidence that self-learning was quite common; for instance
William Cobbett never went to school but became one of the most 'powerful political pamphleteers in English history'.[1]
Oxford and Cambridge Universities became less prestigious during
this century as a result of academic decline and inactivity. Many men
therefore went abroad to study medicine; their subsequent practice,
certainly in midwifery, owed much to Dutch and French influences.
Medical students were, however, still attracted to the Scottish Universities.
It is significant that a spate of books was written in this century for

midwives, with the expectation that many would be able to read and learn from them.

He-midwife or She-midwife?

In the early eighteenth century, many doctors were taking an increasing interest in the complications of labour. They were obviously aware of the nature of the Chamberlen's secret, and in fact several pairs of crude forceps were designed and used by such men-midwives as Edmund Chapman, William Giffard, William Perfect and Benjamin Pugh, all of whom practised in London or the neighbouring counties. William Smellie was the outstanding man-midwife of this century and he used forceps from 1735. Chapman claimed to be using forceps as early as 1723 and Giffard from 1726. Benjamin Pugh described forceps with long handles and a pelvic curve 'joined by a slotted arrangement in each side, which avoided the use of any form of screw or pin'.[12]

Because of the increasing numbers of men who were taking an interest in 'instrumental midwifery', books on the subject were written by several of its experienced practitioners. By 1731 William Giffard, who was a surgeon and man-midwife, wrote about the management of difficult cases, and in 1754 Benjamin Pugh wrote *A Treatise of Midwifery* for young practitioners. Female modesty, which had hitherto excluded men from the birth chamber, was disappearing among the upper and middle classes and so the practice of male accoucheurs conducting the delivery became popular in London and the surrounding towns. By the end of the century the custom had spread to more rural areas. It is known that when Mrs Custance, the wife of a Norfolk Squire, gave birth in 1791 she was attended by a man-midwife.[9] The use of the term 'brought to bed' in accounts of childbirth among the gentry implies that this class abandoned the birth chair for the bed when they abandoned the traditional midwife for the male accoucheur. Some of these accoucheurs were also physicians. Physicians were qualified in medicine by virtue of having obtained a degree (albeit in some cases acquired very easily on the Continent)[13] and were subject to the regulations of the Royal College of Physicians which had been founded in 1518. It appears, though, that in addition other 'medical men' were also practising midwifery; these included barber-surgeons and apothecaries. Barber-surgeons had formed themselves into a Guild as early as the thirteenth century. Membership of this Guild, following successful apprenticeship gave them an exclusive entitlement to perform surgical procedures using instruments. In 1540 this Guild became the Company of Barber-Surgeons. Some men qualified both as surgeons and physicians, others were surgeon-apothecaries, or apothecary-surgeons; some men qualified as apothecaries only. They were all considered able to practise as man-midwives. 'From the Parish Poor Law accounts, it is known that the surgeons or apothecaries employed by the Authority not infrequently "laid a woman" '.[13] The apothecaries formed themselves into a Worshipful Society of Apothecaries in 1617, having dissociated themselves by an Act of Parliament from the Freemen of the Mystery of Grocers.[13] Even some 'non-medical' men set themselves up as men-midwives (see page 104).

The explosion of scientific knowledge, especially in physiology and anatomy, attracted some men of very high calibre to the study and practice of midwifery. With the application of their knowledge as physicians, and their skills as surgeons (using their newly acquired forceps) these men-midwives changed irrevocably the nature and pattern of midwifery practice.

The greatest practitioner of midwifery was **William Smellie**, who was born in Lanark in 1697. He studied medicine in Glasgow and started his medical practice, which included midwifery, in Lanark in 1720. He was called by midwives to assist them with 'preternatural' births, and from 1735, for some of these cases, he used obstetric forceps which later he was to improve and modify. He would have liked to have attended normal labours and natural births, but the midwives excluded him from what they regarded as their cases. He went to London in 1738 and shortly afterwards moved to Paris, specifically to study midwifery. On his return to London he both practised and taught midwifery, giving courses of lectures on reproductive anatomy and abnormal midwifery to *male* pupils. He also published a course of lectures on midwifery in 1742 and wrote his *Treatise on the Theory and Practice of Midwifery* in 1752. With his pupils he delivered over a thousand poor women in the space of ten years; there were in addition to the cases to which the midwives called him when they encountered difficulties. This was a break away from the monopoly of normal deliveries by midwives. Smellie obviously felt that understanding and experience of the normal should precede instrumental practice, and he managed to secure for his pupils what he himself had earlier been denied in Scotland. These particular mothers benefited from his undoubted exceptionally skilled professional attention, and even more mothers would benefit ultimately because his pupils were so thoroughly grounded and trained in both theory and practice.

Many other men around this time took an interest in normal cases and were therefore in direct competition with the midwives, especially in and around London. It would appear that the men-midwives commanded a larger fee than the female midwives and so, as in France, their engagement for a confinement became a status symbol. On the whole the female midwives were left with the less lucrative areas of practice, both in city and country, but nevertheless were still the choice of some women and their husbands who found the idea of an unchaperoned male, for the purpose of labour and delivery, distinctly distasteful.

Although Doctor Smellie became the focus of the midwives' fury, because of their threatened position, his own motivation was to develop midwifery as a science for the benefit of all women, rich and poor alike. He taught the theory of natural and preternatural labour and delivery, and using models or 'dummies' he demonstrated fetal positions and mechanisms of delivery. He was extremely keen to share his knowledge and skills, and so extended his teaching to female pupils. It is interesting, however, that he taught them separately from men, obviously viewing their role as being both different and distinct.[14] Although he expected the midwife to have a knowledge of relevant anatomy and physiology and of the course of both normal and abnormal labour and of methods used to assess its progress, nevertheless his attitude to the female midwife seems fairly condescending, as can be seen from the conclusion of his *Treatise*. In this he expressed the view that

> she ought to avoid all reflections upon male practitioners, and when she finds herself *difficulted*, candidly have recourse to their assistance: on the other hand, this confidence ought to be encouraged by the man, who, when called, instead of openly condemning her method of practice, (even though it be erroneous) ought to make allowance for the weakness of the sex, and rectify what is amiss, without exposing her mistakes . . . These gentle methods will prevent that mutual calumny and abuse which too often prevail upon the male and female practitioners, and redound to the advantage of both: for no accoucheur is so perfect but that he may err sometimes: and on such occasions he must expect to meet with retaliation, from those midwives whom he may have roughly used [our italic].[15]

Despite the fact that Smellie admits that 'no accoucheur is perfect', he implies that it would be the midwife's method of practice, rather than the failure of natural processes, that could cause her to find herself 'difficulted'. Smellie created the Obstetrician, elevated midwifery as a specialty for doctors and in so doing earned himself for perpetuity the title 'Master of British Midwifery'. His skills would be difficult to equal, but despite this and regardless of their ability (or lack of it), all doctor practitioners were subsequently seen as 'superior' to midwives, purely on the grounds of their gender and education, which endowed them with a higher social status.

William Hunter, who was a pupil of Smellie, became the chief surgeon man-midwife at the British Lying-in Hospital in 1749. He was appointed Royal Obstetrician and attracted clientele from the aristocracy but 'his patients ranged from the Queen down to the poorest of her subjects'.[16] Hunter advanced the knowledge of reproductive anatomy but was extreme in his policy of non-intervention and did not favour the use of forceps, stating 'it was a thousand pities they were ever invented, for where they save one they murder twenty'.[17]   .

The antagonism of the female midwives towards men-instrumentarians in general, and towards Doctor Smellie in particular, was most forcibly expressed by **Elizabeth Nihell** (Figure 14). She was a midwife who had had a two-year training at the Hotel Dieu in Paris. She married a surgeon-apothecary and they practised in the Haymarket in London. In 1760 she wrote a book entitled *Professed Midwife. A Man-midwife or a Midwife? A Treatise on the Art of Midwifery*. She dedicated it to 'all fathers, mothers and likely soon to be either'. She openly mocked and ridiculed

> that multitude of disciples of Dr. Smellie, trained up at the feet of his artificial doll, or in short those self-constituted men-midwives made out of broken barbers, tailors or even pork butchers, for I know myself one of this last trade, who, after passing half his life stuffing sausages, is turned an intrepid physician and man-midwife.

She described them as a

> band of mercenaries who palm themselves off upon pregnant women under cover of their crochets, knives, scissors, spoons, pinchers, fillets, speculum matrices, all of which and especially their forceps . . . are totally useless.[23]

Elizabeth Nihell recognised that female midwives were seriously threatened, and much of her argument was both justified and sound. She fully realised that as instruments could only be used by surgeons, and as only men could be surgeons, then women had no place in a set-up where men were increasingly motivated to advocate the use of forceps. Her argument therefore was in the main 'political', but unfortunately because she claimed that instruments, which she regarded as 'pernicious innovations' were *never* necessary, she ruined her case by overstating

Figure 14: Elizabeth Nihell

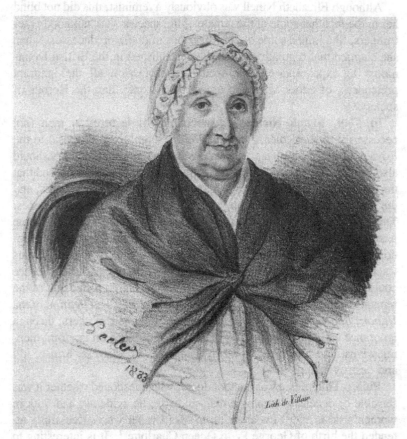

Source: Courtesy of the Wellcome Institute Library, London.

it. Her strong prejudice against male interference was concentrated in a venomous, undignified, personal attack on Dr Smellie. Her most famous phrase was her allusion to his large hands, which she likened to 'the delicate fist of a great horse-godmother of a he-midwife'. A similar comment was made by a doctor colleague, a Dr William Douglas, who sneeringly said that Smellie's hands were 'fit only to hold horses by the nose whilst they are shod by the farrier, or stretch boots in Cranburne Alley'.[14] Elizabeth Nihell was not alone in her criticism of men as midwives. Some doctors, and in particular Frank Nicholls, a physician who practised midwifery, expressed the view that the need for men-midwives was being exaggerated, as were the complaints about the incompetence of female midwives.

Although Elizabeth Nihell was obviously a feminist, this did not blind her to the fact that some of the female of the species were not good practitioners. She joined some of her illustrious midwife predecessors when she claimed that regulations should be established in the British Dominions 'to expel and exclude from the profession all the ignorant pretenders, of either sex, who are in fact, worse than the Herods of society'.[19]

In 1749, **Frank Nicholls** gave courses of lectures to men (not necessarily medical men), and in 1752 he submitted a proposal to the Royal College of Physicians suggesting that lectures on midwifery should also be given to *women* within the College. In addition he proposed that the College ask the Bishops to demand attendance at these lectures, and the passing of an examination, as a prerequisite to granting licences. These proposals were not accepted on the grounds that at this time some female pupil-midwives were already receiving instruction in the London area. It appears that Nicholls was attempting to centralise this teaching in order that an 'official' and therefore more meaningful licence could be granted.[20] Frank Nicholls became a declared proponent of the female midwife and in 1751 he wrote a tract entitled *The Petition of the Unborn Babes*. In it the 'babes' complained that their mothers, through ignorance and fear, were persuaded to place reliance on ignorant men-midwives, and hire them at extravagant rates to 'distress, bruise, kill and destroy' them.

Phillip Thicknesse was another doctor who questioned whether it was sensible or decent to employ a man-midwife; he evidently had faith in women's skills and drew attention to Mrs Draper who successfully attended the birth of George IV to Queen Charlotte.[21] It is interesting to note that the midwife had no duties in the lying-in period — not even in a Royal confinement — because records show that

the usual retinue was appointed:
  Wet Nurse — Mrs Scott
  Dry Nurse — Mrs Chapman
  Rockers — Jane Simpson and Catherine Johnson[22]

A proponent of the man-midwife, for cases of complicated labour, was **John Maubray**, who suggested that instead of calling the doctor a man-midwife he should be called an andro-boethygynist, i.e. man-helper of woman. He lectured to men on midwifery at his house in Bond Street. Dr Maubray felt that English women should be encouraged to

follow the lead given by their European sisters who had readily accepted
the male doctor into the birth room 'in order to secure their own and
their children's safety'. Men, he asserted, were better equipped than
women in every way to assist in complicated births, and his book, *The
Female Physician . . . The Whole Art of New Improv'd Midwifery* (1724),
confirms his confidence in the abilities of men and their new instruments.
In his book he mentions deliveries with the mother lying in bed, sitting
on a chair or simply standing up.[23] Dr Maubray also put on courses of
instruction for female midwives. The positive physical, intellectual and
psychological attributes that he considered necessary for the 'ordinary
midwife' to possess are as follows:

She ought to be a woman of good middle age, of solid parts, of full
experience, of a healthy, strong and vigorous body, with clever
small hands, since nothing can be more agreeable and conducive
to the art of midwifery than slender hands, long fingers and
ready feeling.

She ought to be patient and pleasant, soft, meek and mild in her
Temper, in order to encourage and comfort the labouring
woman. She should pass by and forgive her small Failings and
Peevish Faults; instructing her gently when she does and says
amiss. But if she will not follow Advice, and Necessity require,
the Midwife ought to reprimand and put her smartly in mind
of her Duty; yet always in such a manner, however, as to
encourage her with the hopes of a Happy and speedy
Delivery.

In the like manner, as she ought to be modest, temperate, sober,
so ought she to be faithful and silent; always upon her guard
to conceal those things which ought not to be spoken of'.

Maubray listed the following features as *disqualifying* factors:

She who would discreetly undertake midwifery ought not to begin
the practice too young nor continue it till grown too old.

She ought to be no weak, infirm or diseased person, incapable of
undergoing the fatigue which the business too often requires;
such as watching night and day; turning the infants when in the
wrong posture; or extracting them at length, which act frequently requires the full strength of a strong man instead of a weak
woman.

She ought not to be too fat or gross, but especially not to have thick or fleshy hands and arms or large-boned wrists; which of necessity must occasion racking pains on the tender labouring woman.

She ought not to be a conceived or childbearing woman, because this may be of bad consequence, not only to the labouring woman but also to the conceived midwife herself, and her own infant.

She ought not to be an ignorant, stupid, indolent or dull person . . . neither ought she to be a self-indulgent, slothful, lazy, inconsiderate, passionate, proud or obstinate person, nor peevish, morose, surly, neither ought she to be a tippler, or drunkard, nor a tatler or vagabond nor a covetous or mercenary person.

Maubray expected the midwife not only to be a paragon of all the virtues but also able to turn and extract the fetus: in fact to be able to deal with complicated cases.

Theoretical Knowledge of the Midwife

Maubray thought it was absolutely necessary for the midwife to be instructed in the following:

I.   Of the external or internal parts of generation, and the adjacent parts; together with a competent skill of the respective substance and nature, connection and function of each of these in time of birth.

II.   Of the pelvis, or bason and its contents; together with a true knowledge of its bones, their form or figure, office and connection etc. upon that occasion.

III. Of that wonderful body the MATRIX and its vagina or neck, together with the understanding of its balance and structure, duty, and function in time of labour.

IV.   Of the strange natural qualities and amazing singular faculties of this body in distinguishing all its peculiar properties.

V.   Of the touch, or handling the woman, together with knowing its many various uses and manifold distinct advantages.

VI.   Of the genuine and real, as well as the spurious and bastard, labour pains; how they differ in themselves and are to be carefully distinguished.

VII. Of the method of laying the woman and manner of extracting the after-birth; together with all the heterogenous and preternatural contents of the womb.

Practical Knowledge of the Midwife

Maubray took the view that the midwife ought to have a full and complete knowledge of the following:

I.   Of the various methods to be taken for the present ease and expeditious relief of the labouring woman.

II.   Of the discreet method of turning an ill-situated infant (whatsoever the preternatural posture may be) and drawing it forth safely by the feet.

III. Of her own personal duty (as midwife) both to the mother and child after delivery as also towards all labouring women, to whom she may be called upon critical conjectures.

Maubray obviously recognised that the well-informed midwife, instructed according to his syllabus, had an important part to play.

John Douglas succeeded Dr Maubray. He was in favour of the 'midwoman' for the majority of births and proposed 'an effective method to enable the *midwomen* to perform their office in all cases (excepting those few where instruments are necessary) with as much ease, speed and safety as the most dexterous *midmen* [our italics]'.[24] His radical proposal was as follows:

1.   That a hospital be erected for example in London or Westminster (at public expense, by donation or subscription) for the reception of two or three hundred poor women who are big with child.

2.   That a proper number of midwomen be appointed to attend them.

3.   That two surgeons be appointed to assist these midwomen in all extraordinary cases, and to demonstrate the structure of the parts concerned, explain the art of touching etc. in set lectures, at least three times a week, to all the midwomen and their apprentices who please to attend.

4.   That every young woman, who designs to practice midwifery, shall be obliged to attend these courses during their apprenticeship; and then go and practice for a set time under those expert women in that hospital. Afterwards let them be *examined* as to the skill and knowledge they have acquired in their profession by two surgeons and six or seven other persons appointed by His Majesty and if approved to receive from them a *Certificate* of their fitness to practice in London or anywhere else.

5.   That, until fit hospitals can be built and endowed, a *midman* be appointed in every city or county town, and demonstrate to

them the truth of their doctrines on the poor of the neighbourhood, of which there are plenty everywhere.

Douglas goes on to say that if such a scheme were put into operation in the large towns in England, then he would be satisfied that within a few years 'there would hardly be an ignorant midwoman in England'.[24] Douglas's term 'midman' (literally 'with man') was meaningless in this context.

In 1737 yet another doctor, **Henry Bracken**, wrote a textbook for midwives. He entitled his book *The Midwife's Companion*.[25] His preface is devoted to the berating of 'ignorant' midwives. He defined such midwives as those who were utterly opposed to calling for the assistance of a man-midwife because they felt they possessed skills sufficient to match any complication of childbirth that might present itself to them. He felt strongly that this over-confident attitude was responsible for many infants being destroyed unnecessarily. He advised an investigation into perinatal deaths. 'I wonder', he wrote, 'that there is not a law, to have a Jury appointed, with the assistance of an able and honest man-midwife, to enquire into the circumstances of the case of children born dead, maimed or distorted.'

Thomas Dawkes, surgeon in London in the first part of the eighteenth century, recognised the distinct and important role of female midwives in the practice of *normal* midwifery. He acknowledged that there were educated, expert and able midwives in London and other towns, but he felt that rural 'country' midwives were all too often uneducated, unskilled and ill-qualified for their office. In the preface to his book *The Midwife Rightly Instructed*, published in 1736, Dawkes addressed the married ladies of Great Britain and appealed to them to choose as their midwives *women* of genius and good capacity and to discountenance 'ignorant and daring' women. Mothers, he said, were to expect certain standards of knowledge, proficiency and conduct, and he suggested that the better educated and more able town midwives should be encouraged to extend their sphere of practice. Dawkes felt that among other attributes the midwife should be 'sober and cheerful, tender, able to read and on occasions to write . . . hear easily . . . and have a good acquaintance with the liberal arts and anatomy'. He went on to remark: 'who can say what noble minds and what exalted geniuses the world may have lost by the conduct of rash and adventurous midwives?'. He expressed the view that all midwives should be taught by men who had knowledge of reproductive anatomy and of aberrations from the anatomical normal. He tells the 'married women of Great Britain' that they should assess the capability of their midwives by asking them such questions as 'What is the lie and presentation of the fetus?', or 'How are the waters formed?' — quite an exacting question even for a modern midwife! Although Thomas Dawkes appears to have had limited personal practical midwifery experience, he was keen to instruct midwives in theory and he stressed the necessity of using a skeleton and a dead fetus to demonstrate fetal positions and obstruction, and also for mechanisms and delivery practice. The book concludes with a dialogue between the author and a midwife. During questioning the midwife answered that she had only been instructed in the actual delivery procedure and in the immediate care of the baby but with *very little explanation.*[26]

George Counsell, a contemporary of Thomas Dawkes, also acknowledged the place of the female midwife in the management of *normal* labour and delivery, and he stressed that she must be able to recognise deviation from the normal and *call the doctor* in such cases. He told midwives that they must 'never presume to make use of instruments. It is sufficient to know when they become necessary.'[27] Counsell's writings reveal that he was an experienced man-midwife who aimed to improve the practice of midwifery by sharing with midwives his own proven 'successful' methods. In 1752 he wrote a book which he called *The Art of Midwifery or The Midwife's Sure Guide*. This was obviously aimed at learners as he gives precise details of the clinical course and management of the three stages of labour and the technique of delivery of the baby, placenta and membranes. Counsell deplored the fact that there was no legislation regulating the practice of midwifery, declaring:

> for it is a truth too well known that mothers and children are daily if not hourly destroyed by ignorant wretches . . . How much then is it to be lamented that no care has yet been taken by any law to prevent these cruel and most fatal proceedings? Laws have been enacted for the preservation of the brute species, and shall the human species be neglected? Surely an affair of such vast weight and importance that is now even a national grievance, in which the safety of millions as yet unborn will be concerned, must one day become the subject of a Parliamentary Inquiry.

The book opens with two diagrams, one of a gynaecoid pelvis and the other of a contracted pelvis with explanations of their significance for childbearing. Counsell describes how to perform a vaginal examination, first to ascertain whether labour was established and then to predict the course of labour and to assess its progress from the state of the 'circle or ring i.e. the womb's mouth'. He discusses lie and position of the fetus, engagement of the head in the 'bason' and the significance of head flexion. He describes how delivery usually follows the 'bursting of the water-bag', and how, when the head is flexed and the position occipito-anterior, the labour should be natural so that the midwife would have little to do but to receive the child and deliver the 'after-burden'. Although this is valid teaching, Counsell's technique of delivery of the placenta has not stood the test of time. He gives a perfect description of how to perform manual separation and removal of the placenta, and advises this procedure as a matter of routine. In the case of a post-partum haemorrhage, however, he advised midwives to 'pull the cord in all directions, upwards, downwards and from side to side in order to loosen the womb-cake'. This method, he claimed, would prevent the 'tearing of the after-burden into sundry parts or portions'!

In subsequent chapters Counsell instructs midwives on how to manage difficult cases. For the management of uterine inertia with intact membranes, he advised that the mother should walk about and change her posture, and that light nourishing broths and jellies should be taken along with wines mixed with yolk of egg, spices and sugar. Counsell did not advise the midwife to perform artificial rupture of membranes but he did describe how to perform a membrane sweep using butter, lard or sweet oil as a lubricant. He mentions certain herbal concoctions for the midwife to administer. The basis of these was oil of juniper, which was to be mixed with sugar, water and wine, or with pennyroyal water or with beer, egg and nutmeg. If these 'stimulants' failed to induce contractions, he suggested 30 grains of ipecacuanha or other emetic to cause vomiting in the hope of reflex action on the uterus. He believed also that strong snuff, pepper or raceginger could produce a sneezing attack sufficient to provoke contractions.

To aid recovery of a woman fatigued and weakened by a long or difficult labour, Counsell recommended meat broths with pot herbs added, and that she should drink claret, port or madeira. He also suggested concoctions such as syrup of cowslips or compound peony water sweetened with syrup of cloves or gillyflowers. To this could be added liquid laudanum (tincture of opium), but he warned the midwives that they should not give more than 15 to 20 drops of laudanum without calling for medical aid! It is interesting that laudanum was used as a postnatal 'pick-me-up' rather than as an analgesic.

Counsell felt it quite proper for a midwife who diagnosed a transverse lie to rupture the membranes at full dilatation of the cervix and immediately to perform a podalic version and breech delivery. This is rather surprising, given his instruction that, in the case of an obstructed head, and a full bladder, the midwife was to call for a man-midwife to catheterise the patient and so secure the delivery.

Counsell appealed to midwives to understand that having to send for a doctor was not a sign of failure, nor did it mean a loss of reputation on their part, but that a failure to send for help could both damage a midwife's reputation and cost the lives of mother and baby.

Recognition of Respective Roles

There is evidence that in the middle of the eighteenth century midwives themselves, along with some lay people, realised the need for skilled help from men-midwives in certain cases. An unwritten understanding seemed to develop between some female midwives and some doctor-instrumentarians that when the midwife encountered difficulties she would call the doctor for assistance. *Edmund Chapman*, who was a surgeon/mid-wife and teacher of midwifery, wrote in his *Treatise on the Improvement of Midwifery* that 'the best midwives commonly send for advice when they see the appearance of danger'.

William Perfect in his *Cases in Midwifery*[28] demonstrates the routine involvement of midwives in complicated as well as uncomplicated deliveries. He records many interesting occasions on which he was judiciously called by the midwife. One such call was to a maidservant who had summoned the assistance of the midwife who found her vomiting, bleeding per vaginam and convulsing. The midwife discovered that this woman, who was six months pregnant, had taken 'black powder' in order to procure an abortion. Despite the efforts of the doctor and midwife rigors ensued and death followed. On another occasion he was called by the midwife to a poor woman delivering a breech and where the head was 'stuck fast in the vagina'. He records that the midwife prudently declined to make use of any great force and sent for him. It is interesting to note that this mother was given mulled wine during her labour. Perfect relates that he was unable to respond to the midwife's call for five hours so that all he could do was to deliver the stillborn child using long curved forceps.

On 3 February 1777 Perfect was called by a midwife to a mother with jaundice whom she had delivered of twins, the first of which was a footling but both of which were born jaundiced. He diagnosed 'ideopathic jaundice' and records that both babies succumbed.

A very interesting case to which he was called by the midwife was that of Mrs L. who delivered of her first baby on 2 March 1762. In attempting to deliver the placenta the cord snapped and so the midwife sent immediately for Dr Perfect. He found it impossible to perform a manual separation and removal and so left the placenta *in situ*. It was expelled spontaneously on the third post-partum day. His history of this mother is also very interesting: it shows that retention of the placenta occurred in her five subsequent deliveries and that the placenta delivered between the second and fourth day in every case.

Clearly, in rural England, the traditional delivery by the village midwife and the modesty that allowed only female attendants at births could only be set aside in exceptional circumstances. The following extract, signed by Churchwardens, is taken from the Parish Register of the village of Evercreech, Somerset, and dated 6 May 1759.

> Whereas Jane the wife of Robert Crocker is in a very weak condition and near her time of delivery and her case in that respect being thought very dangerous, therefore we the undersigned whose names are hereto subscribed hereby consent and agree that a man-midwife shall be allowed for attending but at the time only of such labour and delivery.
>
> Witness our hands at a vestry held the day and year above.

Five signatures follow. The calling in of a man-midwife would increase the cost of the delivery considerably. The village midwife, in this case Fanny Rolls, charged 2s 6d (12 pence) for her attendance at the birth. The doctor probably charged one guinea (£1.05).[29]

The distrust between doctors and midwives is mirrored in the fictional case of the birth of Tristram Shandy, which took place on 5 November 1718 at a time when men-midwives were becoming fashionable. The village midwife concerned was a 'thin, upright, motherly, notable, good, old body'. She became the village midwife in her forty-seventh year after being widowed. The local parson and his wife, seeing both the need for a midwife and her potential, saw to it that she was 'a little instructed in some of the plain principles of the business' and thereafter obtained and paid 18s 4d for her licence to practice. She was obviously a person with common sense who let nature take its course rather than interfere. Tristram's father wanted a man-midwife 'by all means' but his mother 'by no means'. So, when labour started, his mother sent immediately for the midwife but his father ordered the servant to saddle a horse and go for Doctor Slop, whom he regarded as an expert operator. The midwife was with the mother during the labour but the doctor stayed chatting in the parlour downstairs and felt it an affront to his dignity when the midwife wished him to come to the birth room to discuss progress. He therefore requested that she came down to him.

Slop questioned the midwife as to the presentation, which she was confident was a head. He tried to shake her confidence and stressed the awful consequences should he apply his forceps to the breech. He said it was difficult to be certain of the presentation but was relying on the midwife's findings. It was obvious that the doctor was not interested in either the alleviation of pain or in the management of labour, his sole object being to extract the child by the use of his forceps. In so doing he crushed the baby's nose so severely that it required a reconstruction of the bridge. Throughout, the doctor asserted his superiority over the midwife and belittled her in front of the Shandy family.[30]

Other references are made in literature to midwives in the late seventeenth and eighteenth century. In Wycherley's Restoration Comedy *Country Wife* (1675), there are passing mentions of her which are of a derogatory nature: 'A quack is as fit for a pimp as a midwife for a bawd'; the same character in the play asks, 'But have you told all the midwives you know, the orange wenches at the playhouses, the city-husbands, and the old fumbling keepers of this end of the town? *for they'll be the readiest to report it* [our italics]'. Unfortunately midwives were seen as gossipy women of low moral character. The Restoration Comedies were noted for their portrayal of the whole political and social scene and there was undoubtedly more than a grain of truth in these fictional references.

Daniel Defoe's *Moll Flanders*, written in 1722, also gives a vivid picture of the social scene and the place of some midwives in it. Moll, a woman of loose morals, needed a midwife on two occasions and she describes how she, as a 'kept' woman, was delivered and cared for at the expense of her 'protector'. It would appear that certain midwives specialised in this sort of practice, from which they obviously made quite a good living because they were able to charge high fees for the confidential nature of their cases. Indeed they exploited the situation. When Moll was in London, she lived in the midwife's house for nearly four months. The house was 'handsome', comfortable and clean, and such houses were unusual in the London of that time. The fee charged by the midwife for her professional services varied; she apparently had three different scales of charges depending on the prosperity of the 'father'. The lowest total paid out for Moll was as follows:

	£	s	d
1. For three months' lodging in her house, including my diet at 10s a week	6	0	0
2. For a nurse for the month, and use of child-bed linen	1	10	0
3. For a minister to christen the child, and to the godfathers and clerk	1	10	0
4. For a supper at the christening if I had five friends at it	1	0	0
5. For her fees as a midwife, and the taking of the trouble off the parish	3	.3	0
6. To her maidservant attending	0	10	0
	13	13	0

The other charges for the same but rather more luxurious services were:

	£	s	d
1. For three months' lodging and diet etc. at 20s per week	13	0	0
2. For a nurse for the month, and the use of linen and lace	2	10	0
3. For the minister to christen the child etc.	2	0	0
4. For a supper and for sweetmeats	3	3	0
5. For her fees as above	5	5	0
6. For a servant-maid	1	0	0
	26	18	0

The highest account of expenses charged by the midwife was as follows:

	£	s	d
1. For three months' lodging and diet, having two rooms and a garret for a servant	30	0	0
2. For the nurse for the month, and the finest suit of child-bed linen	4	4	0
3. For the minister to christen the child etc.	2	10	0
4. For a supper, the gentleman to send in the wine	6	0	0
5. Midwife's fees etc.	10	10	0
6. The maid, besides their own maid, only	0	10	0
	53	14	0

Moll says that during her stay the midwife delivered 'twelve ladies of pleasure' in her house and in addition professionally attended another 32 or thereabouts in similar accommodation. The midwife's income from her practice would therefore be £600 to £1000. This itself would make her a wealthy woman, but this particular midwife had other shady sources of income which included the procuring of abortions and the disposal of unwanted babies of these ladies of pleasure. (It was over a hundred years before the first Infant Life Protection Act was passed in an effort to prevent such practices.) Despite this unscrupulous conduct, Moll speaks fondly of her as a skilled and kindly midwife.

This midwife could be said to be typical of many midwives practising in large towns, who appear to have been experienced and professionally competent and certainly literate and numerate. Of course not all such midwives would provide services for mistresses and prostitutes, but some would see this as fulfilling a social need. The lucrative nature of this insalubrious work would overcome any twinges of conscience the midwife may have had, and would even reconcile her to being called 'Mother Midnight', a title which implied moral opprobrium.

Notable Midwife and Doctor Practitioners and their Writings

Sarah Stone started practising midwifery early in the eighteenth century and became a reputable midwife. Her mother, a Mrs Holmes, was a famous practitioner in her own day, and earned the respect of at least one doctor, who is quoted as saying that she was the 'best midwife that ever he knew'.[31] Sarah Stone was fortunate to have received education and to have seen dissection of female bodies as well as to have had access to books on anatomy; but she gave the credit for her practical skills to her mother to whom she was 'apprenticed' for six years. She appears to have acted in the capacity of a consultant midwife, being called out by other less able midwives to deal with difficulties that were beyond their clinical competence. This was especially so when she practised in the West Country, where men-midwives were in very short supply. Because she was obviously well taught and exceptionally skilful clinically, she was opposed to men-midwives and their indiscriminate use of forceps. 'I cannot comprehend', she says, 'why women are not capable of completing this business when begun, without calling in men to their assistance, who are often sent for when the work is near finished; and then the midwife who has taken all the pains, is counted of little value, and the young men command all the praise . . . I am certain that where twenty women are delivered with instruments (which is now become a common practice), that nineteen of them might be delivered without, if not the twentieth, as will appear in my observations.'[32]

Sarah Stone describes many of her experiences, some of which were harrowing, and the fact that she was able to cope with them speaks highly of her ability and nerve. She declared that she never needed to use instruments above four times in her life, although her case load in Taunton was over 300 a year, but she did occasionally have to perform craniotomy. When called by other midwives she had to travel considerable distances on horseback to outlying villages and she describes arriving on some occasions drenched and exhausted.

Sarah Stone's constitution appears not to have been very strong and the repeated loss of sleep and constant demands for her assistance took their toll. She describes one exacting experience:

> I was sent for to a comber's wife in St. James's Parish, about 8 o'clock at night, but being very ill of the cholick, could not go. About 5 o'clock in the morning, they sent again and told me the woman would die if I did not go to her assistance, for neither of her midwives could deliver her. This obliged me to rise and go with them, although I was so ill as to be forced to hold the woman's husband and another. When I got there I found the child's arm out of the birth. I immediately searched for the feet which I soon found, and in a little time completed the delivery. I was led home and in my bed before the clock struck six.

This particular case finally determined her to leave Taunton and practise in the city of Bristol, where the demands on her physical stamina would be less. She eventually moved again and set up practice in Piccadilly, London, where she published *A Complete Practice of Midwifery*, which contains over forty of her presumably most memorable cases. Though she recognised the need for some theoretical teaching for midwives, Sarah Stone felt that her clinical experience under the guidance of an expert midwife had been of most value to her. She felt that before practising the 'art where life depends', every midwife should be instructed for at least three years.[33]

One of the best textbooks for use by midwives was *The Art of Midwifery Improv'd Fully and Plainly Laying down whatever Instructions are Requisite to Make a Compleat Midwife*.[34] This was originally written in Dutch by an obstetrician, **Henry van Deventer**, and 'made English' for the benefit of English midwives. The book opens, as its predecessors, with a chapter on 'Qualifications which are requir'd to make a woman fit for the practice of midwifery'. Van Deventer deemed it necessary for midwives to be professionally instructed in their 'important art', being convinced that 'Theory ought to go before practice as the body before the shadow'. He considered it a wonder that 'Magistrates are not more solicitous to erect fit schools for the instruction of young midwives in every city . . . so that by this means . . . a great number of women, as well as infants, might be saved who are lost for want of reasonable help'. He admitted, however, that 'A prudent midwife, who understands her business and presently knows what to do in the beginning of a difficult birth and performs her work faithfully, as her duty requires, and her love to her neighbour commands, cannot be too well rewarded for her pains.' Van Deventer wanted the midwives to realise the importance of sending for medical help to prevent a catastrophe in circumstances such as deformed pelves, abnormal lie, and presentation or position of the fetus, especially if she had not learned how to deal with these herself. He fully recognised the onerous and often life-saving responsibility carried by the midwife, and was insistent that successful delivery was not chance or fortune but 'an art which depends on as firm a foundation as a great many others'. He was anxious that the midwife should be sufficiently knowledgeable to recognise signs of deviation from the normal to 'prevent, correct or remove them'. Van Deventer's list of those he considered *unfit* for midwifery include

All women who are very much in years . . .
Young women, such as virgins and new married women
Infirm, diseased or consumptive persons
Women that are too fat or gross
Those who are maimed
Those who have crooked fingers and whose hands and arms are crooked and stiff
Those who are of a stupid and dull sense and incapable of perceiving things distinctly
Those who are not handy
Those who are slothful

It was Van Deventer's contention that

those who would be midwives ought to know how to write and read, they ought to have good books and to read them over and over that they may daily improve their theory and readiness in order to practice, giving a good attention to everything they hear, read and experience in these matters. She should be grave, temperate, sober, considerate, tenderhearted and have presence of mind.

He perceived midwifery as a womanly art and conceded that 'men may undervalue this Office'. He continued:

Nothing can be more useful to Mankind, or more necessary, which a skilful woman can apply her mind to. I doubt not if woman with child, and their husbands know what difference there is betwixt a prudent and imprudent, a skilful and unskilful midwife (and how one, by her assistance, may contribute to the health as well as the saving of the life both of the mother and infant, and how the other may be prejudicial through neglect, nay, by occasioning the death of both) but they would be more cautious and not so easily put their confidence in such.

The chapters of van Deventer's book cover: anatomy of the reproductive organs; internal 'touching' and internal manoeuvres; birth of the baby; delivery of the afterbirth; the qualities of a surgeon who practises midwifery. He describes in detail the secundine, womb-cake or placenta, with its navel-string and its membrane containing the infant and humours (waters). He also mentions the external 'secret parts' of a woman (the privitus or privies) but 'for modesty's sake' does not provide an illustration, believing that such figures 'rather serve to excite impure thoughts and give occasion to obscene discourse'. He instructs on the handling and touching of women and advises that before such internal examinations the fingers should be anointed with fat, butter or oil. He gives a list of indications for internal examination and urges midwives to undertake this procedure in order to foresee danger and so call help. He taught how such examination would reveal true from false pains; how infants are 'seated'; and about progress and prognosis of the labour.

Van Deventer advocated that, during the labour, mothers should 'walk or stand, being held up by somebody til the infant is brought forward for birth'. He advised the chair for delivery — 'that they may rather sit than lye'. He actually listed a birthchair among 'Midwife's utensils'; and described equipment for giving a clyster (enema) as being a bladder fixed to a box or an ivory pipe or a pewter siphon. Herbs or household commodities were used for evacuant or stimulant enemata, for which the midwife was told to prepare, boil and sieve the following ingredients:

Wheat bran — one handful. Boil alone or with flowers of camomile — one handful in a pint and a half of rainwater to one pint of water. Strain them through a linen cloth or sieve. Add 2 spoons of sugar, honey or black syrup and a pinch of salt.

or

Pint of new milk. Let it just boil, then taking it from the fire add 2 spoonsful of coarse sugar, syrup or honey and a pinch of common salt. Mix it well and strain it and it will be fit for use. Add, if you will, some spoonsful of oil of turnips or olives.

If the clyster is not just to purge but to excite pain, prepare with tops of wormwood, the smallest leaves of savin cut small, flowers of motherwort and camomile — of each one handful, seeds of levisticum, fennel, aniseeds — half spoonful. Boil in a pint and a half of rainwater til a 1/3rd part be wasted. Strain and add 1 or 2 spoons of honey or sugar with a little salt.

He describes in detail how to give the enema, how to care for the mother and how to dispose of soiled linen.

Van Deventer gives a detailed description of the intricate design of a birth chair made to his specifications, which, he claimed, would facilitate birth (Figure 15). This wooden chair had a hinged back, to allow the mother to be in a sitting *or* lying position, and hinged side doors. The seat was cut away to allow for support of her thighs. This chair could be dismantled for transportation, 'put into a sack, and easily be carried by any man . . . and it is a thing to be wished for, that every midwife were furnished with such a chair'.

He defines a natural birth as one 'performed by the force of nature without art or other help', and that in such a birth 'a midwife performs her duty if she receives the infant, cuts off the navel-string, takes care of the infant by washing and nourishing it'. He describes difficult or preternatural births, stating that a difficult birth 'owes its origin, either to the mother, or the infant, or the midwife'. From the mother's point of view the contributory factors included structural abnormalities of the pelvis and womb, and also convulsions, fluxes, epilepsy and fainting fits, for which conditions he instructs the midwives to call the physician to prescribe medicine and give advice.

He writes in some detail about the delivery of the placenta and membranes.

Figure 15: Van Deventer's Birth Chair

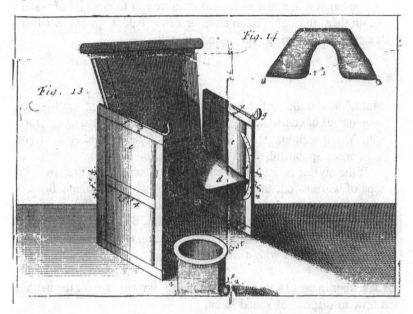

Source: *The Art of Midwifery Improv'd*, H. van Deventer, 1746.
(Photographed from original by the Department of Medical Illustrations,
University Hospital of South Manchester.)

The umbilical cord should be tied with thick linen cloth and the after-birth should be drawn out without delay; to which end the navel-string is to be held in one hand, being turned two or three times about the fingers and the other is to be passed by it into the womb, which yet is open enough, to draw out the after-birth.

He states that this is his preferred and recommended method as against other contentious methods such as 'the woman blowing into her fist, or bathing her belly with warm wine or placing a piece of candle into her throat to make her vomit'.

Van Deventer advised that 'if the child faints at birth the midwife must rub the soles of its feet with a hair-cloth, putting a bruised onion to its nostrils, sprinkling wine upon its face, nostrils, ears and eyes and whatever else is customary to do'.

The last chapter deals with the birth of 'monsters', which he reckon-ed was surgeon's work, but he recognised that the midwife would have to perform this work in the country areas where a skilful surgeon would not be available.

In his 'recapitulation', van Deventer emphasised that it was his earnest desire that those who practised midwifery might exercise their art according to solid foundations of true knowledge.

First, that a midwife, the state of things being known to the woman in labour, or those who are near her, may administer Help with the greatest tranquillity of mind, leaving off when 'tis proper, or working when her work is requisite.

Second, the relations may with the greatest satisfaction, expect and wait whilst the midwife treats the woman in labour, doing whatever is necessary to be done.

He perceived that:

Nothing can be more grievous to a midwife than to be instructed and murmured at, and suspected so that if the labour succeeds prosperously it is chiefly ascribed to Fortune, but if it hath an event contrary to expectation she that works is blamed, though she not only took all the pains she could, but managed with care and prudence. But what I do advise — it is better that a midwife should be exposed in her reputation, than the mother and infant should be exposed to the Danger of their Lives or perish through her ignorance.

Margaret Stephen, another educated midwife, held similar views to Sarah Stone on the potential ability of women midwives. She was the mother of nine children and practised for thirty years in London in the late eighteenth century, becoming a midwife of such repute that she was engaged to attend Queen Charlotte in some of her confinements. In 1795 Margaret Stephen wrote *Domestic Midwife or The Best Means of Preventing Danger in Childbirth Considered*. This book was deemed by Aveling to be 'perhaps the best upon the subject that has been written by any women in our own language'.[35] Her preface indicated her belief that midwifery should primarily be 'woman's work' and that the vast majority of pregnancies would have a successful natural outcome. She therefore deplored the fact that an increasing number of men were regarding childbirth as an unnatural event which required their instrumental assistance.

Her book describes the onset, establishment and course of natural labour. She explains very clearly the technique of vaginal examination and how to recognise the position of the head by identifying sutures and fontanelles. She recognised that pulling on the cord could cause inversion of the uterus, and so she advised the rubbing up of a contraction to assist separation of the placenta and membranes. She describes beautifully the technique of jaw flexion and shoulder traction for delivery of the aftercoming head in a breech presentation, but advocated *sending for a doctor* in the case of obstructed labour because 'should any misfortune happen, which perhaps is unavoidable, people are more readily reconciled to the event, because there is no appeal from what a doctor does, being granted he did all he could on the occasion'.[36]

In her text Mrs Stephen mentions signs and symptoms of pregnancy and also minor disorders, and relates how 'some women love to be delivered in their cloathes'. She remarks that some women were so keen to preserve their figures that they were tightly bound with broad bandages after delivery. It was common practice for mothers to 'lie in' for three days, and she mentions familiar discomforts of the puerperium such as the problems of 'fixing' the baby to the breast, engorgement, afterpains and the more serious problem of puerperal fever.

Margaret Stephen had been taught by a male pupil of Doctor Smellie, and she herself taught the theory and practice of midwifery to females. She used models and mechanical aids to help in the understanding of anatomy and physiology of labour. She recognised the value of the *discriminate* use of forceps in the saving of babies' lives, declaring 'There is none of all the instruments I ever saw so well calculated to save the lives of children.' Indeed, she taught midwives how to apply forceps and how to use other obstetric instruments. She obviously felt that when forceps were necessary it was the midwife who should use them, and was of the opinion that 'so general a use of men in the business of a midwife has introduced a far greater number of deaths amongst society than it has prevented'.

Margaret Stephen gave a reasoned perceptive exposition of the case against indiscriminate employment of men-midwives. She perceived 'the insinuations of designing men who taught mothers to believe they endangered their own lives, and that of their children, by employing women'. She was astute in her recognition of the fact that many men were out to discredit female midwives by using scare tactics in order to 'take over' their role. She claimed that some men-midwives cast aspersions on the character of female midwives, and that others, by 'oblique insinuations', were out to poison the professional reputation of all midwives. Many men who taught midwives, she maintained, deliberately withheld knowledge in order to establish their own superiority. She acknowledged the superior knowledge and skill of the doctor-physicians, but questioned both the motives and capabilities of some men-midwives, especially those who were young and inexperienced (often chosen because their fees were smaller), who were over-anxious to use instruments. Evidently, men were realising that instrumental midwifery could be quite lucrative, and many commenced practice. Mrs Stephen emphasises the point that because it was only necessary to call a man-midwife when difficulties arose, it should be an *experienced* man of known integrity, and that it was a mistake to assume that any man-midwife would do. It is unclear whether there were any 'training' requirements prior to a man setting himself up as a man-midwife, but men were more likely than the vast majority of women to have been educated and therefore able to learn the theory through formal classes or from textbooks. Nevertheless the paradox that had existed from the seventeenth century continued, whereby midwives with ability (but less theoretical knowledge), and even less prestige, were encouraged to consult men who were without practical experience, and sometimes little relevant theoretical knowledge, but greater prestige by virtue of their profession and gender. Margaret Stephen herself had been admirably instructed, and regarded herself as qualified. She therefore claimed that midwives should be taught, and their knowledge and still examined, and that those not thus trained should be regarded as unqualified midwives. She expressed the wish that women of good education and respectable connections would turn their attention to the science of midwifery.

Martha Mears was a London midwife with a different viewpoint. She practised in the period when the 'battle' between men-midwife instrumentarians and the traditional female midwife was waning. She highly praised the contribution of some of the men-midwives and accepted that the doctor-midwife had a place in certain cases. She was a well-read midwife who herself published a book in 1797 called *The Pupil of Nature*. She urged midwives to extend their knowledge by reading books written by the best practitioners. 'Day and night read them', she wrote, 'read them day and night'.[37]

In 1784 an informative book was written by **David Spence**, an obstetrician and gynaecologist. It was entitled *A System of Midwifery Theoretical and Practical*, and the copy in the Radford Collection, Manchester,[38] bears a handwritten inscription 'To Mr Charles White, Surgeon at Manchester'.

The first section of Spence's book contains chapters on anatomy, conception, nutrition of the fetus *in utero*, fetal development, diseases peculiar to pregnant women, management of women during pregnancy and labouring, lingering labour, laborious births, use of forceps, scissors and crochet, flooding, cases complicated with convulsions, twins, and Caesarian section. Inclusion of both 'diseases' and 'management of pregnancy' shows that Spence's interest was in the whole process of pregnancy and childbirth.

The second section is entitled 'The management of women after delivery', and was written as a guide to those who had the care of women in the puerperium. The midwife may well have made some post-partum visits, but the delivered mother would chiefly have been cared for by the 'monthly nurse' or neighbours. The attendants were advised to keep the woman, during her 'short respite', as free as possible from 'everything which might ruffle her mind'. The necessity for clean linen and 'frequent changes of cloths' was mentioned. The genitalia were to be bathed in milk and water, which was also prescribed for lacerated perineums. After-pains were treated with opiates and fomentations, and engorged breasts with bread and milk poultices. The signs and symptoms of the clinical entity which became called puerperal sepsis were described vividly. Despite the mention of 'green and black putrid lochia', there is no mention of any therapy being prescribed. The aetiology was unclear, as the earlier suggestions that it was due either to obstruction of the lochia, or suppression of milk, had been superseded by the idea that it was an inflammatory condition of the omentum and intestines.

The management of newborn babies is also described. They were to be bathed soon after birth, a binder was to be applied, and the baby was to be dressed in slack garments rather than being swaddled. The treatment for severe birth asphyxia was mouth-to-mouth resuscitation or rubbing the baby's body with spirits before a fire, or plunging the baby into a warm bath. He mentions cases of imperforate anus, hypospadias, spina bifida, hare lip, jaundice, thrush, mastitis and colic. It appears that neonatal convulsions were commonplace. Breast feeding was advocated but two possible alternatives for use when it was not possible were described. One was the use of a wet-nurse, whose qualifications were to be cheerfulness, freedom from venereal disease and a good milk yield. The other was hand feeding by the use of a spoon, horn or boat with an artificial nipple. This 'feed' would probably have been of pap or of barley water.

In the final part of his book, Dr Spence recounts 51 obstetric and gynaecological cases to which he was called. It is not always clear from the text who exactly it was who sought his assistance, but he records that in 20 of the instances it was the midwife who sent for his help. The wide range of emergencies to which she called him included self-induced abortion with post-partum haemorrhage, inversion of the uterus with haemorrhage, and two cases of obstructed labour where delivery was achieved with the patient kneeling. Spence mentions that one of the babies thus delivered had excessive head moulding. The midwife also called him for two cases of cephalo-pelvic disproportion, the outcome of which was craniotomy which was performed with scissors; to a compound presentation, and to two breech presentations, both of which had been diagnosed by the midwife early in labour. She called for his assistance for a prolapsed cord and arm, which were successfully reduced and a normal delivery followed. Another case of arm presentation was less easily managed because the mother had drunk a bottle of spirits and was evidently very uncooperative. Although in this case the baby was stillborn, Dr Spence records that the mother was ambulant on the third day. A hand in the vagina occasioned another call to Dr Spence, who attempted an internal version but he was prevented from completing this procedure by the patient's husband who forcibly pulled him from the bedside. During a second attempt following cord prolapse, the husband brandished a weapon whereupon Dr Spence records that he left the scene concluding that the husband was either 'mad or drunk'. He states that the midwife remained with the patient and that he himself returned following an apology by the husband, but that it was then too late to save the baby's life.

Other cases for which his help was required included ante-partum haemorrhage, uterine inertia and triplets. Two cases of eclampsia prompted the midwife to send for Dr Spence, and in one of the cases the patient had ten intra-partum fits before being delivered of a stillborn baby. He records that the mother had bitten her tongue half through and that she remained comatose for 24 hours after the eclamptic fit. Nevertheless she was up on the 12th post-partum day. It is interesting that the doctor prescribed the internal use of opiates in this case. He pays tribute to at least one of the midwives by recognising her knowledge and attention. After describing one case of breech presentation with cord prolapse and compression complicated by post-partum haemorrhage which necessitated manual separation and removal of the placenta, his final entry reads 'she rose on the third day'!

Wherever Dr Spence's practice was, it is clear that there was mutual respect between him and the midwives, which allowed both to fulfil their complementary roles. Unfortunately this was not the case everywhere, despite the plea from doctors that they should be consulted when complications arose.

Hospital Care for Poor Parturient Women

During the eighteenth century at least nine hospitals became involved to a greater or lesser extent in the care of poor parturient women. This involvement varied from out-patient dispensary facilities and out-patient advice, to the provision by Charitable Institutions of midwives for the delivery and care of patients in their own homes. These midwives could call upon doctors from the same Institution to assist them in difficulties arising in the labour. In some cases the care involved admission to hospital of certain women with social, medical and obstetric problems. This practice applied to Liverpool Maternity Hospital and to St. Mary's Hospital, Manchester, where it continued until 1969.

One of the original motives in the founding of these Charitable Institutions was the relief of the extreme social distress experienced by many who had drifted into towns consequent upon the Industrial Revolution. Another motive appears to have been that such Foundations would provide for the training of women and men in midwifery. However, midwifery did not become a compulsory subject for medical students until 1886 in England, and in Scotland until 1833. In general the Institutions excluded unmarried mothers but one or two were set up in London specifically to cater for the needs of this not inconsiderable group of women.

The first lying-in infirmary was started in 1739 in London by Sir Richard Manningham. According to Spencer,[39] the physician and man-midwife Brudenell Exton introduced female pupils into the hospital to study midwifery practice and skills some time before June 1760. At this time the hospital could receive 25 lying-in women. Male pupils were also admitted for instruction. The hospital became called the Bayeswater Lying-in Hospital in 1791, and then, in 1800 (after Queen Charlotte became its patron), the Queen Charlotte's Lying-in Hospital and ultimately, by Royal Charter in 1924, The Queen Charlotte's Maternity Hospital.[40] The Rotunda Hospital, Dublin, was founded in 1745. This was known first as the Dublin Hospital for Poor Lying-in Women. Originally it had ten beds for delivery and lying-in purposes. In 1747 the Middlesex Hospital reserved five beds for lying-in women but fifty years later the maternity section of this hospital disappeared and was not restored until early in this century. Two years later a hospital, later known as the British Lying-in Hospital, admitted women for delivery under the supervision of men-midwives. It served as a training institution for a small number of female pupils who undertook a midwifery course of four months' duration. In 1750 the City of London Lying-in

Hospital was founded, and in 1756, and the year in which the General Lying-in Hospital, London, was founded, Edinburgh Royal Infirmary opened four maternity beds. These had been expanded to eight beds by 1793. However, these beds were closed because the Edinburgh General Lying-in Hospital opened, which provided more facilities and accommodation for maternity cases. In 1938 this hospital again joined up with the Edinburgh Royal Infirmary and became known as the Simpson Memorial Maternity Pavilion.

Charitable Institutions were being set up elsewhere in England. Towards the end of the century, a doctor, George Stebbing, practising in Ipswich, was very concerned about the lack of help available to poor women in labour. He sent his daughter to London to 'train' as a midwife and on her return he managed to persuade the ladies of Ipswich to establish a Lying-in Charity. Every subscriber was entitled to give a card to a poor pregnant woman, which enabled her to call upon the services of a midwife and a surgeon during her delivery and also allowed her the use of a set of baby linen. His daughter continued as a midwife for over fifty years and her services were in great demand, especially for the wives of doctors.[41]

On 5 May 1790 a Lying-in Charity was set up in Manchester for the delivery of poor women in their own habitations and for the building of a lying-in hospital as soon as the necessary funds had been raised. Rules of this Lying-in Charity were drawn up at its inception. One of its primary aims was the training of midwives. Rule XXI states:

> That lectures or instructions be given at the expense of this Charity to the *practising midwives* belonging to the Institution, and to *female* pupils, in order to qualify them in future to be eligible to that office, by one of the men-midwives to this Charity, to be appointed by the Quarterly Board [our italics].

The appointee was in fact the famous Dr Charles White, who delivered his lectures to the midwives without charge to the Charity. This training for pupil midwives was given 112 years before training became compulsory. Indeed in the next century a claim was made in the Annual Report that St. Mary's Hospitals (as it became called) was the first hospital, as far as is known, to make provision for the proper instruction of female midwives. In the first year (1790), ten midwives and six female pupils at this 'School and Nursery for Young Midwives' completed the course of instruction, were granted certificates and had their names published in the Manchester newspapers. The purpose of establishing a School for Midwives was not only to guarantee skilled and knowledgeable midwives for the Institution itself but 'in order that the Town and Country may be supplied with such as have knowledge and experience'.[42]

A Matron, a Secretary, and an Apothecary were appointed to work alongside men-midwives in-ordinary and men-midwives extra-ordinary (Consultant grade). The Weekly Board had power to suspend the Apothecary, the Secretary, the Matron and the Midwives for mis-behaviour. 'Misbehaviour' included the taking of any fee, gratuity or reward from a patient. The Matron could be married but was required *not* to have children. Very little can be gleaned from the Records as to her actual duties and responsibilities except that she kept a register of wet-nurses and of approved monthly nurses and seemed to be in charge of the housekeeping expenses.

Only certain parturient women were eligible for the services of this Charity (that is, those who were married and very poor), and though most of these were delivered by midwives in their own homes, some of them were admitted as emergency cases to the Lying-in Charity Hospital then at Salford Bridge for delivery. One of the Rules stated that the midwives were immediately to call in one of the man-midwives in-ordinary in all cases of danger and difficulty. It would appear that this system did not give rise to any of the competition or animosity bet-ween midwives and men-midwives that had been so very evident in Lon-don. There is no suggestion in the text of the Rules that the midwives already in practice before the setting up of the Institution were ignorant or incompetent.

Liverpool Maternity Hospital first came into being in 1796 with the foundation of the Ladies Charity, the objective of which was to afford medical and other assistance in childbirth 'to reputable married women or widows resident in this town' in their own homes. After 73 years of existence the Ladies Charity amalgamated with another Liverpool Charity, the Lying-in Hospital (which had opened in 1841), to become the Ladies Charity and Lying-in Hospital and later the Liverpool Mater-nity Hospital and Ladies Charity. Midwives are recorded as being in training from 1842.[43]

In Scotland the first Chair of Midwifery was established in Edinburgh in 1726 under Professor Joseph Gibson, and Diplomas were issued to midwives. In 1739 the Faculty of Physicians and Surgeons of Glasgow required midwives to pass an examination and have a licence before be-ing admitted to practice.[44] Below is the wording of a Certificate issued by Dr Thomas Young MD, the third Professor of Midwifery in the

University of Edinburgh.

These are to certifie

That Margaret Reid, Midwife attended 3 courses of my Lectures upon the Theory and Practice of Midwifery, as also the Lying-in Ward in the Royal Infirmary for the space of [blank] months by which means she had the opportunity of operating in all the different sorts of births. Edinburgh, 11th day of June 1768.[45]

It is known that from 1759 James Muir, a Glasgow surgeon, gave courses of lectures to local midwives, and that in the same year a Dr Skene started a similar course in Aberdeen at the insistence of the town's Kirk Session.

It would appear that Scottish Midwives had a definite social status, because as early as 1710 a pew in a new Glasgow church was especially designated for the city's midwives. Moreover, in 1759, *The Scots Magazine*, a publication subscribed to by the upper classes, recorded the death of a 'Mrs. Knox, widow, an eminent midwife'.[46]

He-midwife or She-midwife?

Although female midwives did not win the battle against the male intruders in the eighteenth century, they at least survived. Men-midwives competed against them with some degree of success in the upper classes but the lower classes regarded them with suspicion, finding it difficult to come to terms with the presence of a man during childbirth, and in any case finding their fees prohibitive.

The term man-midwife, which had been in use since 1625, only indicated the sex of the practitioner. He could have been an apothecary, a surgeon, a physician, or a layman choosing to take up the practice of midwifery. The gifted *professionals* of this group, and in particular William Smellie, clearly saw the need for instruction in theory and practice for male and female alike. Because of his academic interest in pregnancy and his keenness to gain clinical experience, Smellie did not discriminate between rich and poor in his clientele. Many of the other male practitioners, however, were now earning their living from this specialty and therefore they were not motivated towards attending the poor.

Men were attracted to using forceps which were becoming generally available, and their improved design made their use even more effective.

Parturient women were also attracted to the idea of forceps being used to shorten their labours and so, because only men were allowed to use these instruments, this new fashion worked against the female midwife and in favour of the male. Mothers were undoubtedly helped if forceps were skilfully used, and yet at the same time were threatened by their indiscriminate application, especially in the hands of inept practitioners. The antagonism of the female midwives was originally against both men-midwives and forceps *per se* but eventually the more discerning midwives recognised that *doctors* and their forceps had a part to play in complicated cases. Others, however, felt strongly that they themselves should be taught and allowed to use forceps. Some midwives, perhaps because of pride and prejudice, remained antagonistic to change and could not, under any circumstances, accept men in midwifery. Ironically, there would, however, be some rural midwives who were unaware that men had entered their business at all.

A number of eighteenth-century midwives were educated, but most were not. Some town and city women were in fact being trained as midwives in the emerging maternity hospitals, and certainly the involvement of doctors, which took away their monopoly, emphasised to these midwives the need for such training for *all* midwives. Unfortunately, only relatively small numbers of female midwives were 'trained' in England whereas in Scotland a thousand such midwives were trained between 1780 and 1818.[47]

Although Episcopal Licenses were still being granted to midwives throughout the eighteenth century in some dioceses, the possession of a Bishop's Licence was of less value now that the belief in the practice of witchcraft had waned. It seems that such licensing, where it occurred, had become a mere formality, and although it might demonstrate that the midwife was 'in love and charity with her neighbours', it certainly did not guarantee clinical competence. It would appear that doctors attached no importance to a licence granted to a midwife by a non-medical, episcopal body, having as a profession freed themselves from the same requirement. In fact by the late eighteenth century the three traditional professions of medicine, surgery and pharmacy had, particularly in London, established legislation whereby they could examine all men who wished to practice, thus theoretically eliminating those not able to prove themselves fit to have in their charge the lives of men, women and children. George Counsell thought that similar legislation should also apply to those practising midwifery, and he claimed that if the Royal College of Physicians were to appoint in London and elsewhere one or more of their members who were skilled in midwifery, then men and women wishing to practice in that subject should be both examined and licensed.[27] There was also serious discussion concerning the doctor-obstetricians as to whether they properly belonged to the body of physicians (who treated diseases of women) or to the body of surgeons (for operative delivery).

By the end of the century there was general agreement that midwives should receive sound theoretical and practical instruction and be examined in their knowledge before receiving a legal licence to practise. Although the proposals for 'training' made by some doctors and midwives were implemented by some institutions, what was lacking was national and official enforcement of these schemes.

References

1. Cole, G.D.H. and Postgate, R. *The Common People, 1746–1946* (Methuen, London, 1946).
2. Carter, E.H. and Mears, R.A.F. *A History of Britain, Section IV* (Clarendon Press, Oxford, 1948).
3. Porter, R.S. *English Society in the 18th Century* (Penguin, London, 1982, p. 164).
4. Porter, R.S. *English Society in the 18th Century* (Penguin, London, 1982, p. 16).
5. Porter, R.S. *English Society in the 18th Century* (Penguin, London, 1982, p. 224).
6. Porter, R.S. *English Society in the 18th Century* (Penguin, London, 1982, p. 27).
7. Porter, R.S. *English Society in the 18th Century* (quoting Daniel Defoe) (Penguin, London, 1982, pp. 67–8).
8. Dewhurst, J. *Royal Confinements* (Weidenfeld and Nicolson, London, 1980).
9. Woodforde, J. *The Diary of a Country Parson, 1758–1802* (Oxford University Press, Oxford, 1935).
10. Porter, R.S. *English Society in the 18th Century* (Penguin, London, 1982, pp. 27, 41).
11. Appleyard, S. 'The Family World of the Wesleys', *This England*, Winter 1984.
12. Radcliffe, W. *The Secret Instrument* (Heinemann, London, 1947).
13. Burnby, J.G.C. *A Study of the English Apothecary from 1660 to 1760. Medical History Supplement No. 3* (Wellcome Institute for the History of Medicine, London, 1983).
14. Johnstone, R.W. *William Smellie. Master of British Midwifery* (E. & S. Livingstone, Edinburgh, 1952).
15. Smellie, W. *A Treatise on the Theory and Practice of Midwifery* (London, 1752).
16. Graham, H. *Eternal Eve* (Hutchinson, London, 1960, p. 171).
17. Graham, H. *Eternal Eve* (Hutchinson, London, 1960, p. 175).
18. Nihell, E. *A Treatise on the Art of Midwifery. Professed Midwife: A Man-midwife or a Midwife* (London, 1760).
19. Aveling, J.H. 'On the Instruction, Examination and Registration of Midwives', *British Medical Journal, i*, 1873.
20. Clarke, G. *A History of the Royal College of Physicians of London*, Vol. II (Clarendon Press, Oxford, 1966).
21. Aveling, J.H. *English Midwives. Their History and Prospects* (Hugh K. Elliott, London, 1967, p. 115).
22. Graham, H. *Eternal Eve* (Hutchinson, London, 1960, p. 170).
23. Maubray, J. *The Female Physician* (London, 1724).
24. Aveling, J.H. *English Midwives. Their History and Prospects* (Hugh K. Elliott,

London, 1967, pp. 140–1).
25. Bracken, H. *The Midwife's Companion* (London, 1737).
26. Dawkes, T. *The Midwife Rightly Instructed* (London, 1736).
27. Counsell, G. *The Art of Midwifery or The Midwife's Sure Guide wherein the most Successful Methods of Practice Are Laid Down in the Plainest, Clearest and Shortest Manner* (London, 1752).
28. Perfect, W. *Cases in Midwifery* (T. Fisher, Rochester, 1737–1789).
29. Lindsay, G. 'Centuries of Controversy', *Nursing Mirror*, 20 July 1978.
30. Sterne, L. *Tristram Shandy*, Book I, Chapter 7 (1760).
31. Aveling, J.H. *English Midwives. Their History and Prospects* (Hugh K. Elliott, London, 1967, p. 105).
32. Aveling, J.H. *English Midwives. Their History and Prospects* (Hugh K. Elliott, London, 1967, p. 109).
33. Stone, S. *A Complete Practice of Midwifery* (London, 1737).
34. Van Daventer, H. *The Art of Midwifery Improv'd*, 4th Edn (London, 1746).
35. Aveling, J.H. *English Midwives. Their History and Prospects* (Hugh K. Elliott, London, 1967, p. 126).
36. Stephen, M. *The Domestic Midwife* (London, 1795).
37. Mears, M. *The Pupil of Nature* (London, 1797).
38. Spence, D. *A System of Midwifery Theoretical and Practical* (1784).
39. Spencer, H.R. *History of British Midwifery 1650–1800* (John Rale, Sons and Danielsson Ltd, 1927).
40. Adams, M. *A Synopsis of the History of Queen Charlotte's Maternity Hospital* (1984).
41. *British Medical Journal*, Feature on George Stebbing, 1747–1825 (5 December 1981).
42. Young, J.H. *St. Mary's Hospitals, Manchester, 1790–1963* (E. & S. Livingstone, Edinburgh, 1964).
43. Bickerton, T.H. *A Medical History of Liverpool from the Earliest Days to the Year 1920* (John Murray, London, 1936).
44. Atkinson, S.B. *The Office of Midwife, Part I, From Bishops to the Central Board* (Bailliere & Co., London, 1907).
45. Walker, A. 'Midwife Services, England and Wales', in *Historical Review of British Obstetrics and Gynaecology, 1800–1950*, J. Munro Kerr, R.W. Johnstone and M.H. Phillips (eds) (Livingstone, Edinburgh, 1954, pp. 332–50).
46. Marshall, R. 'Birth of a Profession', *Nursing Mirror*, 30 November 1983.
47. Donnison, J. *Midwives and Medical Men* (Heinemann, London, 1977).

7 NINETEENTH-CENTURY MIDWIVES AND THEIR STRUGGLE FOR STATE RECOGNITION

Introduction

The social upheaval created by the Industrial Revolution coincided with an enormous and continuous population explosion which must have stretched resources to, or even beyond, the limit in the industrialised areas. Industrialisation and mechanisation, which had begun in the eighteenth century, expanded at a phenomenal rate in the century that followed. Factories and iron and steel foundries sprang up rapidly, as did engineering works, dye works, breweries, distilleries and soap works. Mills for the spinning and weaving of wool, cotton, silk and flax replaced cottage industries almost overnight. All these industries required a large workforce, and this resulted in mass migration of whole families into manufacturing towns from rural areas where poverty had become extreme, partly as a result of the cessation of small, home-based industries and partly because of the Enclosure Acts.

> What is the situation of the hand loom weaver during the parturient effort? She is upon her feet, with a woman on each side, her arms are placed round their necks and in nature's agony she almost drags her supporters to the floor and in this state the birth takes place . . . and why is this the case? The answer is because there is no change in bedclothing.[1]

The date is the mid-1830s and the writer is referring to women living in Lancashire mill towns, many of whom, he records, were destitute of bedding and furniture.

This sudden urbanisation created an acute need for housing, a need that was filled partly by overcrowding of existing substandard property and by cellar-dwelling, and partly by the hasty erection of row upon row of closely crowded back-to-back dwellings near to the mills and works. The shift of population chiefly affected the North of England and the West Midlands, and 'between 1801 and 1911 the populations of Bradford, Halifax, Huddersfield, Wakefield and Leeds grew by 1000 per cent'.[2]

> Thirty or forty factories rise on tops of the hills I have just described

. . . the wretched dwellings of the poor are scattered haphazard around them. Twelve to fifteen human beings are crowded pell-mell into each of these damp repulsive holes . . . You will hear the noise of furnaces, the whistle of steam. These vast structures keep air and light out of the human habitations which they dominate; they envelop them in perpetual fog . . . A sort of black smoke covers the city. The sun seen through it is a disc without rays. Under this half daylight 300,000 human beings are ceaselessly at work.[3]

In London, Lord Shaftesbury discovered a room with a family in each of its four corners and another room with a cesspool immediately below its boarded floor.[4] Such is the environment into which some babies would be born, and 'midwives' must sometimes have come from equally wretched conditions.

Except in heavy foundry and engineering work, women and children were part of the workforce along with men in mines, mills and factories. Long hours among the crashing, clanging, whistling and clattering of machinery, and in heat and steam in an environment often loaded with atmospheric pollutants, were detrimental to the mental and physical health of the workers. Such conditions led to the passing of several Factories Acts which resulted in a reduction to ten hours for all workers in 1867, and an Act of 1842 forbade employment of women underground in mines.

'Annual pregnancies made a permanent job outside the home next to impossible for a married woman even if she could find someone to look after her children and the house.'[5] Even so, large numbers of impoverished women did go out to work, leaving their babies and children at home. In 1849 an investigative journalist wrote: 'It is no infrequent occurrence for mothers of the tenderest age to return to their work in the factories on the second or third week after confinement.' Some babies were left alone, or in the charge of girls or old women, under the influence of an opiate mixture sold as 'Godfrey's Cordial'. 'First the child is drugged until it sleeps, and then too often it is drugged until it dies.'[6] The Education Act of 1870 made schooling compulsory and stopped the employment of young children.

The atmosphere over industrial towns was laden with smoke and chemicals. The water supply was polluted by factory effluents and untreated human sewage, which was the cause of many outbreaks of lethal diseases such as cholera and typhoid. Many workers, condemned to appalling working and living conditions, were also exploited financially, and some suffered such extreme deprivation that they lacked even the bare necessities of life. A few were more fortunate in being employed by men with an active social conscience who built model factories and accommodation for their workers.

Incredibly, some people, the inhabitants of the nineteenth-century workhouses, were even worse off than those employed. Before the Poor Law (Amendment) Act of 1834, each parish had its own poorhouse. They were usually small (often a cottage was used in rural parishes), and some were quite homely. The sick were cared for by the other inmates. The 1834 Poor Law Act allowed for the amalgamation of two or more parishes into a Union with a common workhouse. Large Union Workhouses were built, and housed the unemployed and unemployable together. Numbered among the unemployed were those seen as idle, scrounging layabouts, and among the unemployable the mentally and physically handicapped, the senile, the deaf, the blind and the mentally sick. In addition there were orphans, the families of prisoners, widows, and the elderly.

> There have been few more inhuman statutes than the Poor Law Act of 1834 which made all relief 'less eligible' than the lowest wage outside, confined it to the jail-like workhouse forcibly *separating* husbands, wives and children in order to punish the poor for their destitution, and discourage them from the dangerous temptation of procreating further paupers [our italics].[7]

Dickens describes 'A Walk in the Workhouse' where he saw some of the 1500 or 2000 paupers, ranging from the infant newly born and not yet come into the pauper world, to the old man dying on his bed. He also saw 'groves of babies in arms; groves of mothers and other sick women in bed; and groves of lunatics'.[8]

Each workhouse had its Infirmary. It appears that a large number of births took place there, and that the Workhouse Medical Officers who were part-time took these posts in order to gain experience in midwifery to benefit them in their private practice.[9] In the Liverpool Workhouse in 6 years in the 1870s, 2502 confinements took place.[10] It is known that the 'nurses' came from the ranks of the able-bodied inmates,[9] and it must be assumed that midwives were recruited in the same way.

As the century progressed, the relationship between the working and living conditions of the urban environment and the occurrence and spread of disease came to be recognised by men in public positions, and it became clear to them that to improve those conditions would improve the people's health and lifespan. In consequence the first Public Health Act was passed in 1848, and Medical Officers of Health were appointed in large cities. Thus was preventive medicine born. Edwin Chadwick, a Poor Law

Commissioner, led the movement towards the provision and control of clean water supplies and the initiation of safe sewage-disposal systems.

In the nineteenth century, both death rates and birth rates were high. The infant mortality rate was 150 per 1000 live births (Registrar General's figures) and 'the maternal mortality rate was 5.4 per 1000 registered births in 1847–54 and 4.75 for 1855–64'.[11] Interestingly enough, however, in the Liverpool Workhouse the maternal mortality rate was 3.2 per 1000 at this time and in Liverpool itself was 3.5 in 1873 and 2.9 in 1880.[10]

During the nineteenth century, the population of England and Wales quadrupled from 8 million in 1801 to 32 million in 1901. In 1851 the population of the country was 17.9 million but by 1871 it had risen to 22.7 million.[12] As the population rose dramatically, infanticide was common. Newly born illegitimate and unwanted babies were thrown into the Thames or disposed of, and this practice led to the first Infant Life Protection Act of 1872. The normal Victorian woman spent much of her time producing children or recovering from one birth to prepare herself for the next. For example, the mother of Edward Lear produced 21 children, all from the same marriage. Even women who were financially and socially well-placed were robbed of their sexual attractiveness and prematurely aged by repeated childbearing.[5]

Threats to the Survival of the Midwife

Developing trends such as the numerical growth of the middle class, the establishment of lying-in hospitals, the regulation of men-midwives, the recognition of obstetrics as a specialty, medical advances, and the takeover of childbirth by male doctors (except among the poorest of women) and the 'training' of monthly nurses to assist them, all led to a steep decline in the need for the female midwife. In consequence her future existence as a professional was seriously threatened. Obviously a few doctors agreed in principle to midwives being restricted practitioners, provided that they were trained for the role, but others, perhaps the majority of doctors, were anxious to see the complete extinction of the midwife. This was because they regarded those women who were ignorant and incompetent as a menace to society, and those who were educated and 'trained' as potential competitors.

Ironically, when, towards the end of the century, women were allowed to qualify as doctors, medical men preferred the idea of registered midwives for normal cases to competition from women doctor-obstetricians. As the practice of medicine became regulated, so it became increasingly obvious that for the midwife to survive she needed formal education and training.

It is reasonable to deduce that up and down the country, in cities, towns, villages and hamlets, midwives of varying degrees of skill delivered the babies of the vast majority of women at home, particularly those of the lower social classes, without medical intervention or assistance. So domiciliary midwives in these places had to deal, alone in many cases, with women of very poor physique, often with pelves distorted by rickets. There was also the possibility of such prevalent intercurrent conditions as cardiac disease, tuberculosis or anaemia, in addition to the complications of the pregnancy itself. These multiparous women were often prematurely aged by desperate poverty and heavy physical work. Even domestic work involved scrubbing, hand washing, mangling and carrying coals. If she worked in a factory or mine, she could be pushing, lifting, and carrying, and she could be forced to stand for shifts of up to 14 hours at a loom in a mill. The cost of engaging a doctor for the confinement was prohibitive, but the midwife could, in dire circumstances arising in the labour, call in a doctor providing that she recognised the gravity of the circumstances and provided that a doctor was available and willing to come.

Nursing was also in the hands of untrained women in the first half of the century. 'The immortal character of Sarah Gamp was sufficient to stamp the Nurse, during the first third of this century, as a person who disgraced one of the noblest callings to which womankind can devote themselves.'[13] Mrs Gamp was both self-professed nurse and midwife.

In 1860 Florence Nightingale set up the Nightingale School of Nursing at St. Thomas's Hospital and instituted a three-year training which she hoped would lead to registration. This in fact was not the case until the next century, but the three-year system of training continued. The nursing profession, with the now famous and charismatic Florence as its leader, attracted educated young women to its ranks, and this raised the social status of nursing. As the century progressed, midwifery became a closed occupation to any woman with pretensions to gentility because the subject, with all its connotations, became 'not talked about' in the Victoria era.

Unregulated Practice

It was not only the practice of midwifery that was unregulated in the early nineteenth century. The majority of medical practitioners were plying their trade without instruction or apprenticeship and without authorisation. It appears that the Medical Colleges only exerted their authority over physicians and surgeons practising in or near London. This unsatisfactory and dangerous state of affairs provoked a physician, Edward Harrison MD, to publish a book in 1806 called *Remarks on the Ineffective State of the Practice of Physic in Great Britain with Proposals for its Future Regulation and Improvement.*

> At present physicians without degrees, or at least without properly authorised degrees, surgeons and midwives without instruction, and apothecaries and druggists without having served an apprenticeship, have intruded themselves not only into the Capital but into almost every market town in England. Even in London the Colleges do not take upon themselves to examine the great bulk of persons, who are called apothecaries, but prescribe as physicians on many occasions, hence the community have no defence against the dangerously ignorant, who amount to a large majority of the profession. Unless the profession be subjected to proper regulations and restrictions, ignorant persons will continue to thrust themselves forward . . . Is it fit, that in such an enlightened kingdom as ours, medicine should be suffered to remain any longer in its present *unregulated* state? Is it not disgraceful that hairdressers, cooks, taylors, farriers etc. should for a moment be tolerated in their injurious practices? Surely the legislature is not aware of the mischief, which is daily committed, in every part of the kingdom, by the frauds of these imposters, otherwise it would take measures to prevent them. Midwifery being of great importance, it is much to be lamented, that no previous instruction, or test of ability is required. It is notorious that a great proportion of accoucheurs are very incompetent. Several persons have fallen under the author's notice who practice midwifery without having attended a single lecture of instruction.

Harrison recalled that the Royal College of Physicians some years previously had undertaken to examine and grant licences to midwives. It is likely that he is referring only to men midwives, as his explanation for the discontinuation of this practice was due to 'its having occurred to the learned body that since they are prohibited by their own laws from exercising the art of midwifery, they are not the most proper persons to decide upon the pretensions of obstetrical candidates'. His concern led him to conduct an enquiry into the state of medicine in the districts within his own county of Lincolnshire. A study of the Horncastle District revealed that, of the 144 persons exercising medicine for gain, only one in nine had been educated for the profession, and in the Market Rasen District less than one in nine of the 65 persons who practised medicine for gain had been educated for the profession. These practitioners (209 in total) consisted of 5 physicians, 18 surgeon-apothecaries, 34 druggists, 57 'irregulars' (one of whom was a man-midwife), and 95 midwives (presumably female, and who must each have had a very low case load). He remarks that 'the county of Lincoln contains several uneducated men-midwives. One of them, the son of a cow doctor, is equally a human and veterinary operator.' It is not surprising that his proposal for improvement was 'that the operation of the medical laws be no longer confined within the limits of the metropolis. Their influence ought to be equally felt, in every part of the kingdom, and as much as possible, through the extended possessions of the British Empire.'[14] Such evidence demonstrates that the conflict between *qualified* doctors (be they physicians or surgeons) and self-styled accoucheurs, i.e. *unqualified* men-midwives, that had first come into prominence in the mid-eighteenth century remained unresolved in the early part of the nineteenth century.

Traditional Midwifery Challenged

The challenge to female midwives from men gathered momentum, with the women being overshadowed both professionally and socially. The conflict between women and the Society of Apothecaries seemed particularly pointed, the latter seeing fit, in 1813, to attempt to persuade Parliament to pass a Bill for the examination and regulation of female midwives. They proposed the setting up of 24 committees in 24 medical districts. These committees, which were to consist of one physician to ten apothecaries or surgeon-apothecaries (seven of whom were to be practitioners of midwifery) would license female midwives on an annual basis on payment of a fee. The exception to these regulations would be midwives already in practice. However, this proposal failed as the Committee of the House of Commons would not allow any mention of female midwives.[15] Although they failed to get midwives licensed, the Apothecaries Society succeeded, through the Apothecaries Act of 1815, in laying down the qualifications to be required of all persons intending to practise as apothecaries, and also the penalties for unqualified practice.[15] This created a precedent which the surgeons were keen to copy but they did not attempt to regulate the practice of midwifery. However, the Society of Apothecaries, many of whose members held both the Diploma of the College of Surgeons and the Society's Licence, succeeded in persuading the College of Surgeons to propose that in future only men-midwives who held their Diploma should be allowed to practise mid-wifery. As many Apothecaries did hold this Diploma they would be entitled to act as men-midwives and many of them became triple-role practitioners: apothecary/surgeon/man-midwife. Presumably their aim was to exclude many non-holders of the Diploma, thus increasing their own opportunities to practise midwifery.

The early nineteenth century saw the proliferation of organisations, societies and associations which granted fellowships, licences and/or diplomas. This multitude of licensing bodies created a bewildering state of affairs.

At the turn of the 19th century there were nineteen different Licensing Bodies, the majority of which were concerned with the licensing of surgeons/apothecaries. The multiplicity of licensing authorities permitted the easy expansion in numbers of legitimate medical practitioners — an expansion which was beyond the control of the Royal College and necessarily represented another challenge to its authority and jurisdiction.[16]

There was undoubtedly not only an increase in the number and availability of men-midwives but also in their acceptability to women everywhere, providing they could afford their fee. Even in rural and relatively remote areas such as Cumbria, the accoucheur or male-midwife had established a place in the community. William Fleming, a Furness diarist, records a christening feast after a male accoucheur had delivered a farmer's wife in 1818. Male midwives advertised their services, as Figure 16 shows. The female midwives were called 'houdy-wives' and were expected to cook the celebration feast after the birth.[17] Obviously these midwives were relegated to a partly domestic, partly nursing role.

In the same year as the happy event just mentioned, an obstetric tragedy, which cast a shadow on the growing reputation of doctor-midwives, took place in the Royal family, following a stillbirth of historical significance. Princess Charlotte, an apparently healthy young woman, was attended during her pregnancy by three doctors, two of whom were primarily physicians and the other an obstetrician. They gave her advice on diet, exercise and hygiene. It is recorded that she had a small ante-partum haemorrhage in the last trimester. It is known that a Mrs Griffiths was the midwife appointed for the confinement, and although in residence for the birth, she did not seem to play any significant part in the management of the labour, perhaps because of the

Figure 16: Advertisements by Men Midwives Practising in the Lake District
in the late 18th or Early 19th Century

(a)

WILLIAM ROSS,

BEGS leave to acquaint the Inhabitants of *Ambleside* and its *Vicinity*,
that he practises Midwifery.

W. R. should have thought it unnecessary to have troubled the Public
with the present notice, but that he wished to correct a report which has
been propagated with great industry, for the purpose of injuring him in
the public opinion, that he did not practise Midwifery.—During the four
Years he studied at the University of *Edinburgh*, he attended the Midwifery, in common with the other Medical Professors in that University,
and hopes by a diligent attention, in this, as in every other part of his
Professional Duty, to Merit and Share the Public Favour.

J. Soulby, Printer, Ulverstone.

(b)

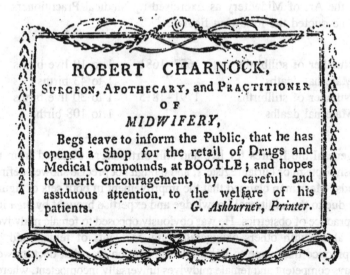

ROBERT CHARNOCK,
Surgeon, Apothecary, and Practitioner
OF
MIDWIFERY,
Begs leave to inform the Public, that he has
opened a Shop for the retail of Drugs and
Medical Compounds, at BOOTLE; and hopes
to merit encouragement, by a careful and
assiduous attention, to the welfare of his
patients.   *G. Ashburner, Printer.*

Source: W. Rollinson, Life and Tradition in the Lake District (J.M. Dent,
London, 1981).
Note: The Bootle mentioned in (b) is a village in Cumbria, not the town near
Liverpool.

presence of three eminent doctors. After the first stage, which was characterised by uterine dysfunction, the Princess eventually entered the second stage of labour. Indecision and poor clinical judgement on the part of the medical attendants resulted in the delivery, unaided, of a large male child, after a protracted second stage of 24 hours. The Princess died six hours later following a complicated and possibly mismanaged third stage.[18] It seems that in this particular period there was a reaction against the use of obstetric forceps and in fact the accepted philosophy was to use them 'only as a last resort'.[19]

One of the original proponents of non-intervention was Thomas Denman, who was an influential practitioner, writer and teacher of obstetrics. He was appointed Physician Man-Midwife to the Middlesex Hospital, and became the 'leader of the London man-midwives'.[20] Sir Richard Croft, who was in charge of Princess Charlotte's labour, was the son-in-law of Thomas Denman. He agreed with the policy of non-intervention, which would account for his inactivity on this occasion; shortly afterwards he committed suicide.[21]

Despite this conservatism, doctors were tightening their grip on the management of childbirth, and statistics were used by Dr Samuel Merriman to support the case of men-midwives. He published an article in the *London Medical and Physical Journal* on 14 March 1816 entitled 'On the Art of Midwifery as Exercised by Medical Practitioners'. In this he quoted the following figures:[22]

Number of stillbirths	1657–1681	1 to 19 live births
Maternal deaths	"	1 to 43 births
Number of stillbirths	1791–1815	1 to 30 live births
Maternal deaths	"	1 to 108 births

In general the figures for live and still births were obtained from the parish baptism or burial registers, and though not precise showed definite trends. Merriman claimed that the improvement in both sets of figures was due to the additional knowledge and expertise brought by *men* into the practice of obstetrics. He was obviously opposed to female midwives, and along with others exaggerated any incidents of female-midwife malpractice that came to light. His implication was that doctors were always competent and female midwives universally incompetent, whereas without doubt there would be some practitioners in each group whose standard of practice left a lot to be desired. Obviously doctors were, and still are, in a much better position to conceal their own failures, both as individual practitioners and as a profession.

Doctors were not only opposed to the idea of the female midwife but were also critical of other unqualified practitioners. In the *Lancet* of 9 November 1844, a surgeon, Henry Oliver, cited the following case:

> I have known a Druggist-Accoucheur sit by the bedside of a woman with placental presentation and allow the stream of life to ebb away without a single well-directed effort to preserve the patient. The case leads me to remark that whatever evils may result from the ignorance of female midwives the druggist-accoucheur is a far greater curse . . . yet they are armed with the fictitious and unmeaning Diploma of the Pharmaceutical Society.

Struggle for Recognition of Obstetrics as a Professional Specialty

Part of the confused state of affairs resulted from the fact that midwifery *per se* was not a recognised profession. Although physicians, surgeons, surgeon-apothecaries and apothecaries included it within their practice, their Colleges, Companies and Societies seemed rather to despise it and not want to 'own' it, yet the practitioners wanted it to be recognised and themselves to have the exclusive right to practice it. In 1828, the Royal College of Surgeons of Edinburgh passed a resolution requiring attendance at two courses on the 'Art and Science of Midwifery' as a preliminary to examination for the Diploma of the College. Those English doctor-practitioners who wanted midwifery to become an identifiable specialty formed themselves into an Obstetrical Society in 1825 and attempted to obtain the regulation of midwifery. Their particular target seemed to be the men who still, as in the previous century, could change overnight from totally unskilled occupations to being self-appointed men-midwives. Some members of the Royal College of Physicians did not approve of the Obstetrical Society. The President of the Royal College of Physicians, Sir Henry Halford, commented in 1827 that the practice of midwifery was 'an act foreign to the habits of gentlemen of enlarged academic education'.[23] Nine years later Sir Anthony Carlisle, a surgeon, said 'It is an imposture to pretend that a medical man is required at a labour.'[24] This Obstetrical Society was short-lived. The physicians claimed that doctor-surgeons were out to change a natural process into a surgical procedure. Although it appears ostensibly that the physicians were in favour of childbearing remaining a natural process, almost certainly an underlying motive was the feeling that professional men were demeaning themselves socially and professionally by participating in an essentially female function traditionally dealt with by females.

Monthly Nurse. A Substitute for the Midwife?

Most doctor-accoucheurs (general practitioners) and male-midwife 'specialists' were selective of their clients, wishing only to attend those who could pay well. As the professional and social status of these men rose, so the professional and social status of the midwife fell. The doctors did, however, recognise how useful it was to have a female around to undertake the care of the woman during labour, as they personally did not want the tedium of being present throughout labour. Rather than work or compete with a midwife, some seemed to favour a nurse who would watch the labour for them and then care for the mother and baby during the lying-in period. To this end the British Lying-in Hospital, London, started the training of 'monthly nurses' (Figure 17) in 1824, and some twenty years later were 'training' three times more of these nurses than midwives.[11] Although these nurses were of use to the doctor, they were not well esteemed by the public. Such a person is described by Leigh Hunt.

> The monthly nurse . . . is a middle-aged, motherly sort of gossip, hushing, flattering, dictatorial, knowing, ignorant, not very delicate, comfortable, uneasy, slip-slop kind of a blinking individual, between asleep and awake, whose business it is under Providence and the doctor to see that a child is not ushered with too little officiousness into the world, not brought up with too much good sense during the first month of its existence. Her charges are infants in laced caps, with incessant thirst, thumpable backs, and red little minnikin hands. She takes snuff ostentatiously, tea incessantly, advice indignantly, and a nap when she can get it and drinks rather than eats. The monthly nurse is not a highly respectable woman . . . but we have known one rare instance — in which the requisite qualifications were completed, and the precious individual (for when can a mother's luck be greater?) was an intelligent gentlewoman. This is what the assistant moulder of the first month of the existence of a human being *ought* always to be.[25]

In 1837 a book written by Thomas Bull (presumably a doctor) appeared on the market written specifically for mothers and for those

Figure 17: Certificate in Monthly Nursing

Certificate in Monthly Nursing.

FROM

St. Mary's Hospital

AND

The Manchester & Salford Lying-in Hospital.

We hereby Certify that

Mrs. Matilda Ford

has attended one *Course of Lectures at this Hospital on Practical Midwifery and Monthly Nursing, and that, having passed a satisfactory Examination, she is now competent to act as a Monthly Nurse.*

Signed

Manchester, 23ʳ *April* 1887.

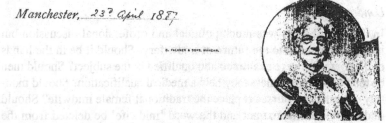

Source: City of Manchester Cultural Services Department.

looking after them and their babies. It was entitled *Hints to Mothers for the Management of Health during the Period of Pregnancy and in the Lying-in Room*. Its readers would be middle- and upper-class mothers who would not only be literate but also able to afford such a book, and so it would be out of reach of those who most needed its advice. It is not clear at what stage of pregnancy mothers booked a doctor or midwife at this time, but Thomas Bull evidently felt that women would find it insuperably difficult to bring themselves to ask the kind of questions he set out to answer. He assumed that the mothers would each have a monthly nurse and addressed much of his advice to her. However, he did comment that 'well would it be for English women if all who undertook this office came from a better educated class of society than they often do as the well doing of the patient during the lying-in month so much depends on the nurse'. Bull recommended that breast-feeding be forbidden if the mother had consumption (tuberculosis), or was of a highly nervous temperament or had a history of nervous or mental disorder, or where the mother was ambivalent towards breast feeding. It is significant that he makes no mention of the midwife in relation to the delivery, and instructed mothers to send for the 'medical man' as soon as labour started. This perhaps highlights the eclipse of the midwife by the medical profession in the first part of this century, especially among the upper classes.

Provisions for Birth according to Location

For most of the nineteenth century there was no uniformity in the provisions for childbirth. The scene in London differed from that in the provinces, which in turn differed from that in rural villages and hamlets.

London

In the capital there was much political and professional discussion but little agreement as to the future of midwifery. Should it be in the hands of doctors who were examined and qualified in the subject? Should men be totally excluded unless they held a medical qualification? Should monthly or maternity nurses replace the traditional female midwife? Should midwifery become extinct and the word 'midwife' be deleted from the language — on the grounds that 'all midwives were a mistake', as Dr Tyler-Smith taught his medical students? One proposal was that 'the office of midwife should be abolished and the very word 'midwifery' done away with on account of its derivation'.[26] It is significant that a Doctor of

Medicine, Michael Ryan, writing in 1841, proposed the use of the term 'obstetrician' because he was anxious to eradicate the 'barbarous and unclassical term midwife'.[27]

During the 1800s the Royal Colleges became more involved in the issue. In 1833 the Royal College of Surgeons desired to appoint examiners in midwifery, but found it was outside the scope of their charter. In 1852 they obtained a supplementary charter which empowered the College to examine persons for the diploma of Licentiate in Midwifery, which, under the Medical Act of 1858, became registrable. In 1861 the Royal College of Physicians were enabled to make midwifery a compulsory subject for their licence. It was almost the end of the century (1886) before the statutory body, the General Medical Council, required qualifications in medicine, surgery and midwifery before a student could be registered as a doctor[24] although some medical schools had already instituted this procedure.

Provincial Towns

Throughout the century, in those cities that had hospital provision, obstetricians who seemed less politically but more practically minded were keen to improve and develop their art, and moreover worked harmoniously with female midwives. It would appear that these doctors with a particular interest in midwifery were genuinely concerned both with the welfare of poor mothers and with helping midwives who faced difficult cases where poverty in the family would preclude sending for medical aid. In Liverpool a scheme for relief had been envisaged in the form of a Lying-in Hospital as early as 1757. At this time a surgeon-midwife, Matthew Turner, who had studied under William Smellie, offered immediate help by offering his services free to married women living in Liverpool who had complicated labours and were unable to afford the doctor's fee. He hoped that

> the gentlewomen who practise midwifery in town, will not look upon anything here mentioned as designed to prejudice or undervalue them; the design being only to give them assistance when 'tis wanted, which I judge may be offered to them in the manner here proposed, without any Impeachment of their abilities, by those who may be allowed to have had better Opportunities of acquiring skill in the Profession than the Practitioners of their Sex usually have.[10]

It was, however, another 39 years before a charitable obstetrical organisation was founded. In the meantime the Ladies Charity, founded

Table 1: Statistics for Labours and Maternal Deaths, Liverpool, 1799–1815[28]

Year	Labours	Deaths	Cause
1799	621	1	No external cause
1803	996	1	Natural and regular causes of indisposition
1811	1515	2	From causes which no human
1812	992	1	hand could have prevented
1813	905	2	
1815	1072	1	In last stages of consumption

in 1796, alleviated suffering by gifts of clothing, food, soap or money, by loans of temporary requisites such as bed linen, and by the provision of a midwife in the patient's home, and if necessary a doctor. Under this scheme there were remarkably few maternal deaths, as is shown in Table 1. This record is attributed to the good health and physique of the country-bred Irish and Scottish immigrants who were attracted to jobs in this developing port.

The Liverpool Lying-in Hospital and Dispensary for the Diseases of Women and Children was opened in 1841. Its birth and mortality statistics for the next three years are shown in Table 2.[28]

Table 2: Birth and Mortality Statistics, Liverpool Lying-in Hospital, 1842–45[28]

Date	Labours	Deaths
January to 9 November 1842	46	1
9 November 1842 to 9 November 1843	73	0
9 November 1843 to 9 November 1844	104	0
9 November 1844 to 9 November 1845	118	0
Total	341	
Stillbirths 18 per 341 births		
Operative deliveries 21		

Instructed Midwives

Midwives who received instruction in the lying-in hospitals either remained in practice there, working under the supervision of the man-midwife specialists, or else worked in the Domiciliary Midwifery Service. St. Mary's Hospital in Manchester (opened 1790) was closed for in-patient deliveries between 1813 and 1853, mainly because of lack of funds, but doctors and midwives based at the hospital delivered some 2000 mothers per year at home. As stated in the Rules of the Charity, the midwives had at their disposal the prompt assistance of medical officers of the Charity 'in all cases of difficulty and danger'.[29] Other midwives practised independently in the city. At Queen Charlotte's Hospital, London, nurses and medical students were received for instruction from 1809 (and probably before that), but it was not until 1851 that a definite period of training, of about three months, was introduced for midwives. They received practical instruction from the matron and sisters, and attended lectures given by the physicians. They took an examination on completion of the training and, if successful, received a diploma and were then qualified to act as midwives.[30]

Uninstructed Midwives

In towns and in country districts, most midwives undertook the office without any formal instruction at all. Many of these women, lacking a general education, would in any case have been incapable of benefiting from any professional education. The sphere of influence from the London and provincial obstetric centres did not reach the remote rural districts and so the provision for birth, particularly among the poorer classes, was the traditional local midwife, who often had only the nearest surgeon upon whom to call for assistance. These local midwives continued to practise, untouched by new knowledge and teaching, but nevertheless some would be capable, skilled, experienced practitioners whereas the standard of practice of others was abysmal. An example of an 'untrained' midwife was cited in the *Lancet* in October 1844. The case in point was conducted by a Devonshire midwife, and a stillborn boy was born before the arrival of the surgeon whom she had called. The midwife explained to him that 'the chield com'd footling, and as soon as he com'd down so fur that I could git at the string, I tied em, and cut em; and that was right wazzun it?'

Advances in Obstetric Care

Chloroform

James Young Simpson, born on 7 June 1811, became one of the outstanding obstetricians of the era. He pioneered the use of chloroform for childbirth, although nitrous oxide and ether had both preceeded it as anaesthetic agents. Simpson first experimented with chloroform on himself, colleagues and friends prior to introducing it into obstetrics. Initially there was opposition to the relief of pain in labour on the grounds that the suffering that the women experienced during childbirth was regarded as one of the strongest elements of the love of the mother for her offspring, and also because suffering was accepted as divinely ordained: 'In sorrow thou shalt bring forth children.'[31] Consequently the teaching of the Church was that pain in labour was inevitable and women should not seek its mitigation. However, claims were being made for the 'magical' effects of chloroform. 'The Lying-in room, from being in a state of gloom, despondency and misery, is instantly transformed, by its means, into one of cheerful hope and happiness.'[32] It is recorded that the first patient to whom Simpson administered chloroform was a doctor's wife, who was so delighted with its analgesic effects that she christened her newborn baby girl Anaesthesia.[20] Arguments continued for and against the use of chloroform but it was used widely after Queen Victoria chose to have it administered at her confinement in 1853 and was very pleased with its effectiveness. Victoria was the first Queen of England to be delivered by a male obstetrician, Sir Edward Locock, who called in a General Practitioner, Dr John Snow, to administer the chloroform at the birth of Prince Leopold. The reaction of midwives to the use of chloroform in labour is unknown. The poorer mothers, for whom they were mainly responsible, were unlikely to demand it or to be able to afford it. It was probably generally administered by doctors to their richer clients at home, in addition to its use in maternity hospitals.

Midwives were eventually permitted by the Central Midwives Board to administer chloroform capsules, but only under the direction and personal supervision of a doctor. This ruling was reiterated in the 1934 Annual Report of the Board. It appears that it was thus used up to 1935 when the College of Obstetricians and Gynaecologists (formed in 1929) considered it unsuitable for use by midwives.[33]

Caesarean Section

James Young Simpson was the first to use chloroform for Caesarean sections and he subsequently claimed that this procedure was life-saving in two-thirds of the cases.[34] Caesarean sections were performed rather reluctantly in the nineteenth century, and then often only as a last resort. This operation was first performed posthumously by command of the Roman ruler, Numa Pompilius, who codified the Roman Law in 715 BC. The purpose was to separate the mother and baby before burial. The medieval Church also made this operation mandatory, either posthumously or when the mother's death was inevitable and imminent, in order to baptise the child which would otherwise, they claimed, be a lost soul.

The first substantiated record of a successful Caesarean section on a living woman was performed in 1500 by a Swiss sow gelder named Jacob Nufer. The midwives told him they could do nothing more to resolve the prolonged labour of his wife and so, using his expertise as a butcher, he opened up her abdomen and delivered a living child, following which he repaired the wound and she survived to produce four more children.[35] However, doctors practising midwifery were divided as to whether this operation was justifiable because the outcome was almost inevitably fatal to both the mother and baby. This may have been because it was not performed electively but only when the labour was obstructed, or the mother *in extremis* from haemorrhage or some other complication. In the late eighteenth and early nineteenth centuries, obstetricians such as Charles White and John Hull of Manchester both advocated, as a matter of principle, this surgical method of delivery over other methods such as craniotomy, which could only result in a dead baby. They were relatively successful at a time when such an operation was fraught with complications such as uncontrollable haemorrhage, shock and infection. Generally these dangers mitigated against the performance of this operation by most obstetricians until the middle of the nineteenth century with the coming of anaesthesia, and even then the number of operations performed was few. The first Caesarean section performed in the Rotunda Hospital, Dublin, was in 1854,[36] and in Liverpool the first such operation was performed by Dr Henry Briggs in 1894.[37] It was not until 1902 that the number of Caesarean sections undertaken in St. Mary's Hospital, Manchester, exceeded double figures for one year, and these were emergency rather than elective operations.[38]

Childbed Fever

In the nineteenth century, only fifteen additional hospitals were established in the British Isles for maternity cases and these were mainly in the big centres of population. One of the reasons for this was that it was considered safer, particularly for uncomplicated cases, for mothers to be delivered in their own homes to avoid the contagion known as puerperal or childbed fever. Its aetiology at that time was unknown (although suspected by White[39] and Semmelweiss[40]), and so it was transmitted unwittingly from patient to patient, and from staff, particularly doctors, to patients because doctors did post-mortem examinations and then internal examinations with unwashed, ungloved hands. Bacteria flourished in the overcrowded, badly ventilated and, in many cases, seldom cleaned wards of those days. Fortunately, hospitals in Britain never suffered such terrible epidemics of this infection as occurred in hospitals in many European countries. Le Fort, a Frenchman living in the mid-nineteenth century reported that 1 in 29 women delivered in European hospitals died from childbed fever, as against only 1 in 212 of those delivered at home.[38] He visited the Maternité, Paris, in 1846 and wrote:

> The principal ward contained a large number of beds in alcoves like English horse-stalls along each side. Ventilation was almost impossible. Floors and partitions were washed perhaps once a month . . . the ceilings had not been whitewashed for many a long year. Lying-in women who became ill were transferred to an isolation room regardless of the nature of the illness; puerperal fever cases and patients affected with diarrhoea, bronchitis, measles or any other eruptive fever. Midwife pupils attend normal lying-in patients and fever cases alike, and perform all the necessary manipulations for every class of case.[20]

The main epidemics in Britain occurred in London in 1860 and 1861, and in Edinburgh in 1873. In Liverpool there were minor outbreaks on a recurring basis from 1874. There were few fatal cases but the problem was sufficient to raise the question of the possible closure of maternity wards. This was also considered on economic grounds as the 'average cost of outdoor maternity services was 8s 10d per head and that of indoor treatment £6 8s 1d'.[10] Although all hospitals experienced a certain number of deaths from this infection, some recorded remarkably few. Collins, when in charge of the Rotunda Hospital in Dublin, implemented the precepts of Dr Charles White of Manchester and managed to keep the hospital completely free from puerperal sepsis for four years. Dr White had advocated, as early as 1763, fresh air, strict attention to cleanliness of patients, attendants and their environment, adequate ventilation, postural drainage and early rising after delivery. Although women were not admitted to St. Mary's Hospital, Manchester, for delivery for 40 years between 1813 and 1853 (partly as a result of the fear of puerperal fever), outbreaks occurred in the domiciliary service. In 1831 there was a severe epidemic of puerperal fever in Manchester, affecting patients delivered by midwives of the Lying-in Charity as well as other patients. Records show that of 30 mothers delivered by one midwife, 16 developed puerperal fever and all died, although at the same time the other midwives delivered 350 women and none were affected by the disease.[39] Isabella Beeton, famous for her *Book of Household Management*, was a victim of this condition. She was one of 17 children born to her mother. Isabella herself had four children, all boys, two of whom died and two of whom lived, but she died of puerperal fever after the birth of her fourth son when she was only 28 years old.[5]

Because of this fatal condition the whole future of maternity hospitals hung in the balance in the mid 1800s. It appeared to be viewed as a national scandal, as an article entitled 'The Harvest of Death', which appeared in the *London Echo*, showed. 'It is worthy of note', it announced, 'that the idea of maternity hospitals, which were once so popular, has been exploded by scientific experience. It has been found that such Institutions are merely nurseries for puerperal fever.' Fortunately, Lister had already laid down the precepts of antisepsis in 1867, and with the discoveries of Pasteur and Koch in the next decade, the science of bacteriology began. The control of the spread of infection thus became possible.

Some Nineteenth-century Antenatal, Intra-partum and Post-partum Midwifery Practices

As a medical journal the *Lancet* commented on current midwifery procedures and issues such as doctors' fees and provision of services. Extracts show that some, albeit limited, antenatal care and preparation were being given. Mothers were being advised to have a daily rest period in a quiet cool room 'in order to keep their sensibilities calm lest the baby became imprinted with harsh passions or disfigurements'.[41] Obviously antenatal influences had credence in the nineteenth century. Vaginal examinations were performed antenatally after the administration of an opiate. Two fingers were lubricated with lard prior to this procedure, 'to feel for the enlargement of the uterus and for the weight of the head of the fetus'.[42]

Although more cases were now in the hands of doctors (and this was particularly true of London and the Home Counties), on the whole there was a belief that interference with the physiological process of labour was wrong and unnecessary. Michael Ryan expressed the view that 'every pregnant woman should obtain the best medical aid for the period of delivery that circumstances will permit, and she should never employ a midwife alone . . .'.[43] On the other hand, Dr Coffin MD (also botanist and herbalist) fervently upheld the view that

> parturition is a natural operation, requiring little, if any, mechanical assistance. We have before observed that no man should act as an accoucheur under any circumstances, but that women should be instructed to do all that is required at the time.[44]

In the first stage of labour the mother was advised to be up and about.[43,44] Ryan recommended nourishment in the form of gruel, arrowroot and sago but forbade alcohol, and for the relief of pain he prescribed liquor of opium. Coffin, on the other hand, had a strong belief in the efficacy of raspberry leaf tea to facilitate labour. Although Ryan advised that 'no attempt should be made to dilate the orifice of the womb, the vagina, or external genital aperture', in ordinary cases of labour[43] he thought it was the duty of the obstetrician to conduct a normal labour and also be prepared to intervene in the third stage.

It appears that most mothers were delivered of their babies in bed. In the Rotunda Hospital, Dublin, the women were generally confined upon a couch and afterwards were carried to a clean bed.[36] The treatment of sepsis, which was the main complication of the puerperium and the inevitable sequel to Caesarean section, varied considerably. In the third decade of the century a Dr Blundell, writing of his management in the *Lancet* (5 April 1828), stated:

> violent practices are uncalled for . . . 30 or 40 leeches, say 30 on average should be applied to the symphysis pubis. Now and then . . . blood to the amount of 16 ounces may be extracted from the arm; laxatives, refrigerants and the antiphlogistic regime for four or five days, will commonly be found to overcome the symptoms.

Later in the century, according to another article in the *Glasgow Medical Journal* (1898), it seems that doctors managed puerperal sepsis by keeping the patients in bed sedated with strong opiates.[45]

Apparently the midwives were keen to get the patient up early, within 24 hours, to help drain the lochia from the uterus, thereby preventing its stagnation.[45] The literal lying-in period was at least 14 days. Ryan advised patients to sit up on the 5th or 6th day if they felt able, but the more delicate were discouraged from doing so until the 9th, 12th or even the 20th post-partum day. A light diet including gruel and beef tea was prescribed for the lying-in period. Camomile tea was prescribed for spasmodic after-pains, hysterical convulsions and for 'windy' babies. It was also used externally to relieve soreness from small lacerations. A solution of carbolic acid in olive oil was used to wash hands and instruments.[46]

Payment for Maternity Services

In the first half of the nineteenth century, doctors' fees ranged from one guinea to one-hundred guineas for delivery plus 5s or 7s 6d per visit including medicine, and 6d or 1s per mile for any journey over two miles, so the lowest fee totalled around three or four guineas. The attending midwife got 'poundage' from the doctor of a quarter of his fee. In some cases the accoucheur refused to pay 'poundage' so the midwife received her half-guinea or so from the family *ex gratia* and separately. After the 1860s the fees payable to doctors rose steeply. These were fixed by medico-ethical associations and were based on the social class of the family, which was judged by the size and appearance of their house.[47] In Stockport in 1842 an account shows payment of 2s 6d to a midwife for her services at the confinement.[48] This was then the average fee but by 1870 it had risen to 7s.[16] At this time working *men* could save for medical fees through Sick Clubs and Benefit Societies but midwives' fees were often excluded from the benefit. Some doctors, especially in country areas, were charitable and would willingly, without expectation of payment, attend a confinement themselves or assist the midwife if called, but this was not always so. Such an exception occurred in 1871 and was recorded in the *Lancet*. In this case a mother in Gloucestershire died while giving birth to illegitimate twins. The midwife engaged by the girl's father found the case difficult throughout the night and so at 7.30 a.m. the girl's father went to fetch the Parish Poor Law Medical Officer who lived about three miles away. The father had no Poor-relief Order and no means of paying privately so Mr Cooke refused to attend. At 5 p.m. the father persuaded a Mr Wood of Ledbury, four miles away, to attend his daughter. When he arrived the mother and both babies were dead. Cooke told the coroner he had frequently attended without payment or a relief order. The *Lancet* concluded:

> Mr. Cooke is a gentleman who has been more than 40 years in practice, and who has reached a period of life at which he cannot be

expected to be at the beck and call of every girl who has the misfortune to have an illegitimate child. The fact is, medical men are far too fearful of claptrap charges of inhumanity.[49]

Changes and Developments Affecting the Role of the Midwife

The great improvements in the science and practice of obstetrics made it a respectable branch of medicine, and where there was doctor involvement, the role of the midwife changed. This she seemed to accept without protest. The new breed of *hospital* midwives, still numbering very few of the total, seemed to accept uncomplainingly their now subservient role alongside the doctors who supervised their practice. Perhaps they perceived that some of the changes and developments were in the interests of the mothers, and in any case beyond their power to alter.

This century did not produce any outstanding or vociferous midwives prepared to campaign to return to their former role as practitioners of normal midwifery, even though they could now claim they were (or at least some were) instructed for that role. However, when Florence Nightingale came on the scene she envisaged the midwife not only regaining her traditional role but rather extending it. She was anxious to widen the scope and raise the standard of the midwife and her practice. She wrote in *Notes on Lying-in Institutions and a Scheme for Training Midwives*:

> I call a midwife a woman who has received such a training, scientific and practical, as that she can undertake *all cases* of parturition, normal and abnormal, subject only to consultation, like any other accoucheur. Such a training could not be given in less than two years . . . no training of six months could enable a woman to be more than a Midwifery Nurse.[50]

Florence Nightingale envisaged midwifery practice as continuing in the hands of women, but intelligent, educated, trained and skilful women, proficient in all aspects of obstetrics, who would consult with physicians only when necessary. She who, by 1862, had established a Nightingale Fund and the Nightingale School for Nurses, started to negotiate for the admission of maternity patients into a new part of King's College Hospital so that pupil midwives could be trained. This particular scheme had to be abandoned when the maternity wing, along with other maternity hospitals, had to be closed because of outbreaks of puerperal fever.

Attempts to Legislate for the Regulation of Female Midwives

By the middle of the century there was an increasing number of educated women, many of whom were daughters of professional men, and many hospitals were accepting such women for 'training'. One such hospital was the Sheffield Hospital for Women, which was founded in 1864 and became the Jessop Hospital in 1878. (Dr J.H. Aveling, who wrote *British Midwives: their History and Prospects*, was one of two men who were instrumental in establishing this Institution and was one of its first Medical Officers.) From its foundation the Hospital provided a midwifery service for the care of patients in their own homes. Training of midwives began at the hospital in 1865. The 1865 Annual Report stated that a prerequisite for admission to the examination was that all midwives had to attend suitable lectures. This presupposed literacy, which was becoming a requirement for midwifery training in hospitals. Minute 29 of the 1868 Report of St. Mary's Hospital, Manchester, stated that 'well educated midwives [must] be attached to this hospital'. It would appear that midwives trained in such centres as St. Mary's Hospital, Manchester, Liverpool Maternity Hospital, Sheffield Hospital for Women, and Queen Charlotte's Hospital, London, were given responsibility for the conduct of normal delivery. It is recorded that, in Queen Charlotte's Hospital in 1885, 'The R.M.O. [Resident Medical Officer] has no duty in connection with a confinement if it is natural . . .'[30]

Other educated women were entering nursing at the instigation of Florence Nightingale, and some of these were forming themselves into the pressure groups of the Female Medical Society and the Ladies Obstetrical College.

After several attempts doctors took a step forward in the regulation of their own profession in the 1858 Medical Act. 'It established a system for the *registration* of practitioners holding qualifications from degree and diploma granting bodies, recognised by the new General Council for Medical Education and Registration, set up under the Act [our italics].'[51] This allowed for the continued practice of midwifery by men not qualified in the subject, and moreover did not require future medical practitioners to study midwifery either. It was the Medical Act of 1886 which required, for the first time, a qualification in medicine, surgery and midwifery before a medical student could be registered as a doctor.[24]

The 1858 Medical Act totally omitted any mention of female midwives, who remained unlicensed and unaccountable to any authority. In the same year a group of London obstetricians founded the London Obstetrical Society. They seemed to have altruistic objectives in that one of their prime aims was the reduction in maternal mortality. They did not envisage the disappearance of female midwives. Indeed they saw clearly that the education of midwives was vital if the objective of reduced mortality was to be achieved, and so one of its members, Doctor Routh, demanded compulsory education for midwives. Nothing came of this worthy resolve at the time.

In 1869 the London Obstetrical Society carried out a survey into the causes of infant mortality. This was instigated by Dr William Farr, who was a statistician in the Registrar General's Department, and who in 1841 had advocated the training of midwives, undoubtedly prompted by the appalling maternal and infant mortality figures which he was analysing. The first question of the survey was into the proportion of births attended by medical men and by midwives. The second asked whether the midwives had been instructed. In 1869, midwives attended births as follows:

	%
In agricultural villages	30–90
In small manufacturing towns	Proportion unclear but suggestion is less than above
Large provincial and manufacturing towns	30–90
London — East End	30–50
London — West End	2

Medical men attended 10–30 per cent of the total births.[22]

These figures show that midwives attended around a million births per year and so obviously were a very necessary workforce. It is ludicrous to think that the doctors who advocated their abolition could manage without them for normal births, and equally ludicrous for them to fear being ousted by the midwives. Doctors were obviously divided in their value judgement of midwives. Some were pleased to approve their training for *normal* midwifery, and others saw them all as the lingering remnants of the old wives' folklore with no place in nineteenth-century society. Dr Farr's Report showed that a considerable number of births took place without a midwife being present. It must be assumed, therefore, that the midwife was, for this investigation, defined as one who habitually and for gain attended births, as the title 'midwife' was sometimes used loosely to apply to anyone — neighbour, friend or relative — who undertook the delivery or assisted at the birth.

The answers to the second question were much less equivocal. The vast majority of midwives had received no proper instruction and were deemed to be ignorant and incompetent. This would have applied to some, but others, although not showing up well in this investigation, may have been possessors of dexterity and clinical acumen. It is not clear how the investigators judged clinical competence. A small proportion of midwives had received some formal instruction but were found to be incapable of dealing adequately with obstetric emergencies. How much better were doctors equipped to deal with these undefined 'obstetric emergencies', which must have included haemorrhage and eclampsia?

Following this Enquiry, the London Obstetrical Society strove, through a Parliamentary Bill in 1870, for the training of midwives and the exclusion from practice of untrained midwives, but they did not succeed in persuading or convincing the Government that this was necessary.[52]

Women in Medicine

It appears that attempts to exclude women from the healing arts began in Britain in 1421 when a petition from Cambridge and Oxford Universities was received and approved by Parliament outlining the dangers of allowing 'ignorant and unskilled' persons to practise medicine and surgery. 'The relative or total exclusion of women from the ranks of the healers seem to have been an integral part of the process of professionalization.'[53]

The Female Medical Society was founded in 1862 'to provide educated women with proper facilities for learning the theory and practice of midwifery and the accessory branches of medical science'.[54] Three years later they had enlarged their ambitions and retitled themselves the Ladies Medical College, the ultimate aim of which was to enable women to study medicine. Women were not, however, admitted to Medical Schools until 1869 when five women were allowed to study medicine in Edinburgh. Prior to this time, two women, Elizabeth Blackwell and Elizabeth Garrett, were already practising medicine. Elizabeth Blackwell studied in New York and practised in St. Bartholomew's Hospital, London, in all wards except the gynaecological ward, from which she was excluded because the Professor of Gynaecology could not approve of a lady studying his subject. Elizabeth Garrett followed in her footsteps. She studied medicine in the 1860s but was not allowed to take the qualifying examinations. She did, however, qualify to become a Licentiate of the Society of Apothecaries and by this means became licensed as a doctor and joined Elizabeth Blackwell on the Medical Register.[53]

In 1873 the Ladies Obstetrical College was established in Great Portland Street, London, with the intentions of producing lady-midwives or obstetrices. They aimed to obtain such amendment to the Medical Acts as would give women access to a registrable diploma for the practice of midwifery, and confer upon properly educated women a defined professional status. In 1875 some of the members of this College sought examination by the Royal College of Surgeons for a licence in midwifery as the Royal College had, in 1872 (in a supplementary charter), gained powers to examine *persons* to become 'Licentiates in Midwifery of the Royal College of Surgeons of England'. Rightly considering themselves as persons, these ladies equipped themselves to meet the criteria laid down by the Royal College of Surgeons so as to enter the examination leading to licence. The Board of Examiners of the Royal College of Surgeons resigned in protest rather than accede to their request, and they had the backing of the London Obstetrical Society in their decision.[52]

Midwives and Midwifery: a Continuing Controversy

Female Midwife or Female Doctor Midwife?

In 1872 the Obstetrical Association of Midwives was formed; this was soon abbreviated to the Midwives Association. The Association was led by Maria Firth, and its members included some London midwives and some women belonging to the Ladies Medical College. This was an interesting amalgam and preceded the Midwives Institute by nine years. Its midwife members appear to have envisaged the type of extended role which Florence Nightingale also advocated. These 'high flyers' saw themselves undertaking the management and delivery of abnormal as well as normal cases. This is precisely what the students of the Ladies Medical college saw themselves doing. They supported the proposed Bill to allow suitably qualified women to be admitted to the Medical Register as 'Licentiates in Midwifery'. Their ideas were favourably accepted by Mr James Stansfield, a supporter of the Women's Rights Movement and President of the Local Government Board. If this proposed Bill had been enacted, it would have created a two-tier structure for midwives, one tier being of superior highly trained midwives, and the other tier of an inferior grade with limited training and restricted function.

Around the same time the British Medical Association and the Obstetrical Society were preparing a scheme for Government approval which would register midwives and allow them restricted clinical practice and a role that included housework and cookery in the patient's home.[11] Implicit in all the discussions and propositions put forward by the medical profession regarding the future role of the midwife was the key issue of her status, a rise in which, they felt, might result in a lowering of their own status in the public estimation. The Midwives Association fiercely contested a part-domestic type of role, but their own proposals did not materialise either. After women were admitted to medical schools, the Ladies Medical College closed and so their support of the Midwives Association ceased. Once women qualified as doctors, they abandoned the midwives' cause, perhaps out of self-interest, feeling that educated female midwives would then be their direct competitors.

The Position of the Midwife. A Question for Professional and Political Determination

In 1872 the General Medical Council took an interest in the position of the midwife and the possibility of her examination and regulation, but it seems clear that the Council was very cautious about taking action for fear of confusing the respective roles of doctors and midwives. It appointed a Committee to look into the matter, and eventually put forward a Bill in 1878 which included reference to midwives. This part of the Bill was soon dropped.[54] Despite the lack of legislation the London Obstetrical Society were determined to upgrade the practice of midwives, and by 1872 they had formulated and implemented proposals for the granting of a diploma to midwives *after examination*. Before a midwife could present herself for this examination she had to meet the most stringent criteria. Dr J.A. Aveling, at this time Chairman of the London Obstetrical Society, sets down the criteria in his book *English Midwives*.[22] These required that the midwife had to provide a certificate of moral character and be between 21 and 30 years of age. She also had to have:

(1) proof of having attended the practice at a lying-in hospital or Charity for a period of not less than six months or of having personally attended not less than 25 labours under supervision satisfactory to the Board of Examiners.

(2) Proof of having attended a course of theoretical teaching by lectures or tutorial instruction, the details of which must be submitted to, and receive the approval of, the Board of Examiners.

With this evidence she could then sit the examination, which required knowledge of reproductive anatomy, normal midwifery, signs of deviation from the normal, obstetric emergencies, the management of the puerperium and the newborn baby, general hygiene and 'the duties of the midwife, with regard to the patient, and with regard to the seeking of medical advice'.

The Government came under pressure the following year (1873) from medical associations including the British Medical Association, the London Obstetrical Society and the General Medical Council regarding the role and practice of the midwife. This provoked a Government Enquiry into the laws and regulations governing the practice of midwifery in other European countries. The Enquiry found that practice had been controlled in France since 1803, since 1810 in Austria, Norway and Sweden, and in Holland since 1865. The information did not, however, goad the Government into action.

In 1874 the Obstetrical Society stated that they approved of midwives conducting normal deliveries but said that they should call upon medical assistance in the event of complications.[55] Again, in 1876, 1877 and 1879, a conjoint deputation from the Medical Associations was made to Government officers urging the education and registration of midwives.[56]

Despite the exacting criteria for entry to the written and oral examination of the London Obstetrical Society, 108 midwives held this diploma within eight years, and the names of 63 of those midwives appeared in a published list in *Work and Leisure* in 1880.[57] The diploma guaranteed that its possessor was a 'skilled midwife *competent to attend natural labours* [our italics]'.[58] Although it conferred a distinction of real value, it was not in any way officially recognised. It helped to make midwifery a little more respectable but a certain stigma still remained.

One of the outstanding young ladies who ventured into midwifery at this time was Alice Gregory, daughter of the Dean of St. Paul's, who, after 'training', practised in a rural district in the early part of the next century. Some of her experiences are related in the next chapter.

Midwives Enter the Political Arena

In the early 1880s some of the elite diploma-holding midwives surveyed the political, social and professional scene and became alarmed at the precarious situation of the midwife. They were made acutely aware of the differences between the social classes in the provision of medical and obstetric care, with the rich now being very well catered for and the poor being almost totally deprived of care. They also perceived that the obstetricians would continue to oppose the upgrading of midwives for fear they should lose their lucrative midwifery practices. These politically aware lady-midwives also perceived that they themselves would need to use 'political' methods and enlist impartial and influential supporters in order to further their cause. There were at this time active social reformers, both men and women, to whom they successfully appealed. The midwives became articulate for their cause and formed the Matrons' Aid Society (or Trained Midwives Registration Society). It was not considered proper to have the word midwife in the main title! Nevertheless, very soon afterwards they added 'Midwives Institute', and before long this became its sole title.

The prime objective of the Society was to obtain legislation to regulate the training and practice of midwives, in order to fulfil their ideal that all mothers, rich and poor alike, should be able to have the services of a trained midwife.[59] Other objectives were the publishing of a list of those midwives from London and the provinces who were now considered professionally 'qualified', and the provision of mutual moral support and association for these women. The chairwoman, who was also the spokeswoman of the original group of eight who formed the Society, was Louise Hubbard, a wealthy single woman already interested in the welfare of women and the feminist cause. She recognised the potential of intelligent, educated women in the upper classes, who had little scope or outlet for useful activity, and she wished to tap their resources of energy and abilities for the benefit of womankind. She aimed to liberate the 'gentlewoman' from her undemanding domestic confines in order that help could be given to women by women. She thought such women would be ideal in occupations such as midwifery and teaching, which would enable them to become financially self-supporting. These concepts ran counter to established Victorian attitudes that marriage and motherhood constituted a woman's only profession.

One of the first members of the Midwives Institute was a non-practising midwife, a Mrs Henry Smith. She had been obliged to give up her midwifery career, because of the prevailing mores of the age, when she married a distinguished surgeon, but she nevertheless remained passionately committed to midwifery. As Miss Veitch, she was the tenth woman to gain the Diploma of the London Obstetrical Society, and had practised in a slum area. Mrs Smith became the first President of the Midwives Institute and wrote an article on the improvement of midwifery standards, which, although it stimulated interest and discussion, could not at this time bring about any radical change.

Membership of the Institute grew rapidly to twenty-four, and regular meetings were held. In 1884, in pursuit of their main objective, they drafted proposals for a Bill to regulate midwifery. This attempt was abortive. In addition to retaining its original objectives the scope of the Institute was enlarged after Rosalind Paget, a newly qualified midwife who also held the Diploma of the London Obstetrical Society, joined in 1885. She was already a nurse and was the niece of William Rathbone who had instituted District Nursing in Liverpool, where she had previously worked. She was dedicated to the Institute's cause but she also saw the need for intellectual stimulus for its members. Rosalind Paget pioneered the setting up of lecture courses and a library for midwives and she also masterminded the regulation of the first-ever journal for midwives.[57] The journal provided the means for professional communication throughout the country. The first issue was a four-page supplement to the magazine *Woman*, and for reasons best known to the editor was entitled 'Nursing Notes'.

New Impetus for Training and Recognition of Midwives

In 1889 the General Medical Council, through whom medical opinion was expressed, made the following resolution:

> That this Council regards the absence of public supervision for the education and supervision of midwives as productive of a large amount of grave suffering and fatal disease amongst the poorer classes and urges upon the Government the importance of passing into law some measure for the education and registration of midwives.[56]

This resolution shows a shift in the 'official' medical viewpoint away from the demise of the midwife and towards a trained practitioner for the benefit of those women in the working class whom they served. It seemed to support the many subsequent Bills put before the Government for the regulation of midwives.

In 1890 the *Lancet* was to point out that it was

> questionable whether doctors would in any sense be injuriously affected by legalised examination and registration of midwives, that midwives as an institution were older than doctors, that a large proportion of the poor were quite unable to pay doctor's fees and that they ran serious risks at the hands of pretended but unauthorised midwives.[60]

In 1890 a second Bill was promoted for registration of midwives and protection of the title 'midwife'. This was a conjoint effort by the Midwives Institute and the London Obstetrical Society. It was opposed on several counts: firstly, because a doctor Member of Parliament, speaking for his medical colleagues, said that the proposed legal status of midwives (who would charge a lower fee than a doctor) would deprive medical men of some of their income from obstetrics; secondly, another Member objected very strongly to the proposed requirement on midwives to produce a certificate of good moral character when this was not required of doctors.

After the failure of this Bill and its successor in 1891, the medical profession, through its various channels, reformulated their views on midwives and their sphere of practice. They agreed to the registration of midwives, but insisted that legislation should precisely define the *limits* of a midwife's practice, and also provide disciplinary measures for breach of such regulations. In 1892 a Select Committee of the House of Commons was appointed to look into the work of midwives. Its first Report in the same year confirmed that there were a large number of 'untrained' midwives whose practice, at its worst, was lethal to mother and baby and, at its best, left a lot to be desired. The Report therefore strongly recommended registration under Act of Parliament.[61] It is unfortunate that the term 'midwife' embraced women at both ends of the social, educational and professional scale and all gradations in-between: some were cultured, educated, strong-minded, idealistic 'ladies' championing all women's causes and particularly midwifery; others were the lowest of the low, being illiterate, unscrupulous, malevolent, gin-drinking characters with dirty hands and undesirable habits, capable of both woman-slaughter and deliberate infanticide, who battened on unfortunate lower-class women in dire need. The 'lady-midwives' must have felt horror at the negligence and misdeeds of their sister midwives.

The Report of the Select Committee the following year highlighted those midwives who were trained and certificated, and who, in contrast to the untrained, were making a beneficial and positive contribution to the welfare of the poor and working classes. This Select Committee made several propositions. First, they saw the need to safeguard existing 'trained' midwives who were to be listed. Secondly, for admission to a Midwives' Register, the passing of an examination was necessary, and those women then registered as midwives would be licensed to practise midwifery but not of course any other branch of medicine. The Committee envisaged that newly appointed County Councils would implement the Act locally.[62] (It is interesting to note that these proposals were almost identical to those enacted in 1902.)

In 1894 the Recorder at the Old Bailey added his views to the controversial issue of midwives. In charging the Grand Jury he said that he greatly regretted that the registration of midwives was not compulsory.[63] There must have been a catastrophe, due to serious negligence, by a midwife to provoke this remark.

In 1893 a group of medical men decided to form an Association which became called the Midwives Registration Association. Four years later the Association for Promoting Compulsory Registration (a lay society which had been initiated by the Midwives Institute) lobbied all coroners in England and Wales, who also had experience of the tragedies caused by midwives unequal to their tasks, and half of the coroners were willing to put their names to a recommendation for registration.[57]

Quite early in this decade some members from the Midwives Registration Association and the Association for Promoting Compulsory Registration formed the Midwives' Bills Committee. The objective of this Committee was to campaign for the introduction into Parliament of further Bills.[11]

Controversy raged over the issue of regulation of midwives and its consequences. Doctors' views differed depending on their rank, specialty and geographical location. Some provincial and rural general practitioners were vehemently opposed on economic grounds. Even nurses, through the British Nursing Association, joined in the fray and their leaders branded midwives as 'an anachronism' and a 'historical curiosity', seemingly jealous that they might achieve legal status before nurses, who were themselves campaigning for registration.[57]

The next Bill was introduced in 1895 by Lord Balfour of Burleigh. This Bill, which was subjected to redrafting, included proposals for a Central Midwives Board, consisting mainly of doctors, to formulate rules relating to the training, examination and practice of midwives. At the same time doctors were still discussing the whole matter of midwives and their control in the local BMA branch meetings. One branch even suggested that midwives should be restricted to working as obstetric nurses and be under the control of doctors locally. Finally the British Medical Association itself drafted a Bill which recognised midwives as such but wanted to secure full control by having only doctors on the Central Midwives Board.

It is interesting to note that the Manchester Midwives Association raised strong objections to any form of registration under medical control. They believed that the interests of the medical men were contrary to those of midwives.[11]

Similar Bills were introduced into Parliament in 1896 (by Mr Cosmo Bonsor), in 1897 (by Sir Tatton Egerton), and in 1898 and 1899 (by Mr J.A. Balfour) and again in 1900 (by Mr Heywood Johnstone). All of these bills were defeated.[64]

During these years of indecision and frustration the Midwives Institute was growing in strength and membership and was widening its scope to include education. It put on courses to prepare midwives for the London Obstetrical Society's Diploma examination, and in consequence many hundreds of midwives gained this Diploma. It is interesting that

> Trained midwives were warned not to use the letter 'L.O.S.' after their names since some innocent — or less innocent and more determined doctors — were claiming that these letters represented not the London Obstetrical Society but 'Licentiate of the Obstetrical Society' and that this must imply that the midwives were claiming to have a 'licence to practice' in rivalry to the medical profession.[57]

The Passing of the First Midwives Act

After eight unsuccessful attempts in eleven years, the Bill introduced in 1902 by Lord Cecil Manners, supported by Sir Tatton Egerton, was successful.

Throughout the nineteenth century the struggle for the registration of midwives had as its focal point the vexed question of status. The inferior social status and professional position occupied by the midwife had much to do with the retardation of registration. However, the first Midwives Act reached the Statute Book in 1902 and ended a decade of 'legislative miscarriages'. The unofficial apprentice system, which had been the accepted method of 'training' midwives for centuries, was thus superseded.

> Like some other medical and social reforms this was slowly constructed amidst the pressures of professional self-interest and militant feminism and the encumbrances of bureaucratic inertia and public ignorance and prejudice. In the meantime the innocent suffered.[64]

This apt statement perfectly encapsulates all the factions that demand to be appeased before change is made that may have unforeseen ramifications.

At long last the hopes and proposals of many midwives such as Elizabeth Cellier, Sarah Stone, Elizabeth Nihell, Margaret Stephen, Martha Mears and Rosalind Paget, and of some of the doctors, for example Andrew Boorde, Peter Chamberlen, Percival Willoughby, John Maubray and latterly Sir Francis Champneys, had been realised in the official recognition of the midwife. However, because the actual change was inevitably slow, unofficial practice continued for some time. In fact most people's mental image of a nineteenth-century midwife is that of Sairey Gamp which is due in no little part to the descriptive genius of Charles

Dickens. He portrays her as an unforgettable character so real that it is difficult to think of her as fictitious. Dickens himself says that she was a 'fair representation of the hired attendant on the poor in sickness'.[65] His flair for description is such that very little imagination is required to visualise this 'midwife' prototype. She was old, earthy, fat, and red-nosed, smelt of spirits and was addicted to taking snuff. She lived in High Holborn but her sister self-styled nurse/midwives could be found in all the poor districts of London. She rented accommodation in the house of a bird fancier, which was identified by her signboard bearing the designation 'MIDWIFE'. Her apartment was a front first-floor room, which was 'easily assailable at night by pebbles, walking sticks and fragments of tobacco pipe'. It is easy to picture anxious fathers-to-be knocking her up in the small hours to attend a labour, and to imagine her waddling along the London streets armed with her umbrella. She also attended the sick and the dead, and 'went to a lying-in or a laying-out with equal zest and relish'. It is little wonder that she needed the solace of her daily half-pint of porter. As she says, 'Whether I sicks or monthlies . . . I hope I does my duty, but I am but a poor woman and I earns my living hard.' In such a populous area she would be kept very busy, and a typical night's work could be to lay out a corpse, and on return to her lodgings then be called out to deliver twins. She emerges as a strong personality, full of vitality, of little or no education but very necessary to the society in which she lived. It is unfortunate that her midwifery experiences are not described, and even more unfortunate that such an unprofessional image of a midwife should be so enduring whereas some of her more professional and factual predecessors have long since been forgotten.

Such is the power of a writer so to caricature a type that the word 'gamp' was, for many decades — in fact almost a century — understood to mean a midwife, but rather curiously 'gamp' is now slang for an umbrella, which she invariably carried. Solly Zuckerman, who became Chief Scientific Adviser to the British Minister of Defence, writes of some of his experiences as a medical student in the mid-1920s.[66] He tells how he set out for his first home delivery armed only with his black bag and with the doctrine learnt from the only book he had read on the subject, the message of which was that 'childbirth was a natural event which doctors should not mar by their ministrations'. The mother, who lived in two rooms on the first floor of a small, run-down terraced house, was in bed when he arrived, and with her was the midwife or 'gamp'. Zuckerman says he let nature take its course and 'after what seemed a long delay, the baby was born, and with the gamp's help, I then did what was necessary'.

In marked contrast to Sairey Gamp is the midwife who is vividly portrayed in the autobiography *Lark Rise to Candleford*.[67] The author, Flora Thompson, was born in 1876 in Juniper Hill, a hamlet on the Oxford/Northamptonshire border and lived there until her mid-teens. Her autobiography contains delightful recollections of village life; she was obviously an observant and intelligent girl who seems to have had an unusual awareness of herself, her family and neighbours, and the society in which they had their being. She describes everyday domestic happenings vividly and presents a very clear picture of the social scene, particularly the customs associated with childbirth, as the following extract shows.

A familiar sight at Lark Rise was that of a young girl pushing one of the two perambulators in the hamlet round the Rise with a smallish-sized, oak clothes box with black handles lashed to the seat. Those not already informed who met her would read the signs and enquire 'How is your mother — or your sister or your aunt — getting on?' and she, well primed, would answer demurely, 'As well as can be expected under the circumstances, thank you, Mrs So-and-so'. She had been to the Rectory for THE BOX, which appeared almost simultaneously with every new baby. It contained half a dozen of everything — tiny shirts, swathes, long flannel barrows, nighties, and napkins, made, kept in repair, and lent for every confinement by the Clergyman's daughter. In addition to the loaned clothes, it would contain, as a gift, packets of tea and sugar and a tin of patent groats for making gruel. The box was a popular institution. Any farm labourer's wife, whether she attended church or not, was made welcome to the loan of it. It appeared in most of the cottages at regular intervals, and seemed to the children as much a feature of family life as the new babies. It was so constantly in demand that it had to have an understudy, known as the 'second-best box', altogether inferior, which fell to the lot of those careless matrons who had neglected to bespeak the loan the moment they 'knew their luck again'.

The boxes were supposed to be returned at the end of a month with the clothes freshly laundered; but if no one else required them, an extension could be had, and many mothers were allowed to keep their box until, at six or seven weeks old, the baby was big enough to be put into short clothes, so saving them the cost of preparing a layette other than the one set of clothes got ready for the infant's arrival. Even that might be borrowed. When the hamlet babies arrived they found good clothes awaiting them, and the best of all nourishment — Nature's own. The mothers did not fare so well. It was the fashion at that time to keep maternity patients on a low diet for the first three days, and the hamlet women found no difficulty in following this regime: water gruel, dry toast and weak tea was their menu. When the time came for more nourishing diet, the parson's daughter made for every patient one large sago pudding, followed up by a jug of veal broth. After these were consumed they returned to their ordinary food, with a half pint of stout a day for those who could afford it. No milk was taken and yet their own milk supply was abundant. Once, when a bottle-fed baby was brought on a visit to the hamlet, its bottle was held up as a curiosity. It had a long, thin rubber tube for the baby to suck through, which must have been impossible to clean.

The only cash outlay in an ordinary confinement was half a crown [nearly 13p], the fee of the old woman who, as she said, saw the beginning and end of everybody. She was of course not a certified midwife, but she was a decent intelligent old body, clean in her person and methods and very kind. For the half-crown she officiated at the birth and came every morning for ten days to bath the baby and make the mother comfortable. She also tried hard to keep the patient in bed for the ten days; but with little success. Some mothers refused to stay there because they knew they were needed downstairs; others because they felt so strong and fit they saw no reason to lie there. Some women actually got up on the third day, and, as far as could be seen at the time, suffered no ill effects.

Complications at birth were rare, but in the two or three cases where they did occur during her practice, old Mrs Quinton had sufficient skill to recognise the symptoms and send post haste for the doctor. No mother lost her life in childbed during the decade. The general health of the hamlet was excellent. The healthy, open-air life and the abundance of coarse wholesome food must have been largely responsible for that.

In these more enlightened days the mere mention of the old, untrained village midwife raises the vision of some dirty, drink-sodden old hag without skill or conscience. But not all of them were Sairey Gamps. The great majority were clean, knowledgeable old women who took a pride in their office [Figure 18]. Nor had many of them been entirely without instruction. The country doctor of that day valued a good midwife in an outlying village and did not begrudge time and trouble in training her. Such a one would save him many a six- or

Figure 18: Midwife Caroline Tarplee, born 1828, died 1925. Village midwife of Cropthorne, Worcester

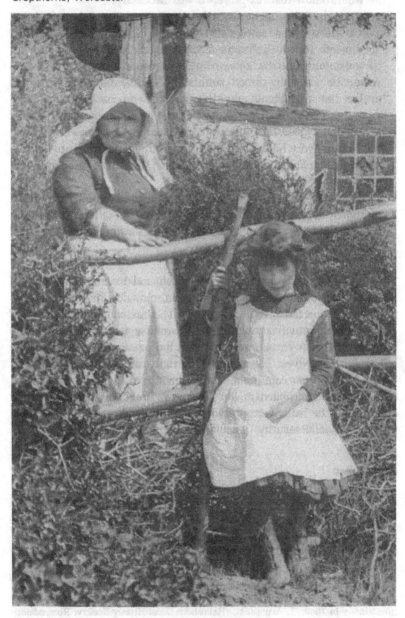

Source: From *The Cropthorne Camera of Minnie Holland*, 1892–1905, by permission of Kawabata Press, Torpoint, Devon.

eight-mile drive over bad roads at night, and, if a summons did come, he would know that his presence was necessary.

The trained district nurses, when they came a few years later, were a great blessing in country districts; but the old midwife also had her good points, for which she now receives no credit. She was no superior person coming into the house to strain its resources to the utmost and shame the patient by forced confessions that she did not possess this or that, but a neighbour, poor like herself, who could make do with what there was, or, if not, knew where to send to borrow it. This Mrs Quinton possessed quite a stock of the things she knew she would not find in every house, and might often be met with a baby's little round bath in her hand, or a clothes-horse, for airing, slung over her arm.

Other days, other ways, and, although they have now been greatly improved upon, the old country midwives did at least succeed in bringing into the world many generations of our forefathers, or where should we be now?

Flora Thompson's comments show insight and understanding into the qualities that go into the making of a good midwife. Mrs Quinton was intelligent, respectable, skilled in diagnosis, conscientious and very kind — and all this for half a crown a time! It would appear from the writer's remarks that such virtues were not rare but possessed by most of the old country midwives. The maternal mortality rate was nil for ten years despite the 100 per cent home-confinement rate. In the country many other factors contributed to the low rates. Food for the mother and clothing for the baby were provided and, although poor, they seemed to have a 'social security' peculiar to such communities.

References

1. Thompson, E.P. *The Making of the English Working Class* (Gollancz, London, 1963).
2. Harvie, C. *The Experience of Industrialisation*, Open University Units 24/25, A101.
3. de Tocqueville, A. *Journeys to England and Ireland*. Quoted in *Nature and Industrialisation*, A. Clayre (ed.) (Oxford University Press, Oxford, 1977).
4. Trevelyan, G.M. *English Social History* (Longmans Green, London, 1944).
5. Phillips, J. and P. *Victorians at Home and Away* (Croom Helm, London, 1978).
6. Reach, A.B. 'When You Could Smell the Opium on the Baby's Breath', *The Guardian*, 21 July 1984 (quoting *Morning Chronicle*, 1849). See also *Manchester and the Textile Districts in 1849*, C. Aspin (ed.) (Helmshore Local History Society, Rossendale).
7. Hobsbawm, E.J. *Industry and Empire* (Pelican, Harmondsworth, 1968).
8. Dickens, C. 'A Walk in the Workhouse', in *Nature and Industrialisation*, A. Clayre (ed.) (Oxford University Press, Oxford, 1977).

9. Davies, C. (ed.) *Rewriting Nursing History* (Croom Helm, London, 1980).

10. Bickerton, T.H. *A Medical History of Liverpool from the Earliest Days to the Year 1920* (John Murray, London, 1936).

11. Donnison, J. *Midwives and Medical Men* (Heinemann, London, 1977).

12. White, R. *Social Change and the Development of the Nursing Profession* (Kimpton, London, 1978).

13. Davies, C. (ed.) *Rewriting Nursing History*.(quoting Margaret Breay, 'Nursing in the Victorian Era', *Nursing Record*, 19 July 1897) (Croom Helm, London, 1980).

14. Harrison, B. *Remarks on the Ineffective State of Physic in Great Britain* (Bickerstaff, London, 1806).

15. Donnison, J. *Midwives and Medical Men* (quoting *Transactions of the Association of Apothecaries and Surgeon Apothecaries of England and Wales*, 1823) (Heinemann, London, 1977).

16. Chamberlain, M. *Old Wives Tales. Their History, Remedies and Spells* (Virago, London, 1981).

17. Rollinson, W. *Life and Tradition in the Lake District* (quoting William Fleming) (J.M. Dent, London, 1981).

18. Dewhurst, J. *Royal Confinements* (Weidenfeld and Nicolson, London, 1980, p. 118).

19. Dewhurst, J. *Royal Confinements* (Weidenfeld and Nicolson, London, 1980, p. 125).

20. Graham, H. *Eternal Eve* (Hutchinson, London, 1960).

21. Dewhurst, J. *Royal Confinements* (Weidenfeld and Nicolson, London, 1980, p. 132).

22. Aveling, J.H. *English Midwives* (Hugh K. Elliott, London, 1967).

23. Clarke, G. *A History of the Royal College of Physicians of London* (Clarendon Press, Oxford, 1966).

24. Walker, A. 'Midwife Services', in *Historical Review of British Obstetrics and Gynaecology, 1800–1950*, J. Munro Kerr, R.W. Johnstone and M.H. Phillips (eds) (Livingstone, Edinburgh, 1954).

25. Hunt, L. *The Monthly Nurse* (1846).

26. Donnison, J. *Midwives and Medical Men* (quoting Dr Tyler Smith) (Heinemann, London, 1977).

27. Ryan, M. *A Manual in Midwifery* (1841, p. 3).

28. Bickerton, T.H. *A Medical History of Liverpool from the Earliest Days to the Year 1920* (John Murray, London, 1936, p. 217).

29. *Rules of the Lying-in Charity* (St. Mary's Hospital, Manchester, 1790).

30. Adams, M. *A Synopsis of the History of Queen Charlotte's Maternity Hospital* (1984).

31. Genesis 2:21.

32. Chavasse, P.H. *Advice to a Wife*, 16th edn, revised by S. Dodd (J. & A. Churchill, London, 1914).

33. *Central Midwives Board Annual Report, 1935*.

34. Simpson, M. *Simpson the Obstetrician* (Gollancz, London, 1972).

35. Dewhurst, J. *Royal Confinements* (Weidenfeld and Nicolson, London, 1980, p. 7).

36. 'An Illustrious Dublin Lying-in Hospital', *Irish Medical Times*, 20 January 1984.

37. Bickerton, T.H. *A Medical History of Liverpool from the Earliest Days to the Year 1920* (John Murray, London, 1936).

38. Young, J.H. *Development of Maternity Hospitals*. Unpublished treatise, 1966 (Archives of St. Mary's Hospital, Manchester).

39. Young, J.H. *St. Mary's Hospitals, Manchester, 1790–1963* (Livingstone, Edinburgh, 1964).

40. Thompson, M. *The Cry and the Covenant* (Doubleday, New York, undated).

41. Smith, F.B. *The People's Health 1830–1910* (Croom Helm, London, 1979, p. 15).

42. Smith, F.B. *The People's Health 1830–1910* (Croom Helm, London, 1979, p. 16).

43. Ryan, M. *A Manual in Midwifery* (1841, p. 167).

44. Coffin, A.I. *Treatise on Midwifery and the Diseases of Women and Children*, 9th

edn (British Medico-Botanic Establishment, London, 1854).

45. Edgar, J. 'Is There Room for Improvement in the Present Mode of Clinical Instruction in Midwifery?', *Glasgow Medical Journal, 50*, 1898, 174–84.

46. Burton, J.R *Midwifery for Midwives* (J. and A. Churchill, London, 1884).

47. Smith, F.B. *The People's Health 1830–1910* (quoting *Lancet* articles of 30 May 1835, 29 July 1865, 19 January 1867, 7 January 1870) (Croom Helm, London, 1979).

48. Bill of Confinement 1842, City of Manchester Archives, Central Library, Manchester.

49. *Lancet*, 1 April 1871.

50. Nightingale, F. *Notes on Lying-in Institutions and a Scheme for Training Midwives* (1872).

51. Donnison, J. *Midwives and Medical Men* (Heinemann, London, 1977).

52. Atkinson, S.B. *The Office of Midwife* (Bailliere & Co., London, 1907).

53. Leeson, J. and Gray, J. *Women and Medicine* (Tavistock Women's Studies, Tavistock Publications, London, 1978).

54. Humphreys, F.R. 'The History of the Act for the Registration of Midwives', *Nursing Times*, 10 February 1906.

55. *British Medical Journal*, 28 February 1874.

56. Atkinson, S.B. *The Office of Midwife* (Bailliere & Co., London, 1907).

57. Cowell, B. and Wainwright, D. *Behind the Blue Door* (Bailliere Tindall, London, 1981).

58. Ministry of Health, *Report on the Training and Education of Midwives* (HMSO, London, 1929).

59. Farrer, M. 'The Royal College of Midwives 1881–1981', *Midwife, Health Visitor and Community Nurse*, July 1981.

60. 'Midwives Registration Bill and the Obstetrical Society of London', *Lancet*, ii (1890), 1149.

61. Ward, A. 'The Passing of the Midwives Act 1902', *Midwife, Health Visitor and Community Nurse*, June 1981.

62. Humphreys, F.R. 'The History of the Act for the Registration of Midwives' Part II, *Nursing Times*, March 1906.

63. Campbell, J. *The Carnegie Report on the Physical Welfare of Mothers and Children, 1917* (Carnegie Trust).

64. Forbes, T.R. 'The Regulation of English Midwives in the 18th and 19th Centuries', *Journal of Medical History, xv* (4), October 1971.

65. Dickens, C. *Martin Chuzzlewit* (Chapman & Hall, London, 1844).

66. Zuckerman, S. *From Apes to Warlords, 1904–1946* (Hamish Hamilton, London, 1978).

67. Thompson, F. *Lark Rise to Candleford* (Oxford University Press, Oxford, 1945).

8 THE TWENTIETH-CENTURY STATE CERTIFIED MIDWIFE

State Regulation

The first Midwives Act received Royal Assent on 31 July 1902 and came into force in 1903 (Figure 19). It was drawn up '. . . to secure the better training of midwives and regulate their practice'.[1] The most important feature of this Act was the setting up of the Central Midwives Board for England and Wales. (The Act did not apply to Scotland and so midwives who 'trained' in Scotland came to England and took the examination of the Central Midwives Board until 1916, when the first Scottish Midwives Act was passed.)

The Central Midwives Board met for the first time at the Privy Council Offices on 11 December 1902. It continued to meet at regular intervals until (in accordance with the provisions of the Nurses, Midwives and Health Visitors Act 1979) the United Kingdom Central Council for Nursing, Midwifery and Health Visiting, in association with the National Boards, assumed statutory responsibility for the education, training and practice of midwives on 1 July 1983.

Initially the Central Midwives Board consisted of nine members appointed as follows:

Four doctors, one representing each of the following: the Royal College of Physicians, the Royal College of Surgeons, the Worshipful Society of Apothecaries, and the Midwives Institute.
Two persons, one of whom had to be a woman, were appointed by the President of the Privy Council for a period of three years. The woman appointed was Miss Jane Wilson, a Nurse and Midwife.
One person, appointed by each of the following, for a term of three years: the Association of County Councils; Queen Victoria's Jubilee Institute for Nurses; and the Royal British Nurses' Association.

Of the two Nursing Bodies entitled to appoint members, the Queen Victoria's Institute chose Rosalind Paget, who was an active midwife, and the Royal British Nurses' Association chose Miss Dorothea Oldham, so all three of the women on the board were midwives. Ironically, though, the member appointed by the Midwives Institute had to be a doctor rather

177

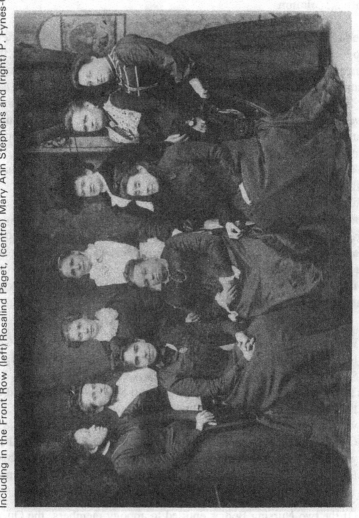

Figure 19: Photograph in Celebration of Midwives Act — Members of Midwives Institute, 1881, Including in the Front Row (left) Rosalind Paget, (centre) Mary Ann Stephens and (right) P. Fynes-Clinton

Source: Courtesy of the Royal College of Midwives, London.

than a midwife. Their choice was Dr Charles Cullingworth, who had actively campaigned for the registration of midwives. A notable omission was any appointee to represent the 600 Poor Law Infirmaries.

The Central Midwives Board was given very wide powers:

I. To frame rules:
    (a) regulating their own proceedings;
    (b) regulating the issue of certificates and the condition of admission to the Roll of Midwives;
    (c) regulating the course of training, the conduct of examinations and the remuneration of the examiners;
    (d) regulating the admission to the Roll of women already in practice as midwives at the passing of the Act;
    (e) regulating, supervising and restricting within due limits the practice of midwives;
    (f) deciding the conditions under which midwives may be suspended from practice;
    (g) defining the particulars required to be given in any notice under Section 10 of the Act. (Section 10 related to notification of intention to practice.)
II. To appoint examiners
III. To decide upon the place where, and the time when, examinations shall be held
IV. To publish annually a Roll of midwives who have been duly certified under the Act
V. To decide upon the removal from the Roll of the name of any midwife for disobeying the rules and regulations from time to time laid down under this Act by the Central Midwives Board, or for other misconduct, and also to decide upon the restoration to the Roll of the name of any midwife so removed
VI. To issue and cancel certificates

and generally to do any other act or duty which might be necessary for the due and proper carrying out of the provisions of the Act.[2]

The rules framed by the Central Midwives Board had to be validated by the Privy Council. Provision was made in the Act for a midwife to appeal to the High Court of Justice against the decision by the Board to remove her name from the Roll of midwives.

Certification under the Act

Admission to the Roll of Midwives

Certain women who already possessed a recognised qualification in midwifery, issued either by the London Obstetrical Society or certain lying-in
hospitals, were automatically admitted to the Roll of qualified midwives
under the Act. The first name on the Roll was that of Mrs Mary Ann
Stephens who had trained at the City of London Lying-in Hospital and
taken the London Obstetrical Society examination in 1881. Her certificate
was dated 29 October 1903. Certificate Number 2 was held by Rosalind
Paget.[3] Also, women of good character who had already been in practice as a midwife for at least one year could apply to the Board for admission to the Roll. These latter were known as *bona fide* midwives.
The Board had to formulate Rules with which to regulate the practice
of their newly acquired force of 'certified midwives', many of whom
were untrained and uneducated.

With the above exceptions, all other women intending to become midwives were required to present themselves for an examination in competence before a certificate could be issued allowing them to commence
practice.

From 1 April 1905 no person could assume the title of midwife unless
she held a certificate issued by the Central Midwives Board, and from
1 April 1910 no person could habitually and for gain attend women in
childbirth, *except* under the direction of a doctor, unless she was certified under the Act. It seems extraordinary that the pre-1900 clamour
for *registration* of midwives should ultimately produce a State *Certified*
Midwife rather than a State *Registered* Midwife.

Training Leading to Certification

In 1903 the Central Midwives Board approved 'period of training' was
three months, and this training period was not extended for thirteen years.

Extracts from First Rule Book, 1903

The examination shall be partly oral and practical, and partly written
and shall embrace the following subjects:

(a) The elementary anatomy of the female pelvis and generative organs.
(b) Pregnancy and its principal complications including abortion.
(c) The symptoms, mechanism, course and management of natural
    labour.
(d) The signs that a labour is abnormal.

(e) Haemorrhage: its varieties and the treatment of each.
(f) Antiseptics in midwifery and the way to prepare and use them.
(g) The management of the puerperal patient, including the use of the clinical thermometer and of the catheter.
(h) The management (including the feeding) of infants, and the signs of the important diseases which may develop during the first 10 days.
(i) The duties of the midwife as described in the regulations.
(j) Obstetric emergencies, and how the midwife should deal with them until the arrival of a doctor. This will include some knowledge of the drugs commonly needed in such cases, and of the mode of their administration.
(k) Puerperal fever, its nature, causes and symptoms. The elements of house sanitation. The disinfection of person, clothing and appliances.

Responsibilities of the Midwife

The midwife shall be responsible for the cleanliness, and should give full directions for securing the comfort and proper dieting, of the mother and child during the lying-in period which shall be held for the purpose of these regulations and in a normal case to mean the time occupied by the labour and a period of 10 days thereafter.

In all cases of abortion, of illness of the patient or child, or of any abnormality occurring during pregnancy, labour, or lying-in, a midwife must decline to attend alone and must advise that a registered medical practitioner be sent for, as, for example, if the following occurs:

(a) In the case of a pregnant woman:

When she suspects a deformed pelvis.
Where there is loss of blood.
Where the pregnancy presents any other unusual feature (as, for example, excessive sickness, persistent headache, dimness of vision, puffiness of hands and face, difficulty in emptying the bladder, incontinence of urine, large varicose veins rupture) or when it is complicated by fever or any other serious condition.

(b) In the case of a woman in labour:

In all presentations other than the uncomplicated vertex or breech, in all cases of breech presentations in primigravidae, in all cases of flooding or convulsions, and also whenever there appears to be insufficient room for the child to pass, or when a tumour is felt in any of the mother's passages.

If the midwife, when the cervix has become dilated, is unable to make out the presentation.

If there is loss of blood in excess of what is natural, at whatever time of the labour it may occur.

If an hour after the birth of the child the placenta has not been expelled, and cannot be expressed (i.e. pressed out) even if no bleeding has occurred.

In cases of rupture of the perineum, or other serious injury of the soft parts.

(c) In the case of lying-in women and in the case of newly born children:

Whenever, after delivery, the progress of the woman or child is not satisfactory, but in all events upon the occurrence of the subjoined conditions in:

1. *The mother:*
   Abdominal swelling and signs of insufficient contraction of the uterus.
   Foul smelling discharges.
   Secondary post-partum haemorrhage.
   Rise of temperature above 100°F with quickening of the pulse for more than 24 hours.
   Unusual swelling of the breasts with local tenderness or pain.

2. *The Child:*
   Injuries received during birth.
   Obvious malformations or deformities, not inconsistent with continued existence.
   Concealed malformations — incapability to suck or take nourishment.
   Inflammation to even the slightest degree of the eyes, eyelids and ears.
   Syphilitic appearance of skin in certain parts.
   Illness or feebleness arising from prematurity.
   Malignant jaundice (icterus neonatorum).
   Inflammation about the umbilicus (septic infection of the cord).

In all cases of the death of women during pregnancy, labour and lying-in.[4]

Approval of Training Institutions

The hospitals wishing to provide training leading to qualification had to apply to the Central Midwives Board, and inspection was a prerequisite for consideration for approval. This was a considerable task, as established maternity hospitals that had undertaken non-statutory training were all anxious to be approved. It was 1905 before two eminent provincial hospitals, the Jessop, Sheffield, and St. Mary's Hospitals, Manchester, were officially approved, and 1909 when Newcastle General Hospital Maternity Unit was approved.

In 1906 the Poor Law Institutions, also anxious for approval as midwifery training schools, complained, through the Poor Law Officers' Journal, about what they felt was discrimination against them by the Central Midwives Board 'in refusing practically to recognise Poor Law Hospitals as Training Schools in midwifery'.[5] In reply the Secretary of the Central Midwives Board published a list, in 1907, of fifteen Poor Law Infirmaries licensed for midwifery training. Fifteen is a small number out of the existing 600, especially in view of the fact that the Minority Report of the Poor Law Commission estimated that 11 000 children were born in workhouses in England and Wales in 1907.[6]

Rules and Regulations and Local Supervising Authorities

There was little point in drawing up rules and regulations unless they could be enforced, and to make sure that midwives followed the provisions of the Act and kept the rules of the Central Midwives Board, *Local Supervising Authorities* (LSAs) were set up. Their duty was to:

(1) Exercise general supervision over all midwives practising within their area, in accordance with the rules laid down under the Act.
(2) Investigate charges of malpractice, negligence or misconduct on the part of any midwife practising within their area, and, if a *prima facie* case was established, to report the same to the Central Midwives Board.
(3) Suspend any midwife from practice, in accordance with the rules under the Act, if such suspension appeared necessary in order to prevent the spread of infection.
(4) Report at once to the Board the name of any midwife practising in their area who was convicted of an offence.
(5) Keep available a list of midwives in their area who notified Intention to Practice, and to supply the names and addresses of midwives

who had notified their Intention to Practice to the Secretary of the Central Midwives Board in January of each year.

(6) Report at once any change of address or death of a midwife so that the Roll would always be up to date.

(7) Ensure that all women using the title of midwife were aware of the Act and of the existence of the Central Midwives Board and of its regulations.

These Local Supervising Authorities were the County Councils and County Borough Councils, who in turn had the right to delegate to District Councils, or to Committees which they themselves appointed. Some of these Authorities were without Medical Officers of Health to undertake supervision but some did appoint a doctor or a midwife as an Inspector; nevertheless, effective supervision was extremely difficult in many areas. Initially, even identification of midwives, especially in rural areas, was either not attempted or impracticable, and so supervision of practice was impossible. It is easy to imagine that quite a number of midwives were blissfully ignorant of the Act for a number of years after it had been passed, so that consequently their practice continued unchanged and unaffected by the Board and its rules and regulations. However, by contrast, midwives in the metropolis could avail themselves of lectures such as one given on 8 March 1904 by Dr Mary Rocke. Her lecture was entitled 'Tokology or Modern Methods to Secure Easy Labour' and for this she advocated 'hot baths in the last month of pregnancy, fresh air, exercise, diet and avoidance of constipation, very hot sitz baths in the first stage of labour, but enema and medication only if strongly indicated'.[7]

Public and Medical Views on the 'Professional' Midwife

Public interest in the midwife continued after the advent of certification and this was expressed by many comments, statements and letters to the general as well as to the medical press. One such comment in *The Hospital*, 7 May 1904, headed 'The 20th Century Midwife' revealed contemporary thinking on the subject.

In future, that is now the Central Midwives Board has regulations, we shall equal continental countries in our arrangements for this ancient and honourable employment of women. Down to the 18th Century accoucheurs were practically unknown, and the midwife always attended confinements, even in the Royal Family, therefore we are only regaining a lost stronghold when we ask that women should undertake this essential womanly work and we are merely protecting the mothers of the nation when we require that our midwives should be thoroughly trained and fairly intelligent and that they should know too much than too little.

Comment in the *County Council Times* (18 May 1904) showed that certification and registration were proving a financial embarrassment to some midwives. The Cerne Rural District Council was perturbed 'that the financial status of many of the midwives acting within their District among the artisan population was such that they were unable to pay the 10 shillings for registration which was required by the Central Midwives Board'. It was felt by this Rural District Council that as midwives gave a vital service to the poor of the District the Council should pay the registration fee on their behalf. However, the County Council advised that the local council had no power to do this and suggested that the problem should be put before the Central Midwives Board and the Rural Midwives Association.

Doctors continued with their prejudice against midwives, which was exacerbated by the fact that midwives now had some professional standing. A note under the heading 'The Midwives Act', which appeared in the *Medical Press* of 26 October 1904, reflected this prejudice.

It seems unlikely that the Midwives Act in its present form will ever become popular with the medical profession. One of its radical defects is experienced in the oft repeated assertion that it calls into being an inferior kind of unqualified medical practitioner.

The focus of their resentment appeared to be the unsatisfactory state of affairs with regard to payment of doctors' fees following the calling in of medical aid by the midwife for complicated cases. Under the Act the midwife was obliged to call medical assistance 'under certain scheduled conditions' (see page 181) but a vital flaw in the Act was the omission of provision for payment of the doctors' fees. The Honorary Secretaries of the Medical Guild had written to the Editor of the *Medical Press* on this matter, stating that the following resolution had been passed at a meeting of the Guild: 'That when medical practitioners choose to attend confinements at the request of midwives the minimum fee charged should be one guinea, to be paid at the time when possible.' They also stated that it was not compulsory for the doctor to obey the midwife's summons.

Publication of the First Roll of Midwives

In 1905 the time allowed for the enrolment of existing midwives had elapsed and the first Roll could be published. It contained 22 308 names, of which 9787 were those of midwives who had undertaken a course of midwifery training and 12 521 were *bona fide*.[8]

The Process of Change. Early Years of Regulation

Bona fide midwives, who constituted the majority on the Roll, therefore continued to make a large contribution to the country's maternity services. In effect, after the Act three sorts of midwives were in practice. One was the 'trained' midwife, who held a hospital Certificate or a London Obstetrical Society Diploma. The second was the *bona fide* midwife, who therefore became certificated by the Board. *Uncertificated* midwives fell into the third category and were allowed to continue in practice until 1905, the year specified in the Act when all those women not certified in any way must cease to assume the title of midwife. It is difficult to estimate just how many uncertificated midwives were in practice between 1902 and 1905, but concern was expressed that their demise might leave the poor in large cities without help. A leader writer in the *Liverpool Courier* of 7 March 1905 asked: 'when the ranks of the midwives are thinned out under the influence of the new law, will enough remain to fulfil the requirements of the lying-in woman?'

Supervision, or the prospect of it, was responsible for the self-elimination of many midwives (the number in Nottingham estimated as high as 60 per cent) who were worried about such simple requirements as having to supply themselves with washable dresses and other basic equipment.[9]

Quality of Practitioners: the Concern of Midwives

As in the past, certain midwives were expressing concern about the quality of midwives collectively and recognised that a large number of women were needed with 'enough education to grasp the responsibilities and scientific requirements of their calling'. Alice Gregory (Figure 20), who wrote this in a letter to the *Morning Post* (23 February 1905), was an interesting character. She was born in 1867 into a cultured professional family and her father, a clergyman, eventually became the Dean of St. Paul's Cathedral. She was an educated, well-travelled girl who 'trained' as a nurse and as a midwife. During her General Nursing Training, circumstances brought her face to face with morbidity and mortality

Figure 20: Alice Gregory (on left)

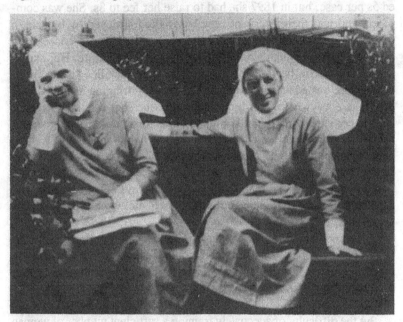

Courtesy: Independent Photography Project, Woolwich, London.

relating to childbirth, which, she perceived, was in no small measure due to the ineptitude and ignorance of 'old gamp' midwives. She was amazed that such practice existed and she resolved to qualify as a midwife and to join the growing number of educated women who were 'trained' and certified to practice. In 1895 she commenced midwifery training in London, which was of three months' duration and cost thirty guineas plus one guinea for board and lodging.

Alice Gregory was a District Midwife for eight years from 1896 in a busy mining area in the heart of rural Somerset. She expressed her enormous satisfaction from her work, which was enhanced by the pleasure she derived from the surrounding countryside. A book on her life emphasises the struggle for existence, both materially and professionally, still being experienced by midwives at the turn of the nineteenth century, and the relief when, in 1902, 'the State became the even-handed patron of the midwife guaranteeing her professional survival'. (In fact, though, the material struggle of the District Midwife was not relieved until she became a salaried employee of the Local Authority in 1936.)

In her first practice as a midwife to nine villages in Somerset, Alice charged 5s per case, but in 1897 she had to raise her fee to 8s. She was competent and was therefore kept very busy; she journeyed by bicycle in the daytime to attend her mothers and very often by pony and cart by night, the cost of which was her major item of expenditure. Her expertise meant that in her area of practice the old, unskilled 'gamp' midwives were ousted and she campaigned towards bringing a similar state of affairs everywhere. Her biographer describes her as a good teacher so it is not surprising that her ambition was to set up a training school for district midwives which she visualised as being annexed to a small general hospital. It was recognised very early that it was all too easy for the average country midwife, whom she described as 'a young woman of the cottage class', to regress to the old bad ways despite training and certification, and she hoped that her scheme would prevent this regression.[10]

Concerned about the lack of supply of adequately trained midwives in rural areas which was mentioned in a letter headed 'For Dwellers in Open Spaces', Alice Gregory replied to the Editor of the *Morning Post* on 23 February 1905 as follows:

But the difficulty of adequately training a sufficient number of women — women with enough education to grasp the responsibilities and scientific requirements of their training is a very great one. A movement is now on foot to establish a training school exclusively for district midwives, and those of a superior class. It is to be opened in Woolwich in May and I shall be delighted to supply particulars to anyone interested in the subject.

Because doctors were few and far between and difficult to contact in the country districts, Alice Gregory's experience had shown her the need for skilled midwives who were able to make clinical judgements and decisions.

An Omission in the Act Identified

In the *Lancet* of 1 April 1905 the following letter appeared.

Society of Apothecaries of London
[21 March 1905] At a meeting of the Court of Assistants the following resolutions were adopted:

(1) That steps be taken to urge upon the Government the desirability of the amendment to the Midwives Act 1902 in the following respects:

    a. by a provision for payment by the Local Authority of members of the medical profession called in by midwives in cases of danger or difficulty as defined by the rules framed by the CMB.

    b. by provision for payment to members of the Board of their reasonable travelling expenses and other disbursements incurred in connexion with their duties.

In the *Lancet* of 20 May 1905 a letter in a similar vein was published as follows:

The Midwives Act and the Payment of Fees to Medical Men

    We have been requested to publish the following resolution of the Islington Medical Society.

    That we, the members of the Islington Medical Society, are of opinion that immediate arrangements should be made under the Midwives Act in the interest of lying-in women of the poorer but not the pauper class for the prompt attendance of a registered medical man in cases of abnormality, and that the payment of such attendance should be made by the Metropolitan Borough Councils, or failing them by the County Council, with powers of recovery where this is possible.

Signed James G. Glover
Chairman

Supervision under the Act and what it Revealed

In August 1904, Manchester Corporation instituted a special committee — the Midwives Supervising Committee — which consisted of twelve members of the Council. It appointed a qualified medical practitioner to act under the supervision of the Medical Officer of Health as the 'Executive Officer' under the Act. Dr Margaret Merry Smith was appointed and was required to visit midwives 'both systematically and irregularly' and to see that their homes were in a sanitary condition, to examine their cases or bags of instruments, to ascertain that their case books were properly kept, and that they understood the use of antiseptics, and also to ensure that they were 'suitably provided in washable dresses'. She was also required to visit the cases attended by the midwives to 'satisfy herself that the requisite procedures' were carried out. A notice to the above effect appeared in the *Lancet* of 18 February 1905.

On 6 May 1905 the *Lancet* carried the Report of a Meeting of the Society of Medical Officers of Health. Dr J.F. Fosbroke, President, read a paper on the Midwives Act 1902. He reported that of 581 midwives in his own county of Worcestershire, every one of whom had been visited by him or his assistant, only 22 (4 per cent) had a certificate of any kind. Fosbroke recorded that 11 per cent were absolutely illiterate, 17 per cent were over 65 years, 8 per cent were very dirty, 16 per cent had no washable dresses, 10 per cent lived in filthy houses and 5 per cent were suspected of drink. He commented that although the CMB Rules and Recommendations were excellent in themselves, they had not been observed. The Medical Officer of Health for the West Riding of Yorkshire reported that 37 per cent of his midwives were 'absolutely illiterate'. He said that 'Numbers of those who had registered did not know what a thermometer was or how to use a catheter', and that their syringes were put away dirty and blood-stained.

In Rotherham 25% of the births in the years 1907 and 1908 were attended by 'old unqualified women'. One such woman, Granny Redman, dismissed the 'new fangled certified midwives' on the grounds that they didn't know much, how could they with only three months training.[11]

It is interesting that in a letter to the *Lancet* of 8 April 1905 the writer claimed that 'Liverpool is well supplied with qualified midwives. 70% have been trained at the Liverpool Lying-in Hospital whilst others hold the Certificate of the Obstetrical Society of London.'

Statutory Examinations for Midwives

The following statement, historical as far as English midwives were concerned, was made in the *British Journal of Nurses* and in *Nursing Echoes* on 4 March 1905.

It is officially announced that the examination of the London Obstetrical Society will henceforth be discontinued and intending candidates are referred to the Central Midwives Board which in June *will hold its first examination of midwives*. Nurses, who desire a certificate which testifies to their proficiency as *maternity nurses* will no doubt avail themselves of the examinations in maternity nursing, instituted by the British Gynaecological Society [our italics].

The *Medical Times* of 25 March 1905 stated that the Privy Council had approved the scheme of examinations prepared by the Central Midwives Board. The examinations were to be partly oral and partly written. The written examination was to consist of six questions and last three hours and the oral examination was to be of fifteen minutes' duration.

Review of the 1902 Act

In 1908 the working of the Midwives Act was reviewed by a Departmental Committee appointed by the Lord President of the Privy Council. Although the report was generally satisfactory, it recognised that the maternal and infant mortality rates were still high, and that there was need for continuing improvement in the training and standard of work of the midwife.

The bulk of the deliveries were still undertaken by midwives, who therefore carried out, almost single-handedly the responsibility for the prevention of avoidable morbidity and mortality. Blame was often laid at the midwife's door when things went wrong, when in fact the mortality or morbidity was frequently unavoidable, arising as it did from social, economic and intercurrent medical conditions. In addition, poverty, bad housing, uncontrolled infectious disease, poor diet and grande multiparity abounded, and in fact there was no significant decrease in mortality until the advent of antibiotics in the early 1950s, despite longer midwifery training, a salaried midwifery service, 'Flying Squads', intramuscular ergometrine, sulphonamides, blood transfusion, antenatal care and gradual social improvement.

Writing in *St. Bartholomew's Hospital Journal* in 1908 under the title 'Midwives in England', Sir Francis Champneys, Chairman of the Central Midwives Board, stated that rivalry between doctors and midwives still existed and that the midwives were in some places regarded as competitors rather than colleagues. The bad feeling was also created by money issues. He discussed the midwife's problems relating to mandatory calling-in of medical aid and the vexed question of payment of the doctor's fee. The midwife in some cases found herself responsible for paying these fees.

The Central Midwives Board brought this matter to the attention of the Privy Council with the recommendation that provision should be made for this payment out of public funds. However, nothing was done, and this unsatisfactory state of affairs persisted.

Attempts to Exclude Unqualified Midwives

The year 1910 was another milestone in the slow but sure evolution of the qualified midwife. From 1 April of that year, women who were not certified midwives were forbidden to attend women in childbirth 'habitually and for gain' *except* under the direction of a medical practitioner. Unfortunately, this effectively allowed many uncertified women to continue to practise with the collusion of doctors who were opposed to the Midwives Act and who were content to continue to allow untrained women to deliver their patients. Such doctors were not usually personally present at the delivery but could claim that handywomen acted under their directions. Where this practice came to light, the so-called midwife suffered a heavy penalty. An item in the *Staffordshire Sentinel* of 29 October 1910 cited such a case. An uncertified woman from Stafford attended three births in one month without a doctor being present. She charged 7s 6d per case, claiming that she did it to get money to pay a previous fine for the same offence! In her defence she stated that she wished to be trained as a midwife but that this was impossible as she could neither read nor write. The verdict was that this case was a 'flagrant breach of the law'.

Newspapers of the time carried stories of many women from different towns and counties, as far apart as Kent and Newcastle, who were fined for acting illegally as midwives. There does not appear to be any evidence of charges brought against colluding doctors.

Supervision of midwives was by now becoming more organised and widespread. The *British Medical Journal* of 20 August 1910 carried this account of supervision in Manchester.

> Inspector Dr Merry Smith paid 341 visits of inspection to examine the midwives' homes, bags, appliances and record books and investigated their mode of practice at the patients' homes. The very poor in the central districts are now sure of skilled care and attendance from midwives working directly in connection with St. Mary's Hospital and the poor women throughout the city can obtain medical aid when required *at the cost of the Corporation* (our italics).

Another letter, in response, stated that doctors' fees were similarly paid in Liverpool and Cardiff and by the Town Council in St. Helens.

Medical Aid — a Moral Dilemma

The payment of fees to the doctor when called by the midwife was, however, still a matter of great concern in many cases. Doctor, midwife and patient were in invidious positions as there was no guarantee that the doctor would receive his payment. Quite a few letters in the press highlighted the fact that some doctors refused to attend unless they were paid first. The problem remained unresolved as to where the money should come from when patients were too poor to pay a fee that far exceeded their weekly income.

The *British Medical Journal* of 3 September 1910 mentions the suggestion that the Boards of Guardians should, in the first instance, pay doctors' fees out of the Poor Rate but that the patient should be held liable for repayment of the fee. This suggestion had been incorporated into a Bill going through the House of Lords. There was, however, great opposition to the Poor Law Guardians having anything to do with midwifery cases and an appeal was successful, thus preventing the passing of the clause in the Bill. It was felt that the thrifty and self-respecting would suffer shame and indignity from any dealings with the Poor Law and the Relieving Officer.

CMB Annual Reports, 1909 and 1910

One of the requirements of the Act was Notification of Intention to Practice by individual midwives to the Local Supervising Authority, which was obliged to send these Returns each January to the Board. However, the Central Midwives Board Report of 1909 stated:

> The greatest difficulty has been experienced in getting these Returns, and it is obvious, that in some of the English counties and in at least half the Welsh, the Act is not being administered at all.

The Report for the year ending 31 March 1910 commented that the Reports of the Local Authority Medical Officers of Health showed, in many cases, a continued improvement in the old type of midwife still practising under their supervision, in respect of cleanliness, carefulness and observance of the rules. Supervisors were active, and the Report mentions 53 cases of malpractice, negligence or misconduct which had been reported to the Local Supervising Authorities. One midwife had been struck off the Roll for drunkenness!

The 1910 Report repeats the statement in the Report of 1909 regarding 'incompleteness of Returns', to the effect that it was 'impossible to estimate the number of practising midwives'. The conclusion drawn, however, was that there was 'no doubt that untrained practising midwives largely exceeded the trained'.

There were at that time 108 Institutions at which midwives could be trained under the rules of the Board, although four of these were in India and one in Hong Kong. Of the 103 in the United Kingdom half were in Poor Law Institutions. Only 57.3 per cent of the successful candidates practised, and 60 per cent of those intended to practise in rural areas.

Safe for Practice?

On 19 May 1911 the Central Midwives Board sent a circular to all examiners, recognised Training Schools, teachers, approved doctors and midwives, and various societies who trained midwives, clarifying the standard required for success in the examination. The examiners were asked to ensure that a candidate did not pass unless they were satisfied that she could be entrusted with the life and health of women in childbirth. This circular was in response to comments by some of the London examiners who were seeking guidance on the standard to be expected of the candidates. They were advised by the Board to ask themselves the question, 'Is she safe?'

The *Oldham Standard* of 4 August 1910 reported a case of a woman of 70 years who was charged with practising contrary to the Midwives Act of 1902. She had been struck off the Roll for negligence in 1908 so was no longer certified to practise. A similar case was reported at Royton. The midwives concerned were fined. Other local reports at the time seemed to highlight the fact that there were inequalities in midwives' skills and abilities. The *Carlisle Journal* of 26 July 1911 quoted the Report of the Inspector of Midwives for Cumberland as having visited all the midwives in the county and finding that the majority had 'no idea of cleanliness or use of antiseptics' and were unable to read a clinical thermometer. It is possible that, in isolated towns without a Midwifery Training School, even certificated midwives lacked incentive to evaluate and improve their standards.

The *Manchester Guardian* of 7 January 1911 reports the findings of an inquest on the body of an infant in Sheffield. It is of interest that the midwife who had been summoned to the case had not attended because she had not been paid her fee beforehand. This was in accordance with a decision made by the Sheffield Association of Midwives. The Coroner commented that 'out of humanity' she should have attended.

This cases focuses attention on the problem of non-payment of fees to midwives as well as to doctors, and the dilemma in which the midwife found herself. A sympathetic correspondent to the *British Journal of Nursing* had more to say about it. In the issue of the 8 July 1911 she wrote:

Midwives and the State

In reading over the Report of the Central Midwives Board I am glad to note that the Committee recognises that midwifery is women's work. There has been a lot of talk about women taking men's work, but in the case of midwifery, men have certainly monopolised the cream of women's work until it is now scarcely fashionable not to have a doctor in attendance at such a time . . .

Their work is most depressing, and to be badly paid makes it a hundred times worse, and they are expected to do a great deal more than any doctor would ever think of doing. In my opinion the Central Midwives Board are most exacting in their rules laid down for midwives, and I sometimes wonder if the same rules are laid down for doctors, because I am sure doctors do not carry these rules out.

M. Atkinson

Training and Clinical Practice

In 1911 the training was still of three months' duration and pupil midwives had to undertake 20 deliveries. They had to care for the mother during her labour and personally deliver her; they had to make abdominal and vaginal examinations during the course of labour; and had to nurse 20 women in the lying-in period and their babies during the first ten days following labour.[12]

The Central Midwives Board introduced a new rule in 1912 which made it obligatory for the midwife to take and record the pulse rate and temperature of the patient at each visit. The Board had been made aware that after repeated instruction by the Local Supervising Authorities some midwives had been found to be incapable of learning how to take a temperature with safety. Therefore, mindful of the fact that this would involve the compulsory removal of a considerable number of untrained women who had been certified under the Act, they deemed it necessary to introduce this rule.

In the Report for the year ending 31 March 1912 the Board mentioned that they were continuing to receive complaints about the prevalence
of midwifery practice by uncertified women. They admitted that difficulties in the way of a successful prosecution were due to the words
'habitually and for gain' which occur in Section 1(2) of the 1902 Midwives Act and which 'however desirable they might have been thought
when the Act was passed in 1902 appear now to be unnecessary and
hampering in the administration of the Act'. Such 'midwives' however
justified their attendance under the emergency-case clause. The Report
also contained extracts of Reports of several County Medical Officers
of Health, each declaring that a much higher standard than formerly had
been attained by county midwives but that there was still room for improvement. Some reported 'distinct signs of improvement'.

Local Initiative on Doctors' Fees

As the matter of payment of doctors' fees was still not resolved, the doctors belonging to the Chesterfield branch of the British Medical Association decided, in 1912, to take the matter into their own hands and to
make a local ruling. This involved sending a memorandum to every midwife practising in the borough, informing them that from 1 August 1912
emergency medical assistance would not be given unless they had prior
confirmation in writing that the midwife had secured, at booking, a retaining fee from the patient for such a contigency.[13] This created a storm
of protest and the midwives naturally contacted the Central Midwives
Board for guidance. The midwives were informed that the CMB had
no control over the medical profession and so were unable to become
directly involved in any attempt to reverse the doctors' directive. The
midwives were advised, however, that their only course of action was
to continue to obey the rule regarding the calling-in of medical aid in
an emergency. This advice would be of little help to midwives in the
practical situation. 'Technical' fulfilment of her legal obligation would
be secondary to the midwife's human concern for the lives of her patients who may not have been able to afford the retaining fee and who
therefore could be denied medical assistance. The midwives were,
however, supported in their appeal to the Central Midwives Board by
one of the Chesterfield general practitioners who asked what right the
doctors had to threaten the midwives and possibly deprive them of a
livelihood.[13] The Executive Committee of the General Medical Council

made a recommendation that the GMC should transmit to the Privy Council an expression of its strong disapproval of the Chesterfield resolution, but added: 'the fact that doctors often had to attend emergency maternity cases without remuneration was the fault, not of the Statutory bodies, but an omission in the law'.[14]

A Glimpse of Midwifery Practice

A contemporary text book[15] reflects the teaching and practice of the day in respect of intra- and post-partum care. Under the heading 'Posture of the Patient', the following advice about the first stage of labour was given: 'Let her please herself, provided no abnormal conditions are present.' Vaginal examination was to be kept to a minimum to avoid infection. It is interesting that there is no mention of pain relief. In the section on the second stage the midwife was instructed to tie a roller towel to the end of the bed and put a footstool or doubled-up bolster at the foot of the bed so that the patient could bend her legs and rest her feet against it. The patient was to grasp the towel during a contraction and press her feet against the footstool. 'The effect of the pain may be helped by the pressure of the midwife's hands or *knee* against the patient's back.' The author stressed that the perineum could be preserved by 'delivering the head *between* uterine contractions [our italics]'. In the section on the third stage of labour the midwife was advised not to ligature the cord until it had stopped pulsating and had 'collapsed'. The pupil midwives were told that uterine contractions would effect the separation of the placenta and its descent into the upper part of the vagina within an hour of birth. Extrusion from the vagina, they were told, would take two or three hours if left to nature, so 'in the majority of cases the midwife herself must express the placenta from the vagina'. They were reminded of the Midwife's Rule that medical assistance must be sent for 'where two hours after the birth of the child the placenta and membranes have not been completely expelled'. After the delivery the midwives were to apply *to the mother* an abdominal binder 'broad enough to reach from trochanters to xiphoid cartilage, and long enough to go one and a half times round the body'.

In the section on the puerperium the teaching was that the patient should remain in bed until the twelfth day. Solid food was generally to be withheld until the bowels had been opened. 'The midwife must give directions for the proper dieting of the patient and should order at first easily digested foods, for example simple soups, beef tea, albumen water, white of egg, gruel, cocoa, weak tea; if solids be allowed thin bread and butter, dry toast and soft-boiled eggs could be given.'

The following advice was given with regard to visiting. 'Patients are always the better for absolute quietude during the first week; it is therefore advisable that the husband only should be allowed to make a visit in the lying-in room'. After the first week, other relatives were to be allowed to see the patient 'but only one at a time'.

Breast and bottle feeding are discussed within the book. All feeding was 'scheduled'. As far as breast feeding was concerned:

> the baby should be put to the breast every *six* hours during the first 24 hour period; every *four* hours during the second 24 hour period; on the third day the two-hourly feeds should be begun. Although the child is only obtaining a little colostrum, yet it is being taught how to suck, and it is receiving its first lesson in discipline and regularity.

Wartime Midwifery

On 4 August 1914 England became involved in the first World War. The absence of male doctors (away in the Medical Corps) made ever-increasing demands on the time and skills of midwives. An experienced Inspector of Midwives at the time felt that her profession was being exploited, and her letter to the *Lancet* of 26 February 1916 included the following statement.

> When one considers there is no profession in the world of more importance to humanity, none on which the future of the race is so dependent, then it is a matter of surprise to find there is no profession more heavily handicapped or which meets with less encouragement in the performance of its duties. The midwife leads an arduous and harrowing existence. In several counties there is still a strong feeling against the midwife who essays to take cases without a doctor. The medical man is jealous of what he believes to be his privilege and will not tolerate any encroachment thereon. At present the midwives who lead the most tolerable lives are those salaried and protected by the Nursing Associations and kindred bodies. Whether a comprehensive scheme on the lines and under the aegis of a nursing organ could be evolved is a matter for consideration.

Inspector of Midwives (5 years' experience)

The need for an increasing supply of well-qualified midwives, as a result of the shortage of doctors and medical students away on active service, was stressed in the *British Medical Journal* of 17 February 1917.

> This journal has always held in high honour the office of midwife believing it to be one of the utmost value to the community when rightly discharged, and which affords useful and satisfying employment for women. The only satisfactory solution for midwives is to be appointed and subsidised by the State and the Local Authorities within measurable distance. This will give the midwife an honourable position and will consequently attract desirable women to enter the ranks.

Longer Training

In the middle of the war, midwifery training was doubled in length from three to six months, although for qualified nurses the training was of four months' duration. The new syllabus for the lengthened training included the following additional subjects:

The elementary anatomy *and physiology* of the female pelvis and its organs.
Pregnancy: its hygiene, its diseases and complications, including abortion (in relation to both the mother and the unborn child).
The venereal diseases (syphilis and gonorrhoea) in relation to their signs, symptoms and dangers in women and children and to the risks of contagion to others.
Elementary physiology, and the principles of hygiene and sanitation as regards home, food and person.
The care of children born apparently lifeless.

By 1917 the Central Midwives Board had recognised 129 Institutions for training in England and Wales. Of these, 16 were in London and 66 were Poor Law Infirmaries. It is interesting that these Infirmaries were not required to fulfil the same conditions for training as non Poor Law Hospitals, which in fact were exempted from the supervision of the Central Midwives Board.[16] This was because they were inspected instead by the Local Government Boards. The Poor Law Institutions in many towns (such as Nottingham, Preston, Rotherham, Stoke-on-Trent, Swansea, Wigan, Wolverhampton, Middlesbrough, Blackpool, Darwen and Blackburn) were the only Institutions with provisions for maternity cases.[17]

Maternity Provision within Hospitals

Up to 1914, with the few exceptions where mothers *booked* a hospital bed (for example at St. Mary's Hospitals, Manchester),[18] almost all the work of maternity hospitals was performed on an emergency basis. Few of the patients would have been seen before and there would be no antenatal records. Only if some major complication arose would patients be sent to hospital, so when they were admitted many would be found to be suffering from such serious conditions as eclampsia, obstructed labour, or massive haemorrhage. Many complications such as pre-eclampsia, anaemia and heart disease passed unrecognised; multiple pregnancies and malpresentations were nearly always dealt with by the midwife in the patient's own home.[19]

Beginnings of Antenatal Care

Early in the century, antenatal care was given at St. Mary's Hospitals, Manchester, following 'booking-in' by the patient. In 1909 a small antenatal clinic was set up in Queen Charlotte's Hospital in London, and in 1915 the first antenatal clinic was started in the Simpson Maternity Hospital, Edinburgh. However, 'the proportion of pregnant women receiving antenatal care in 1915 was incalculably small'.[20] After this date the number of antenatal clinics rose steadily and the concept of antenatal care became commonplace. After the Maternal and Child Welfare Act of 1918, local-authority maternal and child welfare centres, which provided facilities for antenatal clinics, increased in number, and the uptake of antenatal care improved significantly. By 1917 Liverpool Maternity Hospital had an organised ante-natal clinic with nine sub-centres in different parts of the town,[17] but hospital records show 'out-patient' attendance as early as 1869.[21]

Report on the Physical Welfare of Mothers and Children and the Role of the Midwife

In 1917 a Report was commissioned by the Carnegie United Kingdom Trust on the *Physical Welfare of Mothers and Children* (Figure 21).[17] This, written by Dr Janet Campbell, had much to say about the calling, contribution and conditions of service of midwives. The following is an extract from her Report, which sums up the Committee's considered view of the position of the midwife.

Figure 21: Mothers at Mothercraft Class, 1917

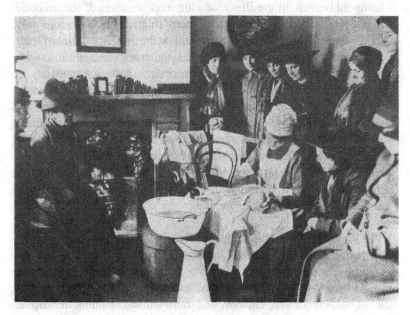

Source: Janet Campbell, *The Physical Welfare of Mothers and Children*.

The midwife occupies an exceptional position in the nursing profession in that she is called upon during her ordinary work to be directly responsible for the lives of two patients, mother and child. The most apparently straightforward case may unexpectedly develop complications, and a safe and satisfactory sequel often depends entirely on the watchfulness, skill, resourcefulness and good judgement of the midwife. Her work makes large claims upon health, time and leisure. For the single-handed midwife there is no such thing as being 'off-duty'. She must respond by day or night, if called; she must never relax her vigilant alertness, must often forego rest, food, relaxation, while always there is the anxious fear of danger to her patient which may result in disaster if she fails to exercise a wise discretion. The highest devotion and self-sacrifice are demanded from her, and she needs a high sense of vocation and a love for her profession for its own sake to enable her cheerfully to meet her numerous difficulties. It is small wonder that many are unwilling to incur these responsibilities, and choose an easier form of service. But apart from the inherent disabilities of the work, the midwife suffers from other disadvantages which are not always fully appreciated, but which serve to

explain much of the disinclination of educated women to become practising midwives. In the first place the relative status of the midwife
is not high. There are admittedly many inferior midwives not only
barely capable of fulfilling what should be the ordinary duties of their
profession, but altogether unable to respond to any demand for a wider
interpretation of these duties. Unfortunately there is a tendency to
regard these women as the typical midwives, and to expect no more
than they can give, instead of looking upon the excellent work of
educated and highly trained midwives as the true standard of attain-
ment desirable, and endeavouring to raise the general capacity to this
level. Greater efficiency and skill will certainly be forthcoming if the
right steps are taken to encourage this. The old stigma attached to
the term *midwife* will disappear, and the title will receive the respect
and recognition which are its due.

The Report therefore highlights the tremendous responsibilities of the
midwife and her long hours and inadequate remuneration. The average
fee charged at this time was 10s 6d to multiparous women and 15s to
primigravidae. Although training had been increased to six months, this
was not considered long enough, and more clinical teaching in hospital
was recommended for such subjects as breast and bottle feeding, baby
care and antenatal care, which required midwives to have more
knowledge of the course of pregnancy, and of palpation, etc. The midwife also had to be aware of wider issues such as social legislation. The
Report pointed out that the training and clinical experience of some of
the pupil midwives was unfortunately entirely district-based. It was realised that in order to practise efficiently in the community, and to be able
to adapt and improvise in the home, the midwife needed to have had
experience in hospital of the diagnoses and management of complications. Without this, it was felt, a newly qualified midwife should not
be allowed to practise single-handed until she had had at least one month's
'protected' practice in hospital. It was also recognised that on-going
education was necessary after certification, and in fact several hospitals
throughout the country were already arranging courses of lectures some
of which were given by experienced midwives. Some of these program-
mes were arranged locally by Midwives' Associations (affiliated to the
Midwives Institute). Midwifery was developing, changing and widening with the advent of antenatal care and antenatal in-patient hospital
facilities, changes in feeding patterns and in infant management; so much
so that it was sometimes difficult for a midwife to keep in touch with
the modern developments in her profession. It was felt that she should

keep up to date with books, reports and government circulars through a library.

The Report showed that there were independent practitioners who could not afford holiday breaks, and that ten-day postnatal visiting by midwives was usual. Midwives' fees in rural areas in Wales varied from 5s to £1 if the midwife undertook monthly nursing also. The Report also revealed that *bona fide* midwives were still in practice, and it mentioned that in rural areas doctors connived with handywomen to defy the Midwives Act; thus totally unqualified lay women continued to deliver women of the poorer classes.

Legislation Affecting Midwives, and a Second Act

A State Insurance Scheme had been in existence since the passing of the National Insurance Act in 1911. This entitled the low-paid worker who made a weekly compulsory payment to the services of a 'panel doctor' and to sickness and maternity benefits. Nevertheless, in many cases if the doctor had to be called, the midwife still had to hold herself responsible for his payment initially.

By 1915, Notification of Birth after the 28th week of pregnancy had become compulsory. Although the midwife was not charged specifically to undertake the duty of notifying the Medical Officer of Health, it nevertheless became the standard practice that she did so, and consequently this created problems for her in terms of the cost of postage stamps.

An Act to amend the Midwives Act 1902 was passed in 1918 and was effective from 1 January 1919. One of the most important principles of the second Midwives Act was to place responsibility for payment of the doctor's fee and mileage expenses on the Local Authority in the first instance, which fee was to be recovered from the patient, if possible. The midwife's finances and expenses received consideration, and as a result of the new Act she was compensated for loss of earnings if suspended from practice, particularly if the suspension was because she was liable to be a source of infection. All forms and books which the midwife was required to possess and complete were provided free under the Act and the postage was paid for all statutory notification forms. This Act also gave power to the Central Midwives Board to suspend midwives for disobeying the rules: previously the only punishment was the severe one of removing their names from the Roll. In cases of alleged misconduct the midwife would be suspended pending the hearing of the case.

The Report on the Work of the Central Midwives Board for the year ending 31 March 1921 recorded that 68 penal cases were heard during the year. These led to 39 names being removed from the Midwives Roll, 25 of which were those of women who had neglected to call medical assistance in cases of inflammation of babies' eyes.

Social and Working Conditions

The effects of World War I were reflected in the social and industrial unrest of the decade between 1920 and 1930 which followed the unfulfilled promise of a post-war utopia. There was anxiety because of the high unemployment, and wages fell as the decade progressed. Conditions were at their worst, and felt the most bitterly, by workers in the coal-mining industry, where, because the Government withdrew its subsidy, wages fell steeply but hours of work were lengthened. This exacerbated the unrest which culminated finally in the General Strike and a miners' strike of six months' duration.

Midwives working in large industrial cities and in rural areas (where farming was also a depressed industry) delivered and nursed women who lived in dilapidated houses and whose famlies were extremely deprived. The diet of the pregnant woman was totally inadequate and lacking in variety and nutriment. As well as sometimes giving their services free of charge, the midwives often provided the bare necessities of life — warmth, clothing and food — for their patients, during the time they were in professional attendance. The Ministry of Health was empowered to make grants to local authorities and voluntary organisations 'in respect of provision of a midwife for necessitous women in confinement' for areas that were insufficiently supplied with midwives.[22]

Enquiry into Training of Midwives

In 1923 Dr Janet Campbell wrote another Report for the Ministry of Health. This time the subject of her enquiry was the training of midwives.[16] The introduction stated that more than 50 per cent of the cases of childbirth occurring in England and Wales were attended solely by midwives. It claimed that more practising midwives were needed possessing a 'higher average of competency' to reduce maternal mortality and morbidity. The mortality rate was almost static in the fifteen years between 1907 and 1922 at almost four per thousand births.

Embodied within the Report were the findings of a survey undertaken by Dr June Turnbull, a Ministry of Health Inspector. She inspected 71 schools of midwifery to investigate how and what pupil midwives were taught, both in theory and in practice, and the equipment and drugs in current use. She found that the use of gloves for internal examinations and deliveries by midwives was rare, and their use even rarer by doctors! Sterilisation of instruments and dressings was 'hit and miss' and it was learnt that in 25 of the schools the material for dressings was 'baked and boiled'. Turnbull reported that the drugs available for use by midwives were ergot, chloral, nepenthe, opium, quinine and pituitrin, but the only drug found to be in common use was ergot. At this time, whereas domiciliary experience was an obligatory part of the training (with very few exceptions), hospital experience was not. In fact 16 out of the 71 training schools could not provide 'intern' experience. This was recognised to be a serious deficiency in the training of midwives.

In addition to these findings it was becoming generally recognised that midwifery training needed to be further lengthened because 'many women are never seen by a doctor', and partly because it was felt that a longer period of training was required in order for the midwife to acquire and retain both the theoretical and practical skills taught. This applied particularly to those midwives who had had limited general education. The extent of the midwife's practice was being enlarged and now included antenatal and more postnatal care, the latter having previously been undertaken in the main by handywomen and monthly nurses. There is substantial evidence in the Report to show that, despite the establishment of antenatal clinics in maternity hospitals, large numbers of women who delivered at home or in nursing homes were not examined even once during pregnancy by either doctor or midwife. In consequence, the number of maternal deaths from infection, which resulted from emergency operative manipulations, remained high. This interference was frequently necessary as a result of such conditions as belated recognition of cephalo-pelvic disproportion.

The cost of training was met by the pupil midwife, but in 1919, for the first time, the Treasury had agreed to make a contribution. A grant of £20 was payable to each pupil midwife who guaranteed to practise on qualification.

Before a decision could be made to change the length and scope of the midwifery course, consideration had to be given to the financial implications: if the training were lengthened, it would mean that the pupil midwife would have to pay double the amount for tuition and board-and-lodging fees, following which she could reasonably expect to receive a higher fee for her professional services. However, this would mean an increased cost to the patient, which many of the poorer women would not be able to afford.

It was apparent that midwifery training at this time was less than uniform and in fact somewhat haphazard. It was being carried out through the following agencies:

Maternity wards of general and lying-in hospitals and their associated extern districts.
Maternity homes subsidised by the Ministry of Health.
Poor Law Institutions (not subject to the supervision of the CMB).
District Nursing Associations.
Practising independent midwives approved as practical teachers by the CMB.

It is obvious that the standard of both practical and theoretical teaching, and the experience available, varied enormously in scope and adequacy, and that the Central Midwives Board regulations for training should apply also to Poor Law Institutions, hitherto exempt. The proposal was to increase the length of training to six months (instead of four) for trained nurses, and to twelve months in the case of direct-entry pupils.

Although the syllabus now included instruction in antenatal investigations and examinations, there was doubt, even at this early stage in antenatal care, as to which professionals should be responsible for the carrying out of the necessary investigations and physical examinations. Such investigations, rudimentary compared with present-day screening, included external pelvic measurements and urinanalysis but not blood-pressure estimations. One view was that every pregnant woman should be examined at least once by an obstetric specialist, but it was realised that this was an unattainable goal. Another view was that whoever was booked for the delivery, whether doctor or midwife, should themselves be held responsible for full antenatal examinations and care. The Central Midwives Board, while agreeing that antenatal investigations should fall within the remit of the midwife, nevertheless laid upon her the duty of reporting certain antenatal disorders to the doctor. It was also recognised that the establishment of breast feeding, the care of the breasts and the management of disorders and feeding difficulties were particularly the province of the midwife, as was the physical care of the normal neonate, although postnatal care was not at this time a statutory duty upon the midwife. Such care was given by midwives who worked in hospital, and possibly in some cases by midwives who had conducted home confinements especially in middle-class areas. Nevertheless, monthly nurses and handywomen (who were still acting as doctors' 'midwifery assistants' at delivery) were also still undertaking postnatal nursing in many cases. The situation of unqualified handywomen conducting the delivery without the doctor being present but with his approval persisted, and such deliveries were often then labelled BBA (Born before Arrival) or 'emergency delivery'. The General Medical Council at this time drew the attention of doctors to the Midwives Act of 1902 and reminded them that attendance at childbirth by unqualified persons, even with their consent, was an offence for which the doctor could face serious professional consequences, even removal from the Medical Register. In spite of this warning, doctors continued to allow unqualified 'midwives' to act as their substitutes. The birth of one of the authors took place at home in the suburbs of a large city in 1922. The doctor had been booked but on the day of confinement he was away at the races and so his totally unqualified handywoman conducted the birth single-handed. The delivery was normal but she left the retained placenta to be removed by the doctor on his return! (This procedure was completed uneventfully at home.)

Maternity nurses were still being trained and allowed to undertake the duties of a midwife under the 'care' of a doctor (Figure 22a). It is interesting that Nurse Annie Clark (Figure 22a) received her training under the auspices of the Cottage Benefit Nursing Association and that this training was three-quarters the length of the course leading to qualification as a midwife (Figure 22b).

At this time, theoretical teaching by midwives varied from the excellent to the barely adequate, and there were no qualified tutors and no courses for prospective midwife teachers. Such courses were being envisaged, and in 1926 courses for selected candidates were held at the Midwives Institute, followed by an examination for a Midwife Teachers Certificate.

In 1923, as in her 1917 Report, Dr Janet Campbell remarked:

> the work of a busy midwife is very hard, holidays and off duty times are difficult to secure, the responsibility is exceptionally grave, and the remuneration comparatively small. Midwifery, more than any other branch of nursing, unquestionably taxes to the utmost professional skill and judgement, physical capacity and endurance, patience and sympathy.[17]

She recommended an improvement in the 'status and position' of the

Figure 22a: Doctor Authorising Maternity Nurse Annie Clark to Undertake the Duties of a Midwife under his Care

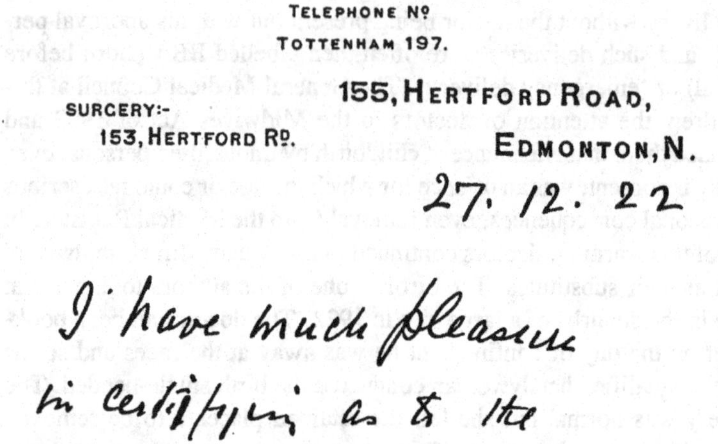

TELEPHONE Nº
TOTTENHAM 197.

SURGERY:-
153, HERTFORD Rᴰ.

155, HERTFORD ROAD,
EDMONTON, N.

27. 12. 22

I have much pleasure in certifying as to the Ability & attention of Nurse Annie Clark in mid wifery attendance under my Care

H Evans
LRCP, S⟍ᵃ

midwife as compensation for her arduous professional life. She commented that 'no doctor is in a position to render to the mothers the many-sided help which the good midwife can offer', and if midwives willing to practice diminished in numbers, we should inevitably 'fall back into the hands of unqualified nurses'.

Figure 22b: Nurse Annie Clark's Certification

Cottage Benefit Nursing Association,

Denison House, 296, Vauxhall Bridge Road, Victoria, S.W.

Telegraphic Address—" ALLATINO, LONDON."

This is to Certify that *Annie Clark*

Fairholme

Middleton Rd, Rotherham

Spinster ⎤
Wife ⎬ born *5 June 1886*
Widow ⎦ was given a course of training in *maternity*

Nursing for a term of *three months* from *18 July 1921*
at *the Maternity Branch 260 Fore St. Edmonton,*
of the Cottage Benefit Nursing association. The
Home is approved by the Central Midwives Board and the
Board of Education
and that she afterwards served as COTTAGE NURSE under the Branch Benefit Nursing Association of
The Cottage Nurses Training Home, Institute
Bury House, Bury St. Edmonton

Further Legislation

The third Midwives Act was passed in 1926. It was known that uncertificated women were still deliberately flouting the law and acting as midwives, sometimes with the agreement of doctors, and very often still
using the pretext that they were called upon in an 'emergency'; therefore
the 1926 Act once more attempted to put a stop to this practice by requiring them to satisfy the court that 'the attention was given in a case
of sudden or urgent necessity'. If this proved not to be the case, they
would be liable to a fine, which could be as much as £10 — a not inconsiderable sum at that time.

The Act also authorised the CMB to divide the Roll of Midwives into
two parts: a Roll of practising midwives and one of non-practising midwives. It also provided, possibly belatedly, for the registration of maternity homes. It is likely that some maternity homes were quite unsuitable
premises with poor-quality staff (probably not certified midwives) giving an inadequate standard of care, and whose record-keeping left a lot
to be desired. The Act aimed to remedy this by requiring maternity homes
to be registered with the Local Supervising Authority, which was empowered to lay down conditions relating to the building itself, to the

amenities, equipment and staff, and to the keeping of records, particularly of births, infections, deaths and causes of death. The homes had to be open to inspection by the LSA.

A Matter of Concern to Independent Midwives

The 1927 Report of the Central Midwives Board stated their policy with regard to midwives advertising their services. Evidently some of the independent district midwives felt a need to do this, which suggests that their livelihood was being reduced by the State system which now provided free antenatal care under the 1918 Maternal and Child Welfare Act, and also by general practitioners 'creaming off' the wealthier clients. It is noteworthy that the Board decided that:

> midwives ought to aim at a standard of conduct which increases, rather than diminishes the dignity of their profession. From this point of view all advertising is to be deprecated and the midwives ought to be satisfied with a plate on their doors, and cards.

Plates outside the doors of domiciliary midwives became commonplace but only for identification purposes (Figure 23).

In 1924, the majority of midwives were district practitioners, attending women, mainly from the lower social classes, in their own homes and receiving fees for their services from those who could afford to pay. Eighty-five per cent of births in 1927 took place at home, and only 15 per cent in institutions.[23] Midwives' annual earnings ranged from £30 per annum to £350 in 1929.[24]

The Training and Conditions for Midwives Considered Again in a Departmental Report

In 1928 a further Government Committee was commissioned 'to consider the working of the Midwives Act 1902–1926 with particular reference to the training of midwives (including its relation to the education of medical students in midwifery) and the conditions under which midwives are employed'. They produced a comprehensive survey and report the following year.[25]

The Committee addressed themselves to the following two vital questions. First, what form of midwifery service should be aimed at in this

Figure 23: Midwife's Plate

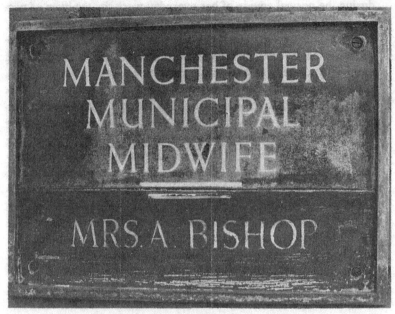

Source: Photographed by J. Towler (author), with permission.

country? Secondly, what place therein should the midwife be given?

In attempting to outline the ideal provision for maternity care they decided that this should consist of a

> comprehensive service organised on a local basis in which the midwife, the doctor and the specialist should each have their part. *The midwife as the person responsible in the majority of cases for the care of the mother throughout pregnancy, confinement and the puerperal period is the one upon whom the main burden would rest*. In all such cases there should be available the services of a doctor, with certain well defined duties towards the mother, to whom the midwife should be able at all times to look for assistance when she is faced with difficulties beyond her ordinary competence and skill, and an obstetric specialist would be called in by the doctor to deal with *exceptional* emergencies [our italics].

The Committee reiterated views expressed in previous reports that

> The midwife occupies an exceptionally responsible position in the life of the community compared with women employed in the allied

branches of the nursing profession, since she is directly answerable during the normal course of her everyday work for the lives of two patients, mother and child. She must at all times, by night and day, exercise untiring vigilance if the trust placed in her skill is not to be betrayed. Night calls, absence of adequate rest and recreation, and often of opportunity to take proper nourishment, are her portion. This is by no means all. There is the ever-present anxiety that failure to exercise a wise discretion may result in not only disaster to her patients, but also in severe disciplinary action, involving possibly the withdrawal of licence to practice, on the part of those responsible for supervising her work. If she is an independent midwife, her practice is in the large majority of cases not sufficiently remunerative to allow her to employ trained assistance, so that she must depend entirely on her own physical resources to carry out the onerous duties that fall to her charge. She can expect no relief when sickness falls upon her, nor can she look to the State for financial assistance on such occasions, in that she is debarred by reason of the conditions of her employment from becoming an insured contributor under the scheme of National Health Insurance.

It seems clear that at this time many women were depriving themselves of professional supervision by only deeming it necessary to make arrangements for the actual confinement, unaware that the outcome of this event depended to a large extent upon investigations, examinations and attention to their general health throughout their pregnancies. The Committee therefore expressed the conviction that the services of the midwife, GP and obstetric specialist should be provided *free of charge* at the time but linked to the National Insurance Scheme.

The Committee was concerned that the maternal mortality rate had not fallen over the past ten years; they recognised, however, that although an improvement in the standard of care given by midwives would be a desirable objective, even the achievement of a perfect standard of midwifery practice would not *per se* materially reduce the high maternal mortality rate. In their opinion, what was required was 'measures of a wider character to deal with the problem, on a broad, even on a national basis'. This would presumably include their 'model' of optimum care, i.e. the involvement of GP and obstetric specialist when appropriate.

The pupil midwife was not at this time required to have attained a specified academic level before being acceptable for training, but the establishment of a common educational entrance test was being recommended by those organisations representing midwives. The Committee also recognised the need to raise the educational standard of the entrants to midwifery training because the quality and capability of the midwives would determine their future status and position. An improved status would itself attract a better calibre of woman into the profession. The Committee stated on several occasions that it would be in the national interest to improve the status and responsibility of the midwife.

Midwife or Nurse Midwife? The question was raised as to whether entrance to midwifery training should be limited to trained nurses or remain open to direct entrants, and this issue is still unresolved today. It was advocated that the 6 months' training for qualified nurses should be extended to a year and that the 12 months' training for non-nurses to two years.

Emerging Deficiencies in Education. Because of the isolation of many midwives and the changing and increasing range of skills and knowledge required, the suggestion of post-certificate courses was made. This proposal was the precursor of the Statutory Refresher Course (1936). It was also suggested that a clinical element should be introduced into the qualifying examination. This is surprising in view of the fact that the CMB Rules had required that 'the examination shall be partly oral and practical and partly written' since 1903. Although a few midwife teachers had taken the examination of the Midwives Institute, many had not had such an opportunity. The Committee therefore felt that the time was ripe to establish a prescribed course, examination and diploma for all potential midwife teachers.

Conditions of Employment, 1929

The midwives practising in rural areas were employed mainly by Nursing Associations such as the Queen's Institute for District Nursing. Prospective midwives were sent for training by this body in return for a year's service in a place determined by the Association. The minimum commencing salary of a Queen's Nurse/Midwife was £68 per year plus £8 per year for uniform and an allowance for accommodation and laundry. Village nurse-midwives were engaged and trained by County Nursing Associations and supplied to affiliated Nursing Associations. They were not fully qualified as Queen's Nurses or even as nurses, but some nevertheless acted in a dual capacity. Their minimum salary was £30 to £40 a year, with allowance for board, lodging, uniform and laundry.

They had to practice in a designated area for at least two years.

Statistics provided by the Ministry of Health to this Committee showed an unevenness in the provision of midwifery care in that 20 per cent of the rural population of England had no access to the services of trained midwives. Perhaps this could be explained by the fact that midwives established themselves primarily in urban areas where there were enough cases to guarantee a reasonable income. This led to a state of affairs in which there were none in some rural area, where, according to the Report (and not surprisingly), doctors were still colluding with handywomen. However, some midwives agreed to practise in certain rural areas, where, for whatever reason, there was no midwife, on condition that the local authority would subsidise their income.

It is apparent that the number of home confinements attended by individual midwives varied enormously between extremes of 250 per year to as few as 10 per year; however, it is obvious that midwives attending so few cases were not dependent upon midwifery as their sole source of income. Returns of the Society of Medical Officers of Health disclosed that in the County Borough areas the average number of home confinements per midwife per annum ranged from 29 to 72. Evidence showed that in some of the smaller boroughs and certain urban areas, e.g. mining districts, mothers were unwilling to engage a midwife, preferring the cheaper services of the traditional uncertified midwife.

Fees charged by the midwives seemed to vary throughout the country between the highest fee of 50s for a primigravida and 35s for second and subsequent confinements, to 25s for a primigravida and 16s for a multipara. On many occasions the midwife working in a poor area received nothing for her services, and although by this time local authorities were empowered to protect the midwife against loss in these circumstances, few did so. Concern was expressed that the better trained and better educated midwives were choosing to return to nursing, which offered better prospects and where they were better paid for less arduous and less responsible work.

At this time midwives were variously employed: in maternity hospitals (voluntary hospitals); in maternity departments of Poor Law Infirmaries (about to be renamed Local Authority or Municipal Hospitals under the Local Government Act 1929); in maternity departments of large Board of Governor Hospitals; and in small maternity homes and newly built small hospitals; or as district midwives employed by local authorities as municipal midwives, by nursing associations, or as independent (self-employed) practitioners, or, finally, attached to large teaching hospitals.

According to the Midwives Institute, who gave evidence to the

Committee, the average earnings of independent midwives (the majority of those 'on the district') was between £90 and £120 per year. For this small sum they worked very long hours with little time off or holidays because of the absence of relief even for sickness. Out of her income the midwife was obliged to buy her own equipment, drugs, dressings and uniform. Should she have to refer her patient for admission to hospital during pregnancy, or transfer her during labour, then she was involved in financial loss. Inevitably, but understandably, some midwives booked more cases than they could actually and properly cope with. It is hardly surprising that few of the better educated women chose district midwifery as a profession because of its very exacting nature.

Several suggestions were put forward with the aim of improving the lot of the independent midwife. One was to impose a limitation on the number of cases each midwife attended to a maximum of 100 per year. This was, however, a difficult problem because a cut in the physical workload would result in a cut in income. However, because in many areas midwives had to compete for cases, not all achieved even this number. Obviously the standard of care given was also of great importance, and so another suggestion was an increase in the minimum fee charged by midwives for their services and possibly a *subsidy* by the Local Supervising Authority. Another reason behind the suggestion of subsidies was to ensure that the very poorest women would not be deprived of the full services of a certified midwife during childbirth. It was hoped that these measures would result in a more even standard of care and to this end the employment of all 'district' midwives by the local authority was also considered. This, perhaps together with a more comprehensive system of insurance, was also seen as a remedy to the use of uncertified midwives, which, despite legislation, had not been eradicated, and was a practice still common enough to cause anxiety.

Although supervision of midwives was being carried out, there was a great lack of uniformity in the way it was executed. Supervisors were employed by county and county-borough councils, and many were physically remote or psychologically distant from midwives and their practice. As there was no defined standard of qualification for supervisors, some were inexperienced and not acceptable to the midwives as an inspector and arbiter of their methods of practice. The Report suggested that in future the chief 'Inspector' of midwives should be the Medical Officer of Health, and his assistant or non-medical supervisor should be an experienced midwife.

It was recognised at this time that no mechanism was in existence to prevent a midwife from returning to practice after she had abstained from work for several years, and the question was raised as to whether she should be required to undertake post-certificate instruction prior to being allowed to notify her Intention to Practice.

Overall the Departmental Committee on the Training and Employment of Midwives saw the midwife as remaining the key provider of maternity care and as carrying the greatest share of the burden.[25]

Duties of the Midwife as Set Out in the Rule Book (1928)

In Pregnancy

The midwife was required to keep notes of antenatal visits 'in a defined form approved by the Board'. At this time it was by no means a regular occurrence for a mother to see a doctor in the antenatal period, and although it had been suggested that a mother should see a doctor in early and late pregnancy, it was recognised that this would encroach 'upon the duties of the midwife in the ante-natal sphere'. It was accepted practice for the midwife who suspected or detected an abnormality or illness during the pregnancy to refer her patient automatically to the doctor. The Rule Book laid down that she *must* send for medical help in pregnancy if and when she found any of the following conditions: deformity or stunted growth; loss of blood; abortion and threatened abortion; excessive sickness; puffiness of hands or face; fits or convulsions; dangerous varicose veins; purulent discharge; sores of the genitals.

In Labour

The midwife had sole responsibility for the conduct of labour unless deviation from the normal arose, when she would again be obliged to send for medical assistance for such complications as: fits or convulsions; a purulent discharge; sores of the genitals; a malpresentation; presentation other than the uncomplicated head or breech; when no presentation could be made out; excessive bleeding; where *two* hours after the birth of the child the placenta had not been completely expelled; in cases of rupture of the perineal body or of other injuries to the soft parts.

In the Lying-in Period

Duties in the lying-in period included 'a blanket bath for the mother each morning for the first week, the making of her bed and attention to the genitals'. Baths were either a luxury or non-existent in a great many homes, hence the necessity for such nursing care. The district midwife generally visited morning and evening for the first three days, daily up to the 10th day and then made single visits on the 12th and 14th day and longer if the circumstances dictated.

Complications in the lying-in period for which the midwife was obliged to call a doctor included: fits or convulsions; abdominal swelling and tenderness; offensive lochia, if persistent; rigor with raised temperature; rise of temperature to 100.4°F for 24 hours or its recurrence within that period; unusual swelling of the breasts with local tenderness or pain; secondary post-partum haemorrhage; white leg.

To the Baby

Her duties to the baby included seeking the assistance of a medical practitioner in the event of: injuries received during birth; any malformation or deformity endangering a child's life; dangerous feebleness in a premature or full-term child; inflammation of or discharge from the eyes, however, slight; serious skin eruptions, especially those marked by the formation of watery blisters; inflammation about, or haemorrhage from, the navel.

Personal Hygiene

Directions to midwives 'concerning their person' including:

when attending to her patients she must wear a clean dress of washable material that can be boiled, such as linen or cotton, and over it a clean washable apron or overall. The sleeves of the dress must be made so that the midwife can tuck them up well above the elbows . . . Before touching the generative organs or their neighbourhood the midwife must on each occasion disinfect her hands and forearms.

Changes at the Central Midwives Board

In 1929 the nine members of the Central Midwives Board were increased to fourteen. The Board was now to be made up as follows:

4 members appointed by the Minister of Health ('two of whom shall be certified midwives on the English Midwives Roll')
4 Registered Medical practitioners (surgeons, physicians, apothecaries)
2 Certified Midwives appointed by the Incorporated Midwives Institute

1 Representative from the Queen Victoria Jubilee Institute for Nurses
1 Representative of the County Councils Association
1 Representative of the Association of Municipal Corporations
1 Representative of the Society of Medical Officers of Health[26]

Medical Advances in the Provision of Care in the 1930s

Social conditions were poor during the 1930s as a result of the worldwide economic depression, which reached crisis proportions. This undoubtedly contributed to the high maternal mortality rate (including abortions) of 4.60 per thousand registered births in England and Wales in 1934. However, the greatest single cause of this mortality was sepsis, which was as likely to follow induced abortion as childbirth. In the course of the next five years the mortality rate dropped to 3.10 per thousand after the introduction of sulphonamides, the use of ergometrine intramuscularly and intravenously, the development of blood transfusion services and increasing provision of emergency obstetric services (Flying Squads). The development of antenatal clinics could well also have contributed to this reduction, because by 1935 approximately 80 per cent of all expectant mothers received antenatal care of some kind.[20] This care was received either from state-aided local-authority maternal and child-welfare clinics, from voluntary and private hospital clinics, and from family doctors and midwives. Half the mothers in large towns and metropolitan boroughs attended the local-authority antenatal clinics, of which by 1932 there were 1060 in Britain. Several Ministry of Health Reports published in the 1920s had recommended that midwives should be encouraged to refer women to the local-authority clinics if they were unable to provide this care themselves, or if they suspected a complication requiring medical expertise. Some midwives were, however, reluctant to do this as such referral could have led to loss of the case and therefore loss of their fee. In 1927 it was recommended that provision should be made for the midwife to be recompensed in such an event.[27]

The care at local-authority antenatal clinics included general physical examination, consideration of obstetric history and general health, pelvic measurement, and abdominal examination/palpation, including measurement of fundal height and abdominal girth and also recording of fetal heart sounds. Urine was tested and blood pressure estimated to detect early signs of pre-eclampsia.[28] These free local-authority clinics were staffed by LA employees including full-time midwives, so the independent domiciliary midwives were booking mothers for delivery who thereafter went to LA clinics for their antenatal care. In consequence family doctors and midwives were becoming unhappy about these clinics on the grounds that they interfered with continuity of care. Moreover, many clinical medical officers had little experience of obstetric practice, and this created intraprofessional bad feeling.

A Department Committee on Maternal Mortality (1932) stated that

there is too little ante-natal supervision by GP's and Midwives, and what there is often too perfunctory to deserve the name. Ante-natal Clinics are too often conducted by those who are not practised obstetricians and there is lack of cooperation between them and those conducting the deliveries.

The Family Doctors wished to give the care themselves, rationally arguing that

in many districts anything that is found out about a patient at the ante-natal clinic is not passed on to the one who is to attend the confinement. To separate the ante-natal supervision of a patient from the conduct of the confinement is simply ridiculous.[29]

On the other hand the number of visits recommended in a Ministry of Health memorandum on antenatal clinics was thirteen, with the first visit at 16 weeks. This suggests more adequate supervision of the pregnancy than could be given by the family doctor or the midwife. It was envisaged that the patient need only see the clinic doctor on three occasions: at the first attendance and again at 32 and 36 weeks, with clinic midwives being responsible for care during the remaining visits.[30]

Growing Problems for Independent Midwives

Free local-authority clinics contributed to the unenviable position in which many single-handed independent midwives, in competition for cases, found themselves during the early 1930s. These clinics were against the financial interests of independent midwives, because they were staffed by local-authority employees, and so part of their livelihood was thereby threatened; in addition, referral of their cases as a result of suspected or detected complications might mean loss of confinement fees also. Moreover, the birth rate was falling whereas institutional confinements were steadily rising, so that the already low income of the private midwife was declining.

Collectively these factors gave the independent midwife justifiable grievance and highlighted the need for a countrywide salaried midwifery service. To compound the problem it seems that these independent midwives were still losing some potential patients to bogus 'qualified' midwives who were still practising illegally 30 years after the passing of the first Act. Some such 'practitioners' were detected by the Supervising Authorities and reported to the Central Midwives Board. An example of this is disclosed in the 1934 Annual Report of the CMB which records that a prosecution on the grounds of falsely claiming a midwifery qualification brought a penalty of a £5 fine or 28 days' imprisonment in default of payment. On the other hand there is no doubt that some midwives enjoyed a reasonable standard of living provided they had sufficient deliveries among mothers who could afford to pay reasonable fees. Below is an example of the tariff displayed by an independent midwife in 1936. She practised in Bury, an average-sized industrial town in Lancashire.

Emma Louise ASHWORTH
Certified Midwife (By examination)
CMB No. 47882
47, Taylor Street, Bury

1st confinement	42/−
2nd confinement	40/−
	1/− per hour charged after waiting 4 hours
Twins	10/− extra
False alarms	2/6d
Nights	5/−
Enemas	5/−
Journeys to Birtle, Walmersley, Jericho, and similar long distances	50/−

The last charge was likely to be the taxi-cab fare. The fact that Emma Ashworth journeyed to outlying districts could mean either that she was one of a very small number of midwives practising in the area or that her reputation was particularly good.

It is interesting that it was appropriate for this midwife to add 'By examination'. This demonstrated that she was trained and had proven herself proficient. She did not, however, avail herself of the right to call herself 'State Certified Midwife', which could be abbreviated to SCM. (This added dignity of title had been allowed by the Central Midwives Board since 1934.) The tariff showed a charge for 'false alarms' but not for antenatal care. Perhaps her confinement fee was an inclusive charge, or maybe she did not undertake antenatal care.

The work of such self-employed midwives, practising in isolation without a colleague, could be demanding and exhausting, and working alone meant that they were never off duty. They would constantly face the difficulties of a workload unpredictable in terms of times of birth so that they could experience severe peaks and troughs. A peak period could very unfavourably affect the quality of care given to mothers and at worst could deprive the mother of professional assistance in her labour. A case in point was reported to the Central Midwives Board in 1935 in which a midwife was unable to attend a confinement because of extreme fatigue. This midwife, when summoned by the husband, told him she was 'too tired to attend' and she suggested to him that he called another midwife. The second midwife was also unable to answer the call and so the confinement took place without a midwife in attendance. The Board upheld the first midwife in her claim that fatigue prevented her from being unable to fulfil her obligation to the patient, but found her at fault in failing to provide a professional substitute.[31] This tells us a lot about the circumstances and conditions of work of midwives who practised independently, and shows the need for midwives to work with a partner or in a team.

Those district midwives employed by Nursing Associations encountered problems of a different nature. The CMB Report of 1935 showed that the Board adjudicated in a complicated ethical issue relating to the booking of abnormal cases by midwives. A Local Supervising Authority wished to uphold a midwife who objected to booking abnormal cases, which her employing association required her to do. The Central Midwives Board informed the LSA that in its opinion the latter 'had no power to instruct a midwife not to undertake work which *by law* she is entitled to undertake [our italics]'. This surprising decision seems to contradict the decision of the midwife in her role as a practitioner of *normal* midwifery, and must have been unwelcome to the unfortunate midwife concerned.

The right of a midwife to refuse to book a case was obviously a topical issue, and the CMB had, on many occasions, been asked to consider this matter. Consistently the Board's view had been (and continued to be) that although she had this right of refusal, as did a doctor, the midwife should not exercise that right when humanitarian issues are at stake. The Board ruled that this also applied to attendance at, and following, abortion. It seems unclear exactly why midwives were expressing their wish to exercise this particular right; it may have been a result of an increasing awareness that their province was normal midwifery and of their wish no longer to bear the responsibility of foreseeably complicated obstetric cases.

Clinical Practice

In the mid-1930s, between 60 and 70 per cent of all births still took place at home and the midwife herself conducted most of these cases. She was still not permitted to offer very much in the way of physical pain relief to the mother. She was 'banned' from using chloroform at the instigation of the obstetricians;[32] she was not permitted to administer 'gas and air', except under the direction and personal supervision of a doctor; but from 1936, using a Minnitt machine, she was allowed to administer inhalational analgesia at her own discretion. (It is not surprising that, in the absence of effective analgesia, the first published work on the psychological approach to pain relief by Grantly Dick Read appeared at this time.) The midwife was also limited in the use of drugs, which were by now available, to control post-partum haemorrhage. It was only 'in circumstances of great emergency' that she was authorised to use even liquid extract of ergot or pituitary extract before the birth of the placenta. Ergometrine, *for injection*, had been in use by medical practitioners since 1932 but midwives were not allowed to use it on their own responsibility at this time.

Maternity hospital labour wards were bare and clinical in the 1930s and could contain two or more beds (Figure 24).

A *Handbook* for midwives published in 1932[33] gives a clear picture of the contemporary management of labour. Castor oil, an enema and a bath were recommended in the early first stage. As a precaution against puerperal sepsis the vulva was washed and shaved. The mother was encouraged to walk about (provided that the occiput was anterior) to facilitate descent of the head and dilatation of the cervix. Sedatives, if given at all, were very mild in their action and included potassium bromide and chloral hydrate. Analgesics were not mentioned but the time-honoured back-rubbing was commended. The mother was encouraged to drink glucose, lemonade and to eat barley sugar. She lay in bed during the second stage of labour but delivered lying in the left lateral

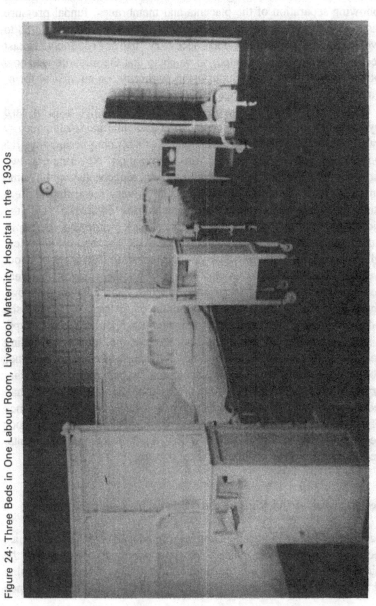

Figure 24: Three Beds in One Labour Room, Liverpool Maternity Hospital in the 1930s

Source: From a collection of historical documents and photographs in School of Midwifery, Liverpool Maternity Hospital.

position. To encourage expulsion midwives were given the following advice: 'a stool or board may be placed at the bottom of the bed for the patient to place her feet against, and a towel may be fastened to a rail at the end of the bed for her to pull on'. To avoid perineal rupture the sound advice of delivering the head *between* contractions was given. Following separation of the placenta and membranes, fundal pressure was used for their expulsion. It stated that midwives were permitted to give ergometrine and ergot when necessary, but not routinely. Breast feeding was strongly advocated, so much so that the midwife was now obliged to notify the Local Supervising Authority, on an official form, if a mother artificially fed her baby.

Midwifery training and practice in the 1930s entailed a lot of hard physical work spread over long hours, strict discipline and small monetary reward. A pupil's allowance during her year's training period was £15 and she had to pay a fee to enter the examination. Nevertheless, two midwives who trained as direct entrants in Manchester at this time remember their training and later practice as very rewarding and exciting. One remembers several forceps deliveries 'on district', with the midwife giving the anaesthetic via an open mask, while she, the pupil, had to press hard on the abdomen! Even so, she recalls very few stillbirths.[34] One of these midwives had to travel a distance of about twelve miles each week to attend a lecture.[35] Another midwife has clear memories of her training experience in 1939, especially in Glasgow, where she spent her sixth and final month, on district. As a pupil she had to provide her own clinical thermometer, two Spencer Wells forceps, scissors, a waterproof apron and fetal stethoscope. However, finding the latter very expensive, she and her colleagues discovered the inner tube of a toilet roll, with certain adaptations, to be a perfectly satisfactory substitute. Many of the women to whom she was called out had had no antenatal care at all, and some had not even had the pregnancy officially confirmed. Nevertheless, she records that no matter how poor the parents' circumstances, and how dirty and infested their tenements, the baby was always welcomed with affection.[36]

Development of the Role of the Midwife in Antenatal Care

During the 1930s, antenatal care was developed and its importance became increasingly recognised. Whereas previously the focus of the midwife's involvement was the labour and delivery, it was being realised that her support and supervision of the mother during her pregnancy was just as much a part of her work as the management of labour and the puerperium. It was seen that the midwife's contribution in the antenatal period should embrace *all aspects* of the mother's welfare. She was encouraged by guidance from the Central Midwives Board in the Rule Book of 1934 to understand that

> her success in practice may be estimated by the proportion of natural childbearing attained with healthy and uninjured mothers and children. Therefore she must make as sure as is humanly possible that no complications occur that can be forseen and/or prevented and that no early signs of disordered function escape undetected.[32]

She was encouraged to 'help the mother by educational and social services to prepare herself and her home for the confinement and for the child'. Because pregnancy was still viewed as a physiological event the mother very often only saw it necessary to book the midwife, and in fact the midwife was only obliged to refer the mother to a medical practitioner if 'some abnormality or suspicion of it' arose. However, the midwife was also being advised by the Central Midwives Board that at least 'one thorough overhaul' by the doctor was desirable to screen for existing medical and obstetric conditions that might adversely affect the outcome of pregnancy.[32] The midwife had to decide whether to refer her mothers to the general practitioner for whose services they might have to pay, or to the hospital or municipal (local-authority) clinic. In 1930 the Ministry of Health had authorised the payment of fees to GPs for the routine examination of pregnant women who had engaged a midwife and who were not insured under the National Health Insurance Act.[37]

Midwives Act 1936

It was accepted by this time that pregnancy care should be a continuum, and yet the prevalence of free local-authority clinics was still being seen to separate antenatal care and thus cause fragmentation. It seemed inappropriate for a private midwifery service to continue because it did not fit into the changing provision and developing structure of health care. It had long been recognised that in order to attract educated women in sufficient numbers into midwifery, major changes would be needed to enable them to practise without considerable personal and financial stress. By 1936 the majority of pupils undertaking midwifery training were State Registered Nurses but few of them practised midwifery after qualification. In the light of this situation, and in accordance with recommendations in Government-sponsored reports, legislative changes were made. The Midwives Act 1936 introduced such fundamental change, in that every county or county-borough council, i.e. the Local Supervising Authorities in England and Wales, was charged with providing an adequate salaried domiciliary midwifery service. They could provide this directly or through voluntary organisations. Those midwives who did not wish to become employees of the local authority, or who were considered to be unsuitable by reason of age, were to be paid compensation on surrender of their certificates. Alternatively, they could chose to continue in private practice. Although under the Act the patient was not expected to pay the midwife directly for her services, she nevertheless was still expected, within her financial resources, to pay the local authority.

The 1936 Act revolutionised the position and standard of practice of midwives. For the first time midwives worked as part of a system which gave them 'off-duty', annual leave and financial security — including pensions, and provided equipment and uniform. Another effect of the Act, which was to the mutual benefit of the mother and the midwife, was the fact that it greatly facilitated her execution of antenatal care in that as an employee of the local authority every midwife could now participate in the LA antenatal clinics. Following the establishment of the Municipal Midwifery Service in England and Wales, under the Act the maximum fees charged for antenatal supervision, confinement and postnatal care for 14 days varied in four areas studied between £2 and £2 12s 6d for a first birth. Less was charged for subsequent births, the lowest fee being £1 10s. The *actual* cost per case was at least double and sometimes treble this amount, and so the service was heavily subsidised by local government.[38] This shows how reasonable the private midwives charges had been and how much she had gained financially, as well as in most other respects, from becoming a salaried professional. However, because of the new Municipal Midwifery Service, the general practitioners tended to see fewer and fewer pregnant women and the erosion of their interest, involvement and skill in 'midwifery' was thus accelerated. This created problems when midwives required medical aid in an intra-partum or post-partum emergency. However, some GPs maintained their interest in midwifery work, and midwives called upon these particular doctors. For example, in London it was estimated that the bulk of the medical-aid calls were answered by about 100 out of 2000 doctors. In fact a body of *general practitioner-obstetricians* was coming into existence spontaneously.[23]

Other provisions of the Act were directed towards the improvement of the basic training and the post-basic education of midwives. It empowered the Central Midwives Board to grant a Midwife Teachers Diploma after examination. Although courses to prepare midwives to teach had been organised in several centres, for some time, there had been no *official* qualification for a midwife teacher. As early as 1924 the Midwives Institute had initiated 'post graduate' instruction for midwives engaged in teaching, and from 1926 special courses for selected candidates were held, followed by examinations, for the Midwife Teachers Certificate. In 1930 the first joint course was arranged with the College of Nursing, and courses soon followed at the teaching centres of Manchester, Liverpool, Birmingham, and Leeds, and at Bristol where, in fact, the University itself awarded a Midwife Teachers Certificate to successful candidates. After the institution of the statutory Midwife Teachers Diploma (MTD), the first residential courses were established in London and Liverpool in 1937 and 1938 respectively. Part-time courses continued during the war years in the major cities. Although a proposal for a national residential Midwife Teachers Training College was formulated by the Central Midwives Board, the Royal College of Midwives and the City of London Hospital, this was not supported by the Ministry of Health. In 1948 two intensive four-month courses were held at the Royal College of Midwives, but both the length and content were judged to be insufficient. Renewed proposals to the Ministry of Health were successful, and in consequence the Midwife Teachers Training College was opened at High Coombe, Kingston upon Thames and received its first students on 13 May 1950. Non-residential courses were also conducted at this time in London, Birmingham, Liverpool and Manchester.[39]

The post-basic education for all midwives was to take the form of residential refresher courses of seven days' duration at five-yearly intervals. Regulations now required midwives returning to practice after a period of abstention to attend a course of instruction the duration of which was to be determined by the Board.

Another provision of the Midwives Act 1936 was the prescription of qualifications for the post of Supervisor of Midwives. The regulations allowed for the appointment of a Medical Supervisor and a Non-medical Supervisor, and it was within the discretion of the Authority to appoint either one or the other, or both. In general, the Non-medical Supervisor was to be a senior experienced domiciliary midwife who was to work with the Medical Supervisor. This definition of the qualifications/requirements for these posts was motivated by an acknowledgement that previously, and in many cases, unsuitable appointments had been made. In some cases Health Visitors with little or no practical experience of midwifery had been appointed and this had had an adverse psychological effect on practising midwives. Moreover, such people were in no position to give advice, instruction and support to the midwives, but rather were seen simply to act as critical inspectors.[40]

The Act also put an end to the engagement of 'monthly nurses', i.e. unqualified persons paid to attend mothers after childbirth, whether or not they were working under the direct supervision of a doctor.

The Scottish equivalent of the 1936 Midwives Act was the Maternity Services (Scotland) Act 1937 which imposed upon the Local Authorities a duty similar to that laid down in the English Act. There was a difference, however, in that it entitled every pregnant mother who was confined at home to the services of a medical practitioner. Practitioners did not, in fact, attend many confinements, on the grounds that their attendance was unnecessary. Hence the professional responsibility of the Scottish midwife was little less onerous than that of her English or Welsh colleagues.[38]

Extension of Postnatal Care

From 1 January 1937 the period for which the midwife was responsible for postnatal care to mother and baby was extended to 14 days. It then became part of the role of the District Midwife to visit those mothers and babies who were discharged from hospital before the 14th day. It was envisaged that this could be difficult to implement because of communication problems between the hospitals and the community midwives. It is unlikely that many midwives had telephones, but even so experience was to prove that such potential difficulties could be overcome.[38]

Extension and Division of Midwifery Training

In 1938 the training for qualification as a midwife was lengthened and divided into two parts.[41] For State Registered Nurses each part was to be of six months' duration; so that the total training period was doubled at a stroke to twelve months. An examination was held after each part. After Part I of the training the examination was written and oral, whereas the Part II examination was clinical and oral. The clinical part included history taking, general and abdominal examination/palpation, urine testing, blood-pressure estimation, examination of placenta and membranes, and use of inhalational analgesia. (Mothers were paid a small sum for acting as 'patients' for the candidates.) The oral part included questions related to the candidate's written case studies, 12 of which were submitted at this time.

The theory of normal and abnormal midwifery and neonatal paediatrics was taught in Part I. The introduction of the new divided training required a complete review of the large number of training schools which had previously been approved. Many of them were found to be quite unsuitable for Part I training and some for any training at all! A complete inspection was carried out by the Educational Supervisor of the CMB (a new post created in 1936), and so for the first time the Board possessed up-to-date information about the Schools it had approved throughout England and Wales. Hospitals subsequently approved as training schools were those that could provide an adequate number and variety of cases for sound practical experience. The pupil midwives were required to conduct ten deliveries in the first period of training. The emphasis in Part II, which included a domiciliary module (*or* was entirely domiciliary based), was on the application of theory to practice, on the acquiring of professional confidence and clinical judgement and skills, and on the widening of the midwife's knowledge. New concepts were introduced, such as the sociological and public-health aspects of practice, and it was also thought desirable for the pupil midwife to gain insight into the psychological needs of mothers and families. The objective was to enable her to put her midwifery knowledge into the context of everyday family and community life.

War and its Effects on Childbirth and Midwives

Between 1939 and 1945 Britain entered the Second World War and this naturally had an effect on the maternity services. Civilian life was disrupted, many husbands were away in the Forces; and older women in the family were working outside their homes replacing the men on the land, in the factories, on the buses and in offices, or were making munitions. This created a lack of help in the home and increased the need for hospitalisation for birth. However, because maternity beds in hospital were in short supply, there were strict obstetric, medical and social criteria for hospital booking. The proportion of babies born in hospital rose from 33 per cent in 1937 to 45 per cent in 1944.

In expectation of war, plans had already been made to evacuate pregnant women from those city areas that were most likely to be bombed;

and emergency maternity homes were set up in large country houses. An emergency maternity service was also inaugurated in seaside towns, using convalescent homes, hotels and boarding houses.[18] Staff from the city hospitals were transferred to these makeshift maternity units, and at times domiciliary midwives could be called upon to help in these circumstances. In the 1940s the birth rate was extremely high and reached an all-time peak in 1946. The minimum number of doctors were left to staff the hospitals, and midwives, working long hours, made up the deficit, bearing with the doctors an exceptionally heavy workload.

Each conventional maternity ward at that time consisted of antenatal and postnatal beds, at least two delivery rooms and a nursery, where babies spent most of the day and night. These wards were often extremely busy, with midwives nursing patients with pre-eclampsia, ante-partum haemorrhage, and severe medical conditions while at the same time conducting labours and deliveries and attending to the needs of parturient mothers who at that time remained in bed between eight and ten days. They also staffed the nursery and in addition undertook a considerable amount of ward domestic work. These were the days when glass syringes and needles were washed and sterilised by midwives on the ward. They also washed, patched and re-sterilised rubber gloves, made dressings, sluiced linen by hand, and washed and dried rubber 'draw' and bed mackintosh sheets. There were no auxiliary nurses to help them, and no ward clerks to assist with the clerical work.

The Rushcliffe Report on Conditions of Service of Nurses and Midwives

In 1941 the Rushcliffe Committee was set up to consider salaries and conditions of service of nurses and midwives, and it reported in 1943. The Midwives Salaries Committee took full opportunity to reinforce the responsible nature of the work of the midwife, and recommended salary scales slightly greater than those granted to nurses of equivalent grade. These recommendations were accepted by the Minister and finally established the professional and social status of the midwife as in no way inferior to that of the nurse. The Report identified midwifery as 'a distinct profession with its own traditions', despite its close relationship with nursing, and it recognised that 'in the main [a midwife's] patients are healthy women discharging a normal physiological function, and the midwife is left to her own knowledge and skill to attend them'. The Committee felt that 'public opinion has been slow to realise the true status and importance of the midwife or the vital part which she plays in the Public Health services'.[42]

At this time (1942), 15 000 midwives were in practice and were employed as follows:

2750	in maternity institutions
2700	in salaried service of local authorities (these midwives could be, and many were, allocated local-authority houses and therefore they lived 'on the spot')
2700	village nurse-midwives
1500	Queen's Nurses
2000	in private practice
3350	others (possibly in nursing or maternity homes or in domiciliary practice attached to a maternity hospital)[43]

The Rushcliffe Committee provided for negotiation between nurses and midwives and their employing authorities until 1948 when it was succeeded by the Whitley Council. In 1945 the Committee recommended that the maximum number of deliveries should not exceed 65 per annum per domiciliary midwife. In the 1948 Rushcliffe Report[42] the term 'District Midwife' was used; this replaced the terms previously used for the same category of midwife, which were 'Domiciliary Midwife', 'County Midwife', 'Borough Midwife', and 'Municipal Midwife'.

Recommended Hours of Work and Caseload. The Committee decided that a District Midwife 'working in favourable circumstances should normally be expected to attend personally about 66 confinements a year without a pupil and 90 a year with a pupil'. Fifty per cent of mothers were still delivered at home at this time. The Committee recommended that District Midwives should be on duty or on call for 132 out of 168 hours in a week for three weeks, but in the fourth week should be given a long weekend of 60 hours consecutive free time.

For hospital midwives: 'A 96-hour fortnight should as soon as conditions permit be brought into national operation'. This 48-hour week was not implemented for almost a decade. The Rushcliffe Committee recommended that the 96-hour fortnight 'should be inclusive of lectures and tutorial classes'. However, in the experience of both writers, pupil midwives were still expected to attend lectures after 11 hours on night duty outside duty hours as late as 1960. The Report further recommended that all grades of Institutional midwives and pupil midwives should be given at least one complete day off a week (implying that not all were).

Shortage of Midwives

The unprecedentedly high birth rate exacerbated the existing shortage

of midwives to a crisis point. At the outbreak of war an Emergency
Powers (Defence) Act 1939 authorised Local Supervising Authorities
to allow women whose names had been removed from the Roll to act
as midwives providing there was a shortage in the area of that Authority. This would include those private midwives who had opted out of
the new salaried midwifery service under the 1936 Midwives Act. This
provision within the Emergency Powers Act remained in force until 1954
although the names were not automatically restored to the Midwives Roll.
Retired midwives were encouraged to return to practice and many did
so. In an additional effort to maintain the supply of midwives, midwifery
was designated as a form of National Service. The Ministry of Labour
and National Service carried out a national Registration of Midwives
in April 1943. The subsequent publicity campaigns drew attention to the
shortage of midwives and a response was aroused, particularly from older
midwives. In September 1943 the Employment of Women (Control of
Engagement) Order required that newly qualified midwives *must* practise for a year.

Reduction in Mortality

In spite of the stresses of the war years on mothers, the maternal mortality rate fell dramatically throughout this time. Many factors were involved besides the purely medical advances. The economic conditions
of families, especially of those in the lower social classes, were much
improved and for the first time many women were able to afford an adequate and healthy diet even though some of it was in the unappetising
form of dried eggs and margarine. Additionally, Government policy was
to supplement the diet of expectant and nursing mothers with extra
rations, vitamins and milk. Although many pregnant women, out of
national necessity, worked in heavy jobs until well advanced in their
pregnancies, their mental and physical health and stamina were obviously
improved and this was reflected in their more successful childbearing
performance.

By 1943 maternal mortality had fallen to half the 1935 rate to reach
2.30 per 1000 registered births. Chemotherapy had been introduced and
there were well-established Flying Squad and blood-transfusion services.
Deaths of babies in the neonatal period had also fallen, though not com-
parably with the maternal rate. Twenty-five neonates died per 1000 live
births and the stillbirth rate was 30 per 1000 births.[43]

Midwives could be justly proud of their contribution towards the improved health of mothers and babies. This achievement was recorded
in a *Historical Review of British Obstetrics and Gynaecology 1800–1950*:

During the war period, and for a year or so after, the midwives had to bear responsibilities greater than at any time since their profession was recognised, and prove their competence by the way they helped to reduce the maternal deaths to a figure hitherto unknown.[23]

Specialists in Normal Midwifery

In discussing the organisation of the maternity services in the 1940s the Goodenough Committee recognised that midwives were 'specialists in normal midwifery'. They appreciated the complementary roles of general practitioner and midwife in the provision of antenatal care, and realised that

the midwife's close association with the patient for as long as possible during the pregnancy provides the midwife with the best opportunity of winning the patient's complete confidence, a factor which may be of the greatest value at the time of her confinement.

As far as the conduct of labour was concerned, they recognised that it would be neither wise nor economical to encourage competition between midwife and medical practitioner for the management of normal labour and birth.

The conduct of a normal confinement is the primary and essential obligation of the midwife to the Community. The medical practitioner has many others which may be urgent and exacting.[44]

Critical Shortage — Peak Birth Rate

At the end of the war the shortage of midwives became critical when the birth rate reached its peak in 1946. This was enhanced by the fact that a substantial number of midwives ceased to practise after their marriage (which at that time prohibited their being employed as hospital midwives) and subsequent motherhood; by the fact that some returned to general nursing, and because of the retirement of those older recalled midwives who had filled the breach during the war years. Another reason offered for the shortage was the lengthening of the lying-in period, which meant more visits had to be made. Also, administration of gas and air, on the midwife's own responsibility, was increasing the time the midwife spent with each labouring mother.

In an attempt to help provide more midwives, courses of midwifery training for State Enrolled Nurses were established in certain centres in 1947. However, the shortage of nurses was also of such national concern that in the same year a Working Party was appointed by the Ministry of Health, the Ministry of Labour and National Service, and the Department of Health for Scotland, to consider the problem. This Working Party was chaired by Baroness Stocks and it presented its Report in November 1948. Its terms of reference were

> To cover any questions which seem to have a bearing on the shortage, including thorough examination of the fields of recruitment and training, the proper duties of a midwife, the steps to be taken to minimise wastage during and after training and the general relationships of the professions of nursing and midwifery.

During the time of the deliberations of this Working Party, the National Health Service Act of 1946 was implemented. Immediately, from July 1948, the Working Party were made aware of a new problem facing midwives and the midwifery service they had hitherto provided. This problem related to complaints received from Medical Supervisors and midwives themselves that, because of the maternity provisions within the NHS Act, general practitioners were seriously encroaching on the midwife's function by taking over the antenatal care of patients, and that, in some cases, midwives were becoming little more than maternity nurses. This brought into prominence once again the persistent underlying conflict caused by the overlapping roles of doctors and midwives in the realms of maternity care. The Working Party recognised that the doctor had responsibility for his patient, but felt that he should regard the midwife as his partner, whose function was 'well established and clearly recognised'. It was documented that the take-over of antenatal care by GPs was an unwelcome trend that could destroy the midwifery service, and that it was in the patient's interest that the role of the midwife and doctor should be complementary, with neither professional having the monopoly. The Working Party's conclusion relating to this matter was that the proper role of the midwife was as a practitioner in normal midwifery, *an expert in all aspects of normal childbearing*, and that her care should continue for at least one month after delivery. This statement was endorsed by the Central Midwives Board in their comments to the Ministry of Health on the Working Party Report.

One of the major preoccupations of the Working Party was the recruitment and retention of midwives. They addressed themselves to the controversial question of whether it was desirable to train as midwives women who were already Registered Nurses or whether non-nurses fulfilled the role of midwife equally well. At the time of State recognition (1902) it had been felt that to attract qualified nurses into midwifery would ensure a minimum standard far above that of the traditional midwife. Registered nurses were attracted, but from the beginning it was shown that only a small proportion of those who trained practised on qualification; this proved to be an expensive exercise, which was eventually remedied by the division of training into two parts, the Part I Certificate proving sufficient for promotion on return to general nursing. On the other hand the number of direct-entrant non-nurses who entered midwifery training had always been comparatively small, but of these a very high proportion practised as midwives, their motivation for training being entirely different. However, direct-entry midwives practising in hospital had traditionally been at a disadvantage as far as promotion was concerned, and so the Working Party recommended that all posts in midwifery should be open to them in future. In discussing this dilemma they focused on the fundamental differences between the midwife and the nurse. They stressed that the midwife was a practitioner in her own right, who spent most of her time caring for mothers and babies during an important but normal period in their lives, whereas a nurse worked under the instruction of a doctor whose right-hand colleague she was, but with her main focus being on illness and the care of the sick. They concluded that although the midwife needed a thorough knowledge of nursing techniques, it was not necessary or desirable for her to be a registered nurse. They proposed, however (20 years before the Briggs Committee met), that nurses and midwives should have a common basic training carrying no qualification, and that this should be followed by specialisation in either midwifery or a branch of nursing. The Committee seemed to consist of people with much insight and foresight in that they could see the disadvantages of a midwifery training divided into two parts, and in fact recommended that the existing divisions should be abandoned in favour of a continuous single-period course of one years' duration.[38]

Social and Economic Aspects of Pregnancy and Childbearing

A tremendous amount can be learnt about the maternity service, its clients and professionals from an objective survey of social and economic aspects of pregnancy and childbirth conducted in 1946 by the Royal College of Obstetricians and Gynaecologists, and the Population Investigation Committee.[45] This gives an overview of the preceding years and the current situation. Fourteen-thousand women in England and Wales were interviewed.

Antenatal Services

It is perhaps surprising to find that, thirty years after the establishment of antenatal clinics and eleven years after an 80 per cent uptake of this service had been documented, no uniform pattern of care existed. Instead care was provided rather haphazardly by a variety of professionals in a variety of places. Some patients attended a private family doctor, an obstetric specialist or more rarely a private midwife. Alternatively, some attended the local-authority antenatal clinic or the hospital antenatal clinic. Of the patients interviewed, 17 per cent stated that they 'attended municipal midwives' (presumably at the midwives' homes), and others received *some* antenatal care when the midwife visited them in their own homes. Some women received care from several sources, whereas a small number of others (0.9 per cent) did not avail themselves of any care at all. This included women of high parity who delivered at home and who did not see the need, describing themselves as 'all right'. The survey revealed that most mothers, then as now, were reluctant to attend for antenatal care in the first trimester of pregnancy.

Although the free and accessible local-authority clinics were popular with patients, their use created a problem for GPs. As was the case in 1936, they meant the loss of GPs' obstetric skills in antenatal diagnosis and overall management of normal pregnancy. Local-authority antenatal clinics were still serviced by appointed medical officers who were prevented, by their role, from prescribing or treating any condition they diagnosed. This necessitated referral of a GP's patient back to him for treatment or hospital consultation. From the midwife's point of view these clinics were ideal, since they provided her with premises and facilities that enabled her to give continuity of care from the antenatal period through to the post-partum period.

Implicit in the Survey Report is the value placed on the role of the midwife and her observed professional competence. Indeed the view was expressed that she should undertake full antenatal examinations and refer patients to a doctor only when she thought necessary.

The Survey's findings showed that midwives working in hospital antenatal clinics were less fortunate than their domiciliary colleagues. This was because hospital doctors tended to see all patients at every visit to the clinic. However, the consultation time with each patient was found to be less than three minutes, and in the view of the Survey Committee 'hurried examinations of this nature could have been avoided if the doctor had left the routine supervision to midwives'. They recommended that, rather than giving superficial attention to all mothers, the doctor should see each mother *once* early in pregnancy, and *once* late in pregnancy, and concentrate on the few high-risk mothers who needed medical supervision throughout pregnancy, and on those patients referred to him with suspected abnormality. This perspicacious Committee recognised that if every patient saw the doctor at every clinic visit, then every pregnancy would be regarded as a pathological rather than a physiological process.

During this decade there was a slight increase in hospital deliveries. The doctor in maternity hospitals was seen as being mainly necessary for antenatal supervision, but he had little opportunity to gain experience in normal deliveries; his role during labour and delivery being limited because normal deliveries were 'competently dealt with by midwives'. At this time 'operative midwifery' was relatively infrequent. The Survey shows that hospital midwives undertook 75 per cent of the deliveries. Hospital in this context included Poor Law Infirmaries, now Municipal Hospitals, voluntary hospitals, and nursing and maternity homes. It is interesting to note that it was frequently the case that the baby could 'only be seen once a week by the father'. It revealed that the majority of mothers chose and preferred home confinement, and one of the main reasons given was fear of separation from close relatives which hospital confinement would inevitably bring. The Report noted that home deliveries, especially of the potential low-risk group, were considered 'extremely safe'. These deliveries were conducted by village nurse-midwives, municipal midwives and midwives working on the districts of teaching hospitals. Delivery at home meant, though, that mothers could be deprived of gas-and-air analgesia. This was because of difficulty in the transportation of machines by the midwives, as they were considered to be too heavy to be carried on bicycles (very few midwives had cars). However, a few authorities sent the inhalational analgesia equipment by ambulance. Objections were raised to this as 'the midwives might well ask that they themselves should be taken to confinements by ambulance'! Only 17 per cent of the women were confined in hospital by choice.

In this Survey it can once again be seen that a doctor was more likely to have conducted the delivery in the homes of the well to do than in the homes of manual workers. It also shows that although the doctor was often nominally in charge, the person undertaking the delivery and carrying the responsibility in the vast majority of cases was the midwife. 'The inference to be drawn . . . is that few GPs have either the time or the interest to undertake domiciliary deliveries.'

The average length of the post-partum stay in hospital was 12 days (although the optimum length of stay was considered to be 14 days). Discharge on the 9th or 10th day was regarded as 'early' discharge, and this was becoming increasingly necessary owing to pressure on the available hospital beds.

Post-natal Examination

At this time there was poor uptake of the sixth-week postnatal examination. The Survey reveals that nationwide only 32 per cent of mothers attended. It is apparent that the majority of those who attended were mothers delivered in hospital or by the general practitioner, and in fact only 12 per cent of those delivered by municipal (local-authority) midwives presented themselves. The quality of the postnatal examination was, however, shown to be extremely variable. In some places it took place during the antenatal clinic sessions, and this, for mothers who had to bring their babies, was altogether too time-consuming and frustrating. The findings of the postnatal examinations demonstrated that a large number of women were suffering from the sequelae of childbirth. This morbidity included backache, vaginal discharges, infections and prolapse. The conclusion was drawn that those women who had distressing symptoms attended for examination, whereas on the whole mothers without any symptoms were more likely not to attend. It is clear, though, that the accepted attitude of the poorer women themselves was that parity and a degree of chronic ill-health went hand in hand. Although it appears that in some authorities it was the duty of the midwife (and in others the responsibility of the Health Visitor) to ensure that the mother attended for postnatal examination, this duty was obviously not performed effectively. This is not surprising when one considers the heavy case load of the midwives, which resulted from the high birth rate at the time and the fact that midwives in those days did their visiting on their bikes or on their feet.

The Survey revealed that 43 per cent of babies were wholly breast-fed at eight weeks and 57 per cent partly breast fed.[45]

New-style Rule Book

In 1939 the Central Midwives Board had commenced the task of revising the section of the Rules that regulated the practice of midwives. It was 9 years before this new Rule Book was issued, and so in 1947 for the first time it incorporated a statement of principles or code of practice *instead* of detailed rules relating to method of work and mode of life. The Rules had changed very little since the original rules were published in 1903 with the *bona fide* midwives in mind. In 1947 it was felt that detailed rules requiring a midwife 'to keep her person clean' were inappropriate and degrading to the well-trained and better educated midwife of this era.

The National Health Service Act

The National Health Service came into being on 1 July 1948 following the NHS Act of 1946 which was a major instrument of social legislation and restructuring resulting from the deliberations of the Beveridge Committee. This Committee, commissioned by the wartime coalition Government, was briefed to consider ways to deal with major social and economic inequalities in British society. One of their recommendations was that a comprehensive National Health Service should be set up

> to ensure that for every citizen there is available whatever medical treatment he requires, in whatever form he requires it, domiciliary or institutional, general, specialist or consultant, and will ensure also the provision of dental, ophthalmic and surgical appliances, nursing and midwifery and rehabilitations after accidents.

The Act provided this comprehensive medical service, which was free at the time of need, although it was to be paid for partly by NHS contributions by all those in employment, partly from local rates and partly from the General Exchequer Funds.

The NHS was organised into three administratively independent divisions. *Executive Councils* were responsible for the organisation and payment of the general practitioner, dental, ophthalmic and dispensing service in their administrative areas. The *Hospitals* were administered by Regional Hospital Boards and Boards of Governors, and *Local Health Authorities*, based on local-government authorities, were established whose function was primarily in preventive and environmental health and in community medicine. This included the provision of a domiciliary midwifery service, antenatal clinics, child-welfare clinics and a school medical service.

A Local Arrangement

In readiness for the NHS 'Appointed Day' the Lancashire County Council decided that the basis of midwifery staffing in urban areas would be one midwife per 66 estimated births, but in rural areas proportionately greater because of geographical considerations and because in these areas the District Midwife was also the District Nurse. Their administrative document stated that 'midwives will undertake ante-natal consultations in their own homes' and that they would be provided with a telephone and be encouraged to use a car.[46]

The Effects of the NHS on the Maternity Services

Maternity medical regulations framed for the NHS provided for the services of both a doctor and a midwife without cost to the patient, and without any obligation being placed on the doctor to be present at the confinement. For his maternity medical services a special fee was payable which varied depending on whether the doctor was regarded as having had enough experience to justify the inclusion of his name on a special Obstetric List. This encouraged a revival of interest in 'midwifery' among GPs, and a gradual wooing away of patients from Local Authority antenatal clinics to the GPs surgeries began. This, as was quickly seen by the midwives, led to lack of continuity for the patient, who was now seeing the GP antenatally (largely without a midwife) but still being delivered at home, most often by the midwife on her own. The home confinement rate at this time was approximately 45 per cent.

Fewer Births, More Maternity Beds — a Change in the Place of Confinement

The birth rate started to fall after 1946, and this coincided with an almost simultaneous but slight increase in the number of hospital maternity beds. By 1952 the percentage of hospital confinements had risen to 64 per cent.

In 1949 the Central Midwives Board in their annual Report were expressing disquiet about the decreasing number of home confinements and the fact that more were being attended by general practitioners, a situation which they felt could seriously affect the experience of future midwives. The CMB identified problems in the training of pupil midwives undertaking Part II training as:

a decrease in the birth rate but no decrease in institutional confinements;

the incursion of the general practitioner into normal midwifery under the National Health Service Act;

economic pressure on mothers to opt for hospital confinement owing

to the provision of an entirely free hospital service;
a housing shortage.

This state of affairs led more Part II Midwifery Training Schools to apply to the CMB for approval to allocate their pupil midwives to only three months 'on the district' and the other three months to hospital midwifery.

The Board's Report included a quote from the Goodenough Report stating that 'in the conduct of labour the pupil midwife has more technical experience than the medical student, and it would be neither wise nor economical to encourage competition between midwife and medical practitioner for the care of normal labour'. The fact that more confinements were being attended by GPs must have precipitated the issue of the circular (No. 1481) by the CMB in October 1948. This states the position of the domiciliary midwife in cases in which a medical practitioner has accepted responsibility to provide maternity medical services within the National Health Service.

the acceptance by the medical practitioner of responsibility for the provision of maternity medical services, and the carrying out of care, does not affect the position of the midwife who is acting as such, but if the doctor has stated specifically that he wishes to be summoned at the onset of labour and that he proposes to deliver the woman himself she is, in that case, acting as a maternity nurse.

Milestones in Pain Relief

The introduction of the National Health Service seemed to raise the expectation of the general public with regard to health care and relief of suffering. This was expressed by mothers who were requesting more relief of pain in labour. Midwives were urged to gain the certificate in administration of gas and air, the equipment for which (Minnitt's machine) had been available since the 1930s. A doctor had to medically certify the patient's fitness to inhale this analgesic. In July 1946 the CMB decided to incorporate instruction and supervised administration of inhalational analgesia in the syllabus of training for a pupil midwife, and this was an examinable subject from October 1947. This was still to be limited to gas and air because trichlorethylene (Trilene), an alternative inhalational analgesia, was not considered by the RCOG to be safe for use by midwives until 1955. Gas and air became more available to mothers having home births when the difficulty of its transportation was overcome by the use of ambulance (in some authorities) or provision of vehicles for the midwives.

In June 1948 the Central Midwives Board, at the instigation of the RCOG, requested the Home Secretary to consider amending the Dangerous Drugs Regulations to permit the use of pethidine by midwives on their own responsibility. They became legally entitled to use pethidine for pain relief in 1950.

References

1. The Midwives Act 1902.
2. The Midwives Act 1902 (2 EDW. 7. Chap 17).
3. Cowell, B. and Wainwright, D. *Behind the Blue Door. The History of the Royal College of Midwives 1881–1981* (Bailliere and Tindall, London, 1981).
4. *Central Midwives Board Rule Book 1903.*
5. White, R. *Social Change and the Development of the Nursing Profession. A Study of the Poor Law Nursing Service 1848–1948* (Henry Kimpton, London, 1978).
6. Oakley, A. *The Captured Womb* (Blackwell, Oxford, 1984).
7. Press advertisement, 1904. Newspaper cutting at Central Midwives Board.
8. Ward, I. *Evolution to Devolution. Milestones in the History of a Statutory Body, 1902–1983* (Central Midwives Board, London, 1983).
9. Letter, 1905. Newspaper cutting at Central Midwives Board.
10. Morland, E. *Alice and the Stork or the Rise in the Status of the Midwife as Exemplified in the Life of Alice Gregory 1867–1944* (Hodder & Stoughton, London, 1980).
11. Mitchell, A. Now we have an Act. Unpublished thesis 1974 (quoted in *Old Wives' Tales* by M. Chamberlain (Virago Press, London, 1981)).
12. Central Midwives Board. *Standing Orders, Instructions and Circulars* (Collected in book form 1917).
13. *The Medical Times*, 7 December 1912.
14. 'Report of the 96th Session of the General Medical Council, 20 November 1912', reported in *The Medical Times*, 7 December 1912.
15. Wallace, A.J. *Syllabus of Lectures on Midwifery* (H. Young & Sons, Liverpool, 1908).
16. Campbell, J. *Reports on Public Health and Medical Subjects No. 21: The Training of Midwives* (HMSO, London, 1923).
17. Campbell, J. *Reports on the Physical Welfare of Mothers and Children. England and Wales. Vol. 2. Midwives and Midwifery* (Carnegie Trust, Tinling & Co., London, 1917).
18. Young, J.H. *St. Mary's Hospitals, Manchester 1790–1963* (E. & S. Livingstone, Edinburgh, 1964).
19. Towler, J. and Butler-Manuel, R. *Modern Obstetrics for Student Midwives*, 2nd edn (Lloyd Luke, London, 1980).
20. Brown, F.J. *Ante-natal and Post-natal Care* (Churchill, London, 1935).
21. Bickerton, T.H. *A Medical History of Liverpool from the Earliest Days to the Year 1920* (John Murray, London, 1936).
22. Ministry of Health, *Report of the Departmental Committee on the Drafting and Employment of Midwives* (HMSO, London, 1929).
23. Walker, A. 'Midwife Services, England and Wales', in *Historical Review of British Obstetrics and Gynaecology, 1800–1950*, J. Munro Kerr and R.W. Johnstone and M.H. Phillips (eds) (Livingstone, Edinburgh, 1954, pp. 332–50).
24. Bent, A. *The Growth and Development of Midwifery in Nursing. Midwifery and Health Visiting since 1900*. P. Allen and M. Jolley (eds) (Faber, London, 1982).
25. Ministry of Health. *Report of the Departmental Committee on the Training and*

Employment of Midwives (Ministry of Health, HMSO, London, 1929).

26. *Central Midwives Board Annual Report 1930.*

27. Campbell, J. *The Protection of Motherhood*, Ministry of Health Reports on Public Health and Medical Subjects No. 48 (HMSO, London, 1927).

28. Oakley, A. 'The Origins and Development of Ante-natal Care', in *Effectiveness and Satisfaction in Antenatal Care*, M. Enkin and I. Chalmers (eds) (Heinemann, London, 1982).

29. Oakley, A. *The Origins and Development of Ante-natal Care* (reference 28, p. 10) (quoting D.D. Logan 'The General Practitioner and Midwifery', *Lancet*, 2, 1141–3).

30. Ministry of Health, *Memorandum on Ante-natal Clinics: their Conduct and Scope* (HMSO, London, 1929; reprinted 1930).

31. *Central Midwives Board Annual Report 1935.*

32. *Central Midwives Board Rules 1934.*

33. Berkeley, C. *A Handbook of Midwifery* (Cassell, London, 1932).

34. Todd, M.A. Personal interview for authors by M. Bane, midwife, 1985.

35. Cotterill, F. Personal interview for authors by M. Bane, midwife, 1985.

36. Baker, M. 'Midwifery by Gaslight', *Nursing Times*, 29 August 1984.

37. Ministry of Health Memorandum 156, 1930.

38. Stocks, M. (Chairman) *Working Party on Midwives, Ministry of Health Maternity Liaison Committee* (HMSO, London, 1948).

39. Stocks, M. *Midwife Teachers' Training College. Report on First Year's Working* (Spottiswoode & Ballantyne, London, 1951).

40. *LSAs under the Midwives Act (England) May 1937.* Ministry of Health Circular No. 1620.

41. *Central Midwives Board Report 31 March 1937.*

42. Ministry of Health *The Midwives Salaries Committee (Rushcliffe Report)* (HMSO, London, 1943).

43. Grundy, F. *A Handbook of Social Medicine* (Gibbs, Bamforth & Co., Luton, 1945).

44. HMSO *Report on the Inter-departmental Committee on Medical Schools (Goodenough Report)* (HMSO, London, 1944).

45. *Maternity in Great Britain* (Survey undertaken by a Joint Committee of the Royal College of Obstetricians and Gynaecologists and the Population Investigation Committee (Oxford University Press, Oxford, 1946).

46. NHS Act 1946. Lancashire County Council Divisional Health Administration Scheme, 1947.

APPENDIX

History and Development of the Royal College of Midwives

The College of Midwives was created out of the Midwives Institute at the Extraordinary General Meeting in 1941 on the occasion of the diamond jubilee of the Institute. The College was then granted the Royal Charter in 1947 and became the Royal College of Midwives.

The College of Midwives is a Company incorporated under the Companies Act 1948. Clause 3 of the Memorandum of Association reads:

The Objects for which the Society is established are to promote and advance the art and science of midwifery and to raise the efficiency of midwives.

It has a UK membership of between 23 000 and 24 000 midwives, most of whom are attached to one of the 212 Branches.

In 1976 the College became the recognised Trade Union for Midwives when it became included in the Special Register for Professional Organisations under the Trade Union and Labour Relations Act which enables it to continue to negotiate salaries and conditions of service for midwives.

Continuing education of the qualified practitioner and consideration of the professional practice of the midwife have been the chief functions of the College. These, together with its charitable activities, are carried out by the Royal College of Midwives Trust.

The College has been affiliated to the International Confederation of Midwives (ICM) since 1931, and congresses in different member countries serve to broaden the outlook and knowledge of individual midwives, allow for discussion on vital issues and for exchange of views and experiences, and also unite and strengthen midwives of all races and creeds in their common purpose of service to mothers and babies.

The Coat of Arms of the Royal College of Midwives (Figure 25), created in 1960, consists of a blue shield surrounded by a black and white border bearing on it an eight-pointed star supported by a pair of hands. The crest is the pomegranate tree, its trunk encircled by an ancient crown, and the supporters are Juno Lucina and Hygeia. Blue is traditionally the colour for the midwife; this colour signifies chastity, loyalty and fidelity. The black and white border represents night and day, as the midwife's

244

Figure 25: Coat of Arms of the Royal College of Midwives

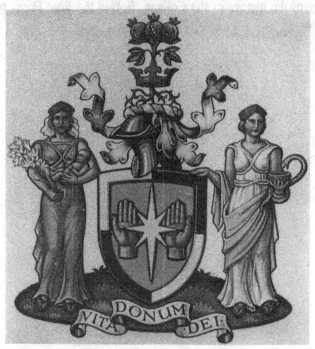

Source: Royal College of Midwives Archives Department.

work is never done. The star is the Morning Star or Star of Bethlehem, the sign of birth, surrounded and supported by the hands of the midwife. The pomegranate tree is an ancient symbol of fertility, and the crown encircling it signifies that it is a royal college.

Juno Lucina was the Roman Goddess of Light and the protectress of womanhood, marriage and childbirth. She is often depicted (as here) holding a sheaf of white lilies in one hand and a young child in the other. Hygeia was the goddess of physical and mental health, and was one of the six daughters of Aesculapius, the God of Medicine. She is depicted with a serpent entwined around her left arm. Not only was the serpent the sign of wisdom and knowledge, but it was also the sign of eternal life, as it appears reborn when it casts its old skin. The motto of the Royal College of Midwives is *Vita Donum Dei* — Life is the gift of God.

In 1981 the Royal College of Midwives celebrated its 100 years of existence with a service in Westminster Abbey. Midwives from every corner of Great Britain assembled for this historic occasion, which took place in the presence of Queen Elizabeth the Queen Mother. The centenary year was also marked by the publication and presentation of a copy of the history of the College, *Behind the Blue Door*, to every member.

9 THE MIDWIFE'S RENEWED BATTLE FOR SURVIVAL

Changes and Challenges of the 1950s

After State recognition of the midwife in 1902, the purpose of training was primarily to improve basic knowledge and practical skills in order to raise the standard and competence of the 'delivery woman' — which term sums up her role at that time. From time immemorial, however, it has been acknowledged that the importance of the midwife to such a major life event as birth far transcended the mere fundamental physical task of performing a safe delivery. Historically and ideally she has been required to possess attributes of cheerfulness, sympathy and empathy in addition to high moral qualities. Such qualities could potentially make a significant contribution to the short- and long-term future of mothers and their babies, which in turn would have its effect upon the health of the nation. In striving for the primary aim of safe birth it gradually became obvious that from conception the health and well-being of the mother had to be considered, safeguarded and improved. It seems incredible that prior to this century so little interest was taken in the mother until she went into labour. As the pregnancy period itself increased in importance, so the role of the midwife expanded. Although initially her attendance on the mother generally did not continue after the birth, it gradually came to be recognised that her role should include not only postnatal nursing care of the mother and baby for 14 days, but also guidance and advice for the puerperium.

In the 1930s and 1940s there was a rapid expansion in the role and training of the professional midwife, and her ability to fulfil that role assumed increasing importance. Events such as the advent of the National Health Service, with its increased hospitalisation, and the envisagement of earlier, and ever earlier, discharge, forced the Midwives Board and the Ministry of Health to consider the place of the midwife in this changing society, and to examine the problem of how to retain such a valuable and key care provider as the midwife when circumstances and policies were fragmenting her vital role.

In 1950 the CMB included within a document on the training of midwives,[1] their view that the psychological aspects of the midwife's function were as important as the provision of physical care. They stated: 'The importance of a good and friendly relationship between the mother and the midwife was seen as vital to the subsequent and long term relationship between the mother and her child.' Indeed they claimed that

> In no other branch of medicine is the attitude of the attendant to her
> patient so productive of positive results as in midwifery . . . the foun-
> dations of a fitter Britain can be well and truly laid by the midwives
> of the country. Midwifery is concerned with the start of a genera-
> tion. Its part is to secure a maximum of new lives at the minimum
> cost in loss and damage to the mother and to give a good start to those
> lives.[1]

More Changes at the Central Midwives Board

In 1952 the membership of the Board was increased to 16.[2] The Society
of Apothecaries and the Queen's Institute of District Nurses were no
longer entitled to appoint members, but the Royal College of Obstetricians became an Appointing Body for the first time. The Royal College
of Midwives had been allowed to appoint two midwife members from
1921 and from 1952 four midwives. The new composition of the Board
was:

  6 members appointed by the Ministry of Health
  4 members appointed by the Royal College of Midwives
  1 member appointed by the Royal College of Physicians
  1 member appointed by the Royal College of Surgeons
  1 member appointed by the Royal College of Obstetricians and
    Gynaecologists
  1 member appointed by the County Councils Association
  1 member appointed by the Society of Medical Officers of Health
  1 member appointed by the Association of Municipal Corporations

Changes in the Place of Birth Affecting the Practice of Hospital Midwives

The hospital confinement rate was continuing to rise as the trend of having a baby in hospital gathered momentum. Consequently the turnover
of patients increased and this meant that more mothers were being
discharged on, or in some cases even before, the tenth day, which was
earlier than in the past. The CMB viewed this trend with some concern
as they considered discharge home before the tenth day to be 'undesirable

practice' for two reasons. The first of these was the fact that this limited the hospital postnatal experience of Part I pupil midwives (hence the Board threatened to withdraw approval for training from any hospital that persisted in this practice). In this connection the Ministry of Health sent a circular to Regional Hospital Boards, Boards of Governors and Hospital Management Committees requesting that patients be kept at least ten and preferably 14 days after birth. A second reason for the CMB's concern was the fact that the midwife had a *statutory* obligation to nurse the mother for the duration of the lying-in period, which was then 14 days, but the hospital midwife was being rendered unable to fulfil this obligation. A solution was reached by providing a continuum of care by midwives, so when the mother was discharged home before the 14th day, responsibility for her care was transferred from the hospital to the domiciliary midwives.[3] From the mother's point of view, earlier transfer home was welcomed because it allowed for a shorter period of separation from their families.

Hospitalisation and its Effects on Domiciliary Midwifery

By 1954 the CMB was increasingly preoccupied with the effects, particularly on domiciliary midwives, of the continued rise in the number of hospital confinements. The Board took a long-term view of the situation and after considering statistical estimates of the future trends of population, and in particular the predictable 'bulge' of women who would reach childbearing age by 1961, they concluded that it was essential that a well-organised domiciliary service be maintained. They recognised that retaining the number of midwives necessary to cope with this future contingency might mean that the immediate workload of the domiciliary midwives would be lessened for a year or two. The Board sought to impress this considered view on authorities concerned with the maternity services.

In a memorandum to the Guillebaud Committee,[4] which had undertaken a review of the cost of the first five years of the National Health Service, the Board made the following statement under the heading of 'Proportion of Institutional and Domiciliary Confinements'.

The Board supports the view that Institutional confinements should be provided *only* for patients for whom it is justified on medical and social grounds . . . Pregnancy and childbearing are physiological processes and apart from financial and economic considerations it is psychologically undesirable to associate such processes too closely with establishments for treating the sick.

Unfortunately, the flood of change was unstoppable and no amount of pressure, even on very sound grounds, could turn back the tide: in the years 1947 to 1957 the national home-confinement rate dropped from 47.2 to 35.4 per cent.[5] However, it appears that, in some places at least, home confinement was still an option. A Lancashire County Council Health Services handbook of the early 1960s stated:

> Midwives are available for home confinements in all parts of the Division to ensure that every mother shall have the necessary advice and attention. Midwives may be engaged by the mother contacting the *midwife of her choice* at her home address or at one of the Ante-natal Clinics, or by enquiring at the Divisional Health Office [our italics].

There follows a list of the names, addresses and telephone numbers of ten midwives.[6]

Inclusion of Mothercraft in the Syllabus of Training

Although it has for a long time been recognised that the teaching of mothercraft is integral to the role of the midwife, the teaching of this subject had never been included in the syllabus of training. Undoubtedly, midwives had taught mothers on an individual basis in their homes and during clinic attendances, but there had been very little systematic development of this aspect of childbearing since Schools for Mothers had been started in 1910. To remedy this, and to satisfy a growing though small demand, the Central Midwives Board included mothercraft, infant care and the principles of nutrition in the syllabus of training in 1955. With less intra-partum involvement, domiciliary midwives were now able to give more time to this neglected area of their work, but this was short-lived because the birth rate rose dramatically in the 1960s and both the hospital and domiciliary midwife became extremely busy with purely practical midwifery.

However, there is evidence that organised mothercraft talks and demonstrations and relaxation classes were provided by some health authorities in the early 1960s.[7]

Investigations into the NHS and the Maternity Services

In 1956 the Guillebaud Committee, set up to review the present and prospective cost of the National Health Service, declared that the maternity
services were in a state of confusion and recommended that a review
of these services be undertaken. In response, the Cranbrook Committee[5] was formed in 1956. Its terms of reference were 'to review the present organisation of the Maternity Services in England and Wales, to
consider what should be their content, and to make recommendations'.
The Report of this Committee was comprehensive, endorsing the view
that the maternity services, as provided through the tripartite structure,
were indeed in a state of confusion. In reviewing the existing provisions
for maternity services they attempted to evaluate the advantages and
disadvantages of the trend towards hospital confinement, and in so doing
gave a very clear picture of the disorganised state of affairs. At that time
it was beginning to be mooted that hospital confinement was safer and
that the criteria for hospital booking should include both medical and
social factors. However, the Committee found that the restricted number
of available beds and poor selection meant that some mothers who certainly qualified for hospital delivery were obliged to have their babies
at home. Although the mothers themselves had a certain amount of
freedom of choice, their choice could not always be respected in areas
where a shortage of maternity beds existed. Many women in the high-
risk group insisted on having their babies at home, and many who, for
a variety of reasons, wished to have a hospital confinement had to stay
at home. In terms of costs, hospital confinement was more expensive
to the State and cheaper to the patient. Proponents of institutional confinement claimed that mothers got more rest in hospital, but in fact the
mothers reported that because of noise and activity, confinement in
hospital resulted in their getting less rest. They complained also of 'casual
treatment' in hospital and disregard for their personal dignity and emotional needs. Other arguments against birth in hospital were the risk of
infection and the loss of the psychological benefit derived from the
familiar surroundings and the support of close relatives at home and the
continuum of personal care previously received from the midwife.
Women's organisations which gave evidence were generally in favour
of home confinements, and the Cranbrook Committee expressed the view
that the advantages of home confinements for the apparently normal case
outweighed the slight risk of unforeseen complications (para. 57). The
Committee also highlighted some of the confusion that existed in the
maternity services at that time because of overlapping and division of

responsibility for patients. Some of the patients were found to be receiving antenatal care from the hospital, the midwife, the local-authority clinic and from a general practitioner-obstetrician, while at the same time receiving general medical care from their own general practitioner. This same situation had existed as an unresolved problem for the preceding 30 years.

The Cranbrook Committee also attempted to evaluate the effects of discharging the mother home early in the postnatal period to relieve the shortage of hospital beds. Because there were no official regulations concerning the length of stay for a mother in hospital, the day of discharge had become extremely variable. This was despite the fact that the Minister of Health was advocating a stay of not less than 10 days. Early discharge was a source of dissatisfaction to both the hospital and the community midwife.

This decade suffered from a chronic overall shortage of midwives, but even so those in practice in 1956 conducted 80 per cent of all deliveries. The shortage was particularly acute in the hospital service and this could only be exacerbated by the planned increase in hospital maternity beds and by the predicted rise in the birth rate. Because domiciliary midwives in the 1950s were still delivering 35 per cent of mothers at home, to whom they gave complete care, their job satisfaction was greater than was that of the hospital midwife. Even so, midwives in some areas were beginning to express dissatisfaction at providing just post-hospital postnatal care.

The Status of the Midwife

Realising the serious consequences that relegation to 'maternity nurse' could have, the Cranbrook Committee were at pains to secure the midwife's continued and unaltered professional place within the maternity service. They emphasised that 'Nothing should be done to lessen the importance of the midwife' (para. 107). They stated that they agreed with the view of the Working Party on Midwives (1949) that the midwife's three assets of time, skill and attitude of mind were of immense value to her patient. They believed that a mother who proposed to have her baby at home should book a midwife and a doctor and that all necessary maternity care should be shared between them (para. 106). Although they confirmed 'the state of confusion' in the maternity services, the Committee nevertheless felt that the tripartite structure would have to be retained in spite of suggestions to the contrary. They saw that to change the structure for the benefit of the maternity services would necessitate a comprehensive restructuring of the entire National Health Service, and that the time for that was not yet ripe. The Committee recommended that there should be more liaison between the three sets of providers of maternity services, and to encourage this they suggested the setting up of local Maternity Liaison Committees.

The Committee advocated that the hospital maternity service should be further expanded, and proposed a 70 per cent hospital confinement rate. However, they stressed that the domiciliary midwifery service should also be maintained. This led to further discussion and disagreement about the advantages and disadvantages, primarily to the mother and baby, of home versus hospital birth. Under discussion also was the effect that such a high hospital delivery rate would have on the domiciliary midwife, in that her role would change to such an extent that she might be in danger of losing her delivery skills. The Committee recommended that there should be close co-operation between the midwife and the general practitioner-obstetrician booked for a home confinement. Doctors who were styled general practitioner-obstetrician had to be on the Obstetric List, and to qualify for this list they were required to have had six months' post-registration experience in a Consultant Obstetric Unit. The doctors on the Obstetric List were paid the full fee if they gave ante- and intra-partum care but the fee was reduced if the patient was transferred to hospital before the onset of labour. It was therefore recommended that in future the full fee should be paid regardless of the transfer as it was thought that financial considerations might well override the mother's interests in some cases (para. 204).

The Central Midwives Board had given evidence and concurred with the Committee's Report. In concluding their evidence, on 22 November 1956, they stated that, in their opinion,

the main purposes of the 1902 Midwives Act have been fulfilled. These purposes were to secure an adequate standard of training for midwives fitting them to conduct normal confinements on their own responsibility, and to provide for an effective supervision of their standards of practice. The Board are confident that the history of the midwifery service over the last 50 years, which shows a steady reduction in the maternal and perinatal death rates, and a vast improvement in the services provided for the expectant and nursing mother, reflects great credit on the midwife, whom the Board firmly believe must *always* form an essential foundation of any good maternity service.[8]

CMB Report 1959

In 1959 Part I midwifery training was reduced from 18 months to 12 months for: qualified State Enrolled Nurses, Fever Nurses, Mental Nurses, Mental Defective Nurses, Tuberculosis Nurses, and Orthopaedic Nurses. A widespread shortage of both hospital and domiciliary midwives was reported in 1959 and this coincided with the sharp rise in the number of births in England and Wales.[9]

CMB Penal Cases Covering a Decade

In the 10 years between 1950 and 1960 a new cause for removal of midwives' names from the Roll was made very apparent in the CMB Reports issued during the decade. Of 31 names removed, 17 were those of midwives committing offences connected with the theft, procuring and misuse of pethidine, and in some cases falsification of drug records. Most of the other 'removals' were for civil offences such as theft and drunkenness and 'fraudulent conversion' (?)

The 1960s Birth Boom

Early Discharge from Hospital

A combination of factors brought about an acute shortage of hospital beds in the early 1960s. The birth rate was consistently rising, the proportion of hospital births was also rising, in accordance with the Cranbrook recommendations, and there was a general tendency towards hospital admission for complications of pregnancy. In certain parts of the country, where the shortage of beds was acute, the only solution was to transfer healthy mothers and babies home 48 hours after birth. This greatly increased the workload of the domiciliary midwives, often in the very places where the home-confinement rate had not fallen to the lower national average. Most domiciliary midwives still had some home confinements although delivery was generally now the lesser part of their role, the greater responsibility being the provision of postnatal care to mothers who were previously unknown to them. Such mothers and babies often presented a variety of problems which were exacerbated by the lack of continuity of professional care. Early discharge created an additional and onerous task for the domiciliary midwife as she was now required to visit in the antenatal period all patients booked for hospital confinement to assess their suitability for early discharge on housing and social grounds.

The pattern of discharge was inconsistent throughout the 1960s, and a ten-day hospital stay following vaginal delivery became a rarity. The time of discharge was sometimes as little as 36 hours after delivery, but could be 10 days. Early discharge led to a very rapid throughput of hospital patients, which was unsatisfying to the hospital midwives in terms of an enormous increase in their workload, a very brief encounter with each mother and a general lack of continuity of care. This very early discharge (36 hours) from hospital by ambulance, with the mother and baby escorted by a hospital midwife, was revolutionary. It soon became evident, taking into account the physical and psychological interests of the mother and baby, that discharge at 36 or 48 hours was preferable to discharge on the third, fourth or fifth post-partum day.

The Emergence of Central Delivery Units

The innovation of Central Delivery Units (as against delivery rooms attached to each ward) at the beginning of the 1960s brought a complete change in the continuum of care given to mothers in hospital in that they were either admitted directly to these large impersonal clinical delivery units staffed by midwives unknown to them, or transferred from their antenatal ward into unfamiliar surroundings to be cared for by staff to whom they were strangers. This conveyor-belt system obviously fragmented the care for the mother, and contracted and specialised the role of the individual midwife in that she became a ward midwife giving antenatal or postnatal care, or a Delivery Unit midwife concerned with labour and birth. This decreased the job satisfaction of midwives, and some of those who worked in very busy hospitals with Central Delivery Units left to seek posts where they could use their whole range of skills.

Recognition of Services Rendered!

In their Report, for the year ending March 1962, the CMB considered it appropriate to 'direct attention to the devoted and faithful service that practising midwives give to the community'. This statement was probably provoked by the fact that in the last six years the birth rate had risen steadily from 664 954 in 1955 to 804 120 in 1961.

Introduction of Obstetric Experience for Student Nurses

In 1961 the General Nursing Council and the Central Midwives Board approved the provision in schools of midwifery of a 12-week course in obstetric nursing for student nurses, after which they would be granted a certificate.[10] Statutory recognition was given to this course in the following year, and the 1964 Board Report showed that 85 hospitals were approved to provide the experience. At this time the obstetric module was one of four options for student nurses, and if they chose this module and obtained the certificate, their Part I midwifery course was reduced to 4 months.

Addition to Midwifery Syllabus

Although the psychological aspects of pregnancy had long been recognised as important by the Central Midwives Board, and by midwives themselves, this subject had not been included in the theoretical part of the training programme. However, in 1961 it was added to the syllabus for the first time, under the heading 'The emotional needs of the mother'.[10]

New Parameters of Midwifery and Obstetrics

During the 1960s midwifery came to embrace genetics, embryology, pathology, endocrinology, biochemistry and ante- and perinatal paediatrics. New knowledge, with its new vocabulary, revolutionised obstetrics and created an enormous increase in the volume of work in every obstetric unit. New diagnostic tests became available, forms and charts proliferated, new concepts had to be grasped and had hardly been assimilated before there were more to be learnt and evaluated. The need for post-basic and continuing education for midwives was highlighted. On the clinical front a new obstetric inhalational analgesia was marketed in the form of Entonox; a new oxytocic drug (syntometrine) was introduced, which midwives were allowed to use on their own responsibility; and syntocinon replaced pitocin as a uterine stimulant. Induction and acceleration of labour, using this oxytocic drug, then became a routine procedure. In hospital the greater involvement of the doctor in the labour ward led to the almost routine performance of a surgical incision or episiotomy for primigravidae. So, in 1967, midwives were for the first time authorised to infiltrate the perineum with local anaesthetic prior to performing an episiotomy, and from 1968 were permitted to intubate the newborn. In the same year the Guthrie test, and then the Scriver test, were introduced for the diagnosis of phenylketonuria, and midwives were trained in how to obtain the blood specimen for these tests. Midwives were also expected to take blood from babies for serum bilirubin estimation and for the measurement of blood glucose. These new, time-consuming techniques challenged the clinical skills of the midwife as well as increasing her responsibility for initiating the test and understanding the implications of the result, and often for ensuring appropriate action was taken. In addition, many non-nursing duties were still being undertaken by midwives, such as domestic cleaning, sluicing of soiled linen and all clerical work. Indeed, the amount of paperwork had multiplied as a result of the rapid turnover of patients and the documentation of new data.

The nursing care of the mother in the lying-in period was changed by the theory that earlier ambulation was more beneficial than the prolonged bed rest previously prescribed. In consequence the post-partum length of stay in bed fell from 9 days, through 6 days, to 3 days, and to the present 6 hours, within a few years. Bidets and showers replaced bed baths and three-times-daily vulval swabbings by midwives, and this significantly saved nursing time. Mothers started to play a greater part in looking after their own babies, and since 'rooming-in' became approved practice in the 1970s, mothers have virtually taken over the routine care. The consequent interaction of the mother with her baby can confer on both of them certain important psychological advantages. It can, however, be argued that if having the baby with her by day and by night exhausts the mother, then it nullifies the potential psychological benefits.

The midwife's work became easier to some extent in that in the mid-1960s CSSD (Central Sterile Supply Department) services were being set up. No longer was she expected to wash, test, repair and pack rubber gloves, pack drums of pads, or sterilise stainless-steel equipment. Gamma-irradiated pre-packed plastic disposable syringes and needles came on the market at this time and proved to be the greatest single blessing to the midwife. Disposable 'plastic' catheters replaced rubber catheters, and disposable paper caps and masks also became available.

Shortage of Midwives

The population explosion of the late 1950s and early 1960s afforded very little time for the midwife to provide psychological support for the mothers delivered in hospital. This provoked the Ministry of Health to issue a leaflet in 1961, which urged that consideration be given to 'human relations in obstetrics'. However, at the same time this document recognised the basic problems of 'overwork and understaffing'. In 1962 the working week of the midwife was reduced to 44 hours and annual leave was increased. In consequence the shortage became critical. In a research document[11] of the time, it was noted that less than 30 per cent of district midwives had a night rota system: in other words 70 per cent were 'on call' almost every night and yet were obliged to undertake their normal duties during the day. Despite the shortage of midwives, 27 per cent of those who completed the survey's questionnaire for newly qualified midwives gave 'interest and job satisfaction' as the reasons for choosing midwifery as a career.

Shortage of Maternity Beds

The rising birth rate resulted in a maternity-bed shortage which, according to obstetricians at a BMA Annual Meeting in 1963, created 'a grave emergency', the essential solution to which, they felt, was the building of new and bigger maternity units. In 1962, the Government, itself aware of the serious deficiencies of outdated maternity hospitals, drew up a programme of hospital building to be started within the next ten years.[12] In consequence, many new large maternity hospitals/units were built, and in years to come the need to occupy all these beds was in part responsible for the almost 100 per cent hospital confinement rate.

Changes in Training to Meet a Changing Role

In the early 1960s the Central Midwives Board began a complete reassessment of the training and practice of midwives in the future maternity service and at the same time a revision of the rules was commenced. It was being realised that a two-part training for a professional qualification was unsatisfactory on several counts, not least of which was the fact that a considerable number of Registered Nurses only took Part I training. This partial training would either quality them for promotion in general nursing or permit them to undertake the Health Visitors' course. The concept of a single period of training was being discussed at this time, but its content would be dependent on the foreseeable changes in the maternity service and the role of the midwife within that service.

Before reaching any conclusions about changes in training, the Board sought the views of the Ministry of Health. In a paper that formed the basis of discussion with the Ministry, the CMB stated:

> The fundamental problem is to decide whether an attempt should be made to revise the professional status of the midwife by restating her responsibilities throughout the whole range of the maternity service which in itself would encourage recruitment; or alternatively seeking to attract a large number of recruits to work of a more limited character.[13]

Had the decision to follow the latter course been made, the post-mortem on the demise of the midwife would have been held long ago.

The Role Defined

In 1966 the World Health Organisation defined the role of the midwife and set out in detail the duties deemed to be within her competence. They defined the midwife as a person who is qualified to practise midwifery. She is trained to give the necessary care and advice to women during pregnancy, labour and the post-natal period, to conduct normal deliveries on her own responsibility, and to care for the newly born infant. At all times she must be able to recognise the warnings signs of abnormal or potentially abnormal conditions which necessitate referral to a doctor, and to carry out emergency measures in the absence of medical help. She may practice in hospitals, health units or domiciliary services.[14]

This definition was adopted by the Central Midwives Board.

Further Changes in Obstetric and Midwifery Practice

The late 1960s saw the introduction of a new phenomenon in the form of 'shared care'. Previously, most mothers who were booked for hospital confinement received all their antenatal care at hospital antenatal clinics. When the care became *shared*, the general practitioner 'officially' undertook antenatal examinations during the second and early third trimesters of pregnancy. *If* the domiciliary midwife was attached to a GP's practice, she would share the care. However, a large number of domiciliary midwives remained geographically based (i.e. operating from within a circumscribed area) and so most of them had no clinical contact during the pregnancy with mothers booked for hospital confinement. Not only was care fragmented for the mothers, but this exclusion of the midwife from antenatal care, together with the still-rising hospital confinement rate, brought about an under-utilisation of the midwife's skills. Her role in antenatal care and mothercraft teaching became limited to the small number of mothers booked with her for home confinement, whereas her role in providing postnatal nursing care for mothers sent out of hospital increased.

Midwifery/Obstetrics in the 1970s

The role of the midwife in the 1970s must be seen against a background of continuing technological advances and increasing obstetric intervention. A *childbirth revolution* took place in the late 1960s and early 1970s which not only significantly affected the mothers, but also so profoundly changed the clinical role of the midwife that by the end of the decade her demise was predicted. So great was the change in hospital practice that a midwife who trained during this period was conditioned to seeing her role as that of assistant to the doctor, a machine minder or technological handmaiden.

Induction of labour became almost routine; the change from pitocin to syntocinon as the induction agent made this procedure easier and relatively safer. Artificial rupture of the membranes was performed following the setting up of the syntocinon infusion, and together these techniques confined the mother to bed for the remainder of the labour. In 1970 IVAC machines began to be used which electronically delivered a predetermined dose of syntocinon intravenously. This was accurate and time-saving, but it meant that less and less of the midwife's time was actually spent at the mother's bedside.

Up to this time progress of the labour, together with the objective and subjective responses of the mother and fetus, were recorded in words, but in the early 1970s *partograms* were introduced by obstetricians, with whom they became very popular. A partogram provides a graphical recording of the physical data related to the labour. Thus physical progress can be demonstrated clearly and can be seen at a glance, but the subjective responses and psychological state and needs of the mother cannot be recorded on this chart. Space was not allocated on the chart for such vital information, and so the assumption must be made that this was seen as irrelevant by the obstetricians who adapted this chart (originally designed for use in what was then Rhodesia).

Technological Developments: Pros and Cons

Pharmacologically controlled labours were relatively rapid, and machines such as the Cardiff pump, to monitor the effect of oxytocin and regulate the dose, were invented and used. Also *cardiotocographs* began to be used, which recorded uterine activity and could record the fetal heart pattern either via an external transducer or by means of an electrode attached to the presenting part. With the advent of these monitors the mother was 'wired' to the machine and so became completely immobilised in a supine position on the delivery bed. Midwives had to become experts in setting up and operating these machines and in interpreting the tracings.

The nature and pattern of the labour following oxytocin induction was different from that of a physiological labour. 'Syntocinon contractions' were sharp and acutely painful from the outset and the necessary increase in momentum was dependent on a regular increase in both the strength of oxytocin and the drip frequency. Such stressful labours called for increased pain relief for the mothers, continuous monitoring of fetal heart rate and frequent estimation of fetal blood gases. The 'Astrup test' was introduced to measure fetal blood gas levels. This involved the taking of a specimen of capillary blood from the fetal scalp, which procedure was technically very difficult and time-consuming (defeating the object) and was a very unpleasant experience for both mother and fetus. Lumbar or sacral epidural analgesia came to be used and 'pain-free' labour was offered. A prerequisite for an 'epidural' is an intravenous infusion. This, and the anaesthetic, absolutely precluded mobility, and immobility and anaesthesia brought their own effects, complications and hazards. The need for forceps delivery with episiotomy increased considerably because of the loss of sensation and urge to push. This proportionately reduced the number of normal deliveries, and the midwife's role moved even further away from assisting the mother to give birth towards the subordinate role of assistant to the obstetrician and anaesthetist. This was recognised by a consultant anaesthetist who suggested that 'an epidural rate of 40% might be considered as really necessary'. That being so, he acknowledged that 'midwives might feel cheated of their role', and so he advised that to help them achieve a 'normal' delivery they should use 'judicial application of fundal pressure and digital rotation of the fetal head'.[15] As anaesthetists became more skilful in the technique of epidural analgesia and with the timing of 'topping-up' doses, so the incidence of forceps deliveries declined. In 1971 the Central Midwives Board extended the role of the midwife by sanctioning her active participation in epidural blocks. Experienced midwives became licensed to introduce local anaesthesia into the epidural space via the catheter *in situ* so as to maintain the analgesic effect. In 1977 the Board approved the removal of the epidural catheter by the midwife, providing she had been instructed and had proved herself competent in the technique.[16]

All these technological innovations increased medical intervention and demanded a greater obstetric presence on the labour ward. Clinical observation and judgement, on the part of midwives and doctors, came to be much less exercised and therefore less valued. The traditional clinical skills of the midwife were denied to the mother by the mechanisation of birth. Attention was focused primarily on the machinery and on the uterus, which was no longer being allowed to perform 'according to its cellular intelligence',[17] but was made obedient to machine-delivered drug stimulants.

So nearly did physiological labour disappear in many hospitals that the CMB in 1974 issued a statement of policy on the subject. It stressed that pupil midwives must receive instruction in the management of natural birth in addition to active management techniques.[18]

Re-assessment of the Midwife's Role

That the midwife's skills were underutilised as a result of a falling birth rate, a hospital confinement rate of over 95 per cent, and unprecedented doctor involvement was recognised nationally as a matter for concern. Accordingly the Department of Health and Social Security produced a consultation paper, 'The Future Role of the Midwife'.[19] The document highlighted certain aspects of care and viewed them as an extension of the midwife's role. These included pregnancy testing, fitting of contraceptive devices, advice and counselling in family planning, abortion and sex education. Emotional and psychological support, 'increasingly needed during technological childbirth', was emphasised, in addition to physical care, and also the midwife was to be aware of and involve herself more fully with the increasing number of psychosocial problems with which mothers were presenting. Health education and parentcraft teaching were to become a specific part of the midwife's role, and she was to give structured group teaching as well as the longstanding one-to-one teaching. The hospital midwife was described as part of the 'obstetric team' and the community midwife became part of the 'primary health care team' of GP, District Nurse, and Health Visitor, with whom she had to relate to ensure continuity of care for mother and baby. This 'political' document sidestepped the main issue of the midwife as a professional practitioner trained and able to provide antenatal, intra-partum and post-partum care on her own responsibility in normal cases, and introduced 'fringe' activities as a substitute.

Because the number of home confinements was relatively small and the number of early discharges from hospital relatively high, the community midwives were more clearly to be seen as being in danger of becoming *maternity nurses* giving post-partum care only. Community midwives were responsible for only 11.4 per cent of the total births in 1972, 9.3 per cent in 1973, 8.4 per cent in 1974 and 7.5 per cent in 1975. The proportion of home births was less than 5 per cent, the remainder being conducted by the community midwives in general-practitioner units.[20] Their antenatal care-giving was of necessity minimal, because of the closure of local-authority maternity welfare clinics under the 1974 NHS Reorganisation Act. In an attempt to counteract this serious situation the Reorganisation Act provided the opportunity for 'integration' of hospital and community midwifery services under one Midwife-Manager who would in future be responsible for the total midwifery service. In effect the intention was that community midwives should work on occasion in hospital in order to update their knowledge on current obstetric practice, maintain their antenatal and delivery skills and provide the necessary workforce; and the hospital midwives would transfer to the community service for short periods. This concept, though sound in principle, was impracticable to implement. For various financial, administrative, geographical and personal reasons it proved to be unacceptable to the midwives themselves — with very few exceptions.

Obstetric Trends Affecting Domiciliary Training

As early as 1970 the decreasing number of home births made it necessary to reduce to six the statutory number of domiciliary deliveries to be conducted by pupil midwives. However, even this small number could not be achieved in some areas and concessions had to be made. In fact in the following year the CMB decided against specifying the exact number of domiciliary deliveries to be undertaken by a pupil midwife but rather emphasised that the pupil should have experience in all aspects of postnatal care up to and including the 28th day (CMB Report, 31 March 1971). This was the first time that such extended visiting of the mother and neonate had been required and it gave the pupils valuable insight into the longer-term problems encountered by some mothers.

CMB 'Approvals'

The time-honoured 'gas-and-air' analgesia was withdrawn in 1970 in favour of Entonox (nitrous oxide and oxygen). The analgesic drug pentazocine (Fortral) was approved for use by midwives without medical prescription. In 1970 the CMB also officially authorised midwives who had been taught and adjudged competent to suture the perineum. This procedure had been carried out by midwives in some hospitals and districts for many years prior to this.

Because, in the 1970s, the traditional skills of the midwife were being replaced by more technical tasks, and extended to cover some medical skills, the Board were asked to define the limits of practice in respect of the setting up of intravenous infusions by midwives. In their reply, quoted on the 1978 Annual Report of the CMB, they gave the following advice.

> In the Board's view the giving of intravenous injections is a procedure *within* the province of a midwife provided she has been properly instructed, and her employing authority is satisfied as to her competence. Similarly the setting up of an intravenous infusion *on medical authority* would be regarded as being *within the proper sphere of the midwife*, although the Board would not expect her to initiate such a procedure on her own behalf [our italics].

As intravenous infusions were a standard part of almost every labour at this time, the routine task of setting them up greatly increased the work of doctors. It is therefore understandable that consideration was given to the midwife's undertaking the procedure. Although the Board sanctioned it as an extended duty of the hospital midwife, it is surprising that they had reservations about her doing so on her own initiative. Having agreed to authorise her to do this, it would then seem logical for them to allow her to carry it out when she found herself in an emergency situation where such an act could be a life-saving measure.

Perceptions of the Changing Role

Because of the widespread concern that the midwife might, by force of medical, economic and political circumstances, lose the vocational and personal-care aspects of her work that have motivated her historically, midwife teacher students were asked how they perceived the changing role of the midwife. Their comments revealed a polarisation of views. Some saw midwives as 'losing status, becoming handmaidens to obstetricians, in a job rather than a vocation, affected by trade union influences, losing identity, no longer practitioners in their own right and enjoying less job satisfaction'. By contrast others saw technology as an extension and a new dimension to the midwife's repertoire. They perceived midwives as 'mini-obstetricians needing greater expertise in advanced technical matters, as becoming one of a health team and moving freely between hospital maternity unit and community'. They would need 'expertise in management and in the behavioural and social sciences and in genetic counselling'.[21]

Advanced Courses for Midwives

From September 1972, courses for the Midwife Teachers' Diploma were lengthened to a full year of three academic terms. A new course in preparation for an Advanced Diploma in Midwifery was set up, which was clinically orientated and designed to deepen the knowledge of senior midwives in clinical practice.

Community Midwives Ignored

A document entitled *Reorganisation of Group Practice* was published in October 1971. This included the Health Visitor, the District Nurse and the State Enrolled Nurse as comprising the community nursing team, but it excluded any mention of the midwife. The Central Midwives Board was concerned about this omission, as they saw the midwife as being an integral part of the group-practice team. It is possible that rather than including her as a professional with a separate identity, the midwife was included in the category of 'nurse'. The Report mentions, for example, that care of discharged mothers and babies would be given 'by the doctor and nurse of the group practice'.[22]

Midwife Chairman of the Board

For seventy years the Chairman of the Central Midwives Board had been a male obstetrician, but in April 1973 Miss Margaret Farrer was elected as its first Midwife Chairman. Miss Farrer held this office until she retired. Then, for the second time, a midwife (Miss N.M. Hickey) was elected, and she continued as Chairman until the CMB handed over its functions to the new statutory bodies in 1983.

The Reaction of the CMB to the Briggs Concept

The Committee on Nursing published its report in 1972 (the Briggs Report). This concluded that in the interest of the profession there should be one single statutory organisation for shared policy making to replace the existing statutory and non-statutory bodies. This concept would bring about fundamental and far-reaching changes in the whole professional structure of education, control and government of all nurses, midwives and health visitors. Such a concept immediately engendered dismay among midwives. In their response to the Report the Central Midwives Board stressed that in their view it was imperative that the professional identity of the midwife should be maintained and that the present statutory differences between nurses and midwives should be observed. They emphasised that midwifery was not, and should not be, merely a branch of nursing, but was a separate and distinct profession. They considered that 'the unique position of midwives, who have a greater degree of clinical responsibility and independence in their "limited form of practice" than that given to nurses' should be recognised.'[20] In 1978, through their representative on the Committee set up to consider the implementation of the Briggs recommendations, the Board repeated their 'growing concern' that 'the independence of the midwifery profession is likely to be engulfed in the statutory framework that is being proposed and that this may contribute to deterioration in the standard of care provided for mothers and babies'.[23]

The Nurses, Midwives and Health Visitors Act was finally passed late in 1979, but earlier in that year, when the Bill was going through the Committee stages in the House of Commons, the CMB still upheld their original opposition to the Briggs concept of the merger of the profession of midwifery with that of general nursing.[24]

Social Legislation and the Midwife

In the 1970s there were significant changes in social legislation, which arose from changing social conditions and affected all health professionals including midwives. The Local Authority Social Services Act was passed in 1970, and in consequence all aspects of child care, including adoption and fostering, were transferred to the new local-authority social services departments. The Chronically Sick and Disabled Persons Act, which provides for services for the handicapped, including children, was also passed in 1970. The Adoption Act of 1976 revoked all previous Adoption Acts. The implementation of this latter Act was also the responsibility of Social Services Departments, and therefore the social aspects of health were now separated from the physical and psychological aspects. Hence liaison between local-authority social services departments and the health authorities was now required in order to provide holistic care. The Congenital Disabilities (Civil Liabilities) Act passed in 1976 required that all maternity and paediatric records should be kept for 21 years instead of the much shorter time of 7 years. This created storage and administrative problems, solved in some areas by microfilming.

In evidence to the Committee of Inquiry into the regulation of the medical profession[25] the Central Midwives Board highlighted what they considered to be a deficiency in the training of medical students, the inadequate coverage given to social legislation. Moreover, they stated that problems arose because increasing numbers of overseas doctors, provisionally and temporarily registered, were attached for clinical experience to both hospitals and general practice. The concomitant problems were related to the fact that the midwife might call a doctor for assistance who not only was 'unable to understand or communicate in colloquial English' but also 'lacked even a rudimentary knowledge of the facilities available within the National Health Service, or his legal responsibility having very scanty knowledge of law relating to viable and non-viable fetuses and stillbirths'.[25] The Board also expressed the view that the attitude and clinical decisions made by such doctors could be influenced by their cultural backgrounds, and they pointed out that all this greatly added to the clinical and legal burdens of the midwife.

In addition, the changing social climate, in which marital instability, illegitimacy, and abdication of parental responsibility were becoming commonplace, gave rise to extraordinarily difficult and complex human situations which could have far-reaching effects on the baby. Midwives, more than ever before, had to become expert amateur psychologists, counsellors and front-line social workers, and had to bear the extra burden of communications with family doctors, community midwives, housing agencies, social services departments, gas and electricity boards and religious agencies, in order to obtain support for a growing multitude of women in dire circumstances.

The Midwife and Post-partum Care down the Years

In the nineteenth century, midwives working in villages gave post-partum care to mothers and their babies, but in towns and cities this care was more likely to have been non-professional and given by handywomen, monthly nurses, grandmothers or sisters. During the present century, the part played by the midwife in the post-partum period has developed and changed considerably. It has been influenced by many factors including the place and mode of confinement, prevailing social mores, and changing paediatric fashions and attitudes towards care of the neonate. For the first sixty years of this century, labours were regarded as physiological events, but the postnatal period was regarded as potentially pathological. Medical attention and interest were therefore focused on this period in particular. In the last twenty years, following the advent of antibiotics, this state of affairs has been reversed, with medical control and presence very much concerned with labour as potentially pathological, but with the puerperium as physiological and therefore meriting very little medical attention. Previously hospital midwives nursed delivered mothers according to the policy of the obstetrician, but cared for normal neonates without intervention from the then small number of paediatricians. As babies at this time were separated from their mothers in ward nurseries it was the midwife who bathed and changed them and took them out to their mothers are scheduled feeding times. In the 1970's the great expansion in the knowledge of the physiological and pathological processes of the newborn enabled the now growing number of paediatricians to deal with conditions which could be attributed to the pharmacological/technological obstetrics of that time. Paediatricians therefore took over the routine management of almost all babies.

Up to 20 years ago the main emphasis in maternal care was on the physical aspects so the midwife had a nursing role to perform. This involved routine vulval swabbing at 8-hourly intervals, bed-bathing, bed-panning, making and changing of beds, and serving of meals. Nearly all of this direct care has disappeared because the mother is not now being viewed as an invalid requiring two to three weeks' enforced bedrest, but as a healthy woman capable of early mobility. The checking of vital signs, uterine involution, perineal healing, and satisfactory establishment or suppression of lactation remains central to the midwife's post-partum role. However, her attention and time are now being directed much more towards the psychological and social needs of the mother, baby and family, and this care is now more individually orientated and given. Great emphasis is placed on the emotional attachment between the mother and her baby, and it is recognised that the attitude, example and actions of the midwife can help or impede this process. Rooming-in and demand feeding are now the accepted norm, and the mother takes a much greater share in the care of her baby by personally changing nappies, 'topping and tailing' and bathing, usually within two to three days after giving birth.

Teaching, counselling and demonstration of practical skills are dimensions of her role that the midwife has found to be of increasing importance in an era in which mothers are theoretically knowledgeable but lacking in actual practical experience and know-how, and at a time when the help and support of the extended family are often missing. The midwife has also had to become adept at detecting signs of social or emotional stress and instability, which can have adverse effects on the baby.[26] Emotional deprivation is a feature of the present age and is much more common than material deprivation and much less easy to counter.

The Midwife and Trends in Infant Feeding and Management down the Years

Throughout the twentieth century, statutory regulations have obliged the midwife to endeavour to promote breast feeding. The majority of midwives, however, did not need this official prompting because they favoured this natural form of feeding, instinctively recognising its physiological and psychological value to the mother and baby.

At the turn of the century mothers had very little choice and consequently 90 per cent breast-fed their babies for 18 months to 2 years.[27] By the 1940s the incidence of breast feeding had fallen to 65 per cent and the duration was much decreased. This fall was related to the introduction of formula milks in 1908, to a rise in the number of babies born in hospital, and to the emancipation of women. By 1965 only 26 per cent of women were breast feeding. This was chiefly because many doctors were not convinced of the benefits of breast milk and were willing to respect the mother's wishes, or to suppress lactation if the mother encountered even minor difficulties. Mothers were encouraged to give their babies the extra nutriments claimed to be present in formula milks, and both mothers and midwives were discouraged in their efforts to establish breast feeding because early transfer home from hospital tended to reduce the yield of milk. Moreover, mothers were by this time being prescribed a high-dose oestrogen contraceptive pill on leaving hospital. Many mothers bottle-fed simply because it was a paediatric vogue in the mid-1960s to give a feed of formula milk by bottle on the day of birth and thereafter, and they reasoned that the baby had already been 'started' on formula cow's milk. This early formula-milk feeding, of amounts and strengths greater than had previously been advocated, gave rise to early and consistent gain in weight which gratified the mothers and doctors.

The mothers who chose to breast feed were mainly from the middle class. They were advised by paediatricians to give routine complementary feeds to ensure that the baby received sufficient protein and carbohydrate. By 1971 the incidence of breast feeding reached an all-time low of between 12 and 20 per cent, but since the mid-1970s has shown a slow but steady increase. This is due in part to the demonstration of the dangers of excessive weight gain and long-term obesity due to infantile over-nutrition.[28] Despite further modification of formula milks, the trend towards breast feeding continued because breast milk was scientifically proven to be in certain respects superior to cow's milk, however modified. Paediatricians therefore suddenly began to recommend and support the idea of breast feeding, and advised the discontinuation of routine complementary feeds. In the 1980s the pendulum swang towards demand feeding and away from complementary feeding of any kind. However, mothers can now make an informed choice about the method of feeding.

Philosophy of the Management of the Newborn

Paediatricians have been responsible for swings of the pendulum with regard to management of the newborn, and midwives have been obliged to conform to these trends sometimes against their natural and professional judgement. Management has been polarised between the two extremes of a very strict, almost impersonal regime to a personalised flexible baby-orientated system of care.

At the turn of the century, pupil midwives and mothers were warned that 'On no account must a crying baby be offered the breast unless the proper feeding time be due'. (See reference 29, and also Chapter 8 of this book.) In 1928, J.B. Watson, writing in *Psychological Care of the Infant and Child*, advised mothers to treat their babies 'like young adults and not in a sentimental way'. He advocated 'a handshake or a pat on the head', rather than kissing or hugging which, he said, would 'spoil the child'.[30] In 1929, mothers in Lincolnshire were advised as follows:

> From the day of birth the baby should be fed every 4 hours during the day, with 5 feeds in all during the 24 hours. The feeds should be given regularly by the clock and the baby should be waked if asleep at feeding times. No night feeds should be given from the first.[31]

This advice was reinforced by New Zealand paediatrician Truby King, whose policies were adopted and became fashionable in this country in the 1930s. He emphasised the dangers of spoiling a baby with too much attention, and he warned against undue affection and insufficient firmness.

Schedule feeding remained in vogue in the 1950s and 1960s. The Cow and Gate *Motherhood Book* (1952), which would conform to the then current paediatric teaching, advised 'precision in every detail of baby's care'. The timetable in the manual gave precise instructions: at 10.30 p.m. mothers were ordered to 'pick up, feed and change but do not talk to baby'. But at 5 p.m. 'mothering and exercise time' was permitted. It seems that natural inclinations were not to be indulged. Such feeding, to a schedule, favoured bottle feeding and was a positive discouragement to breast feeding.

John Bowlby, writing in the 1950s, was the first to draw attention to the importance of the psychological and emotional needs as well as the physical needs of a baby. The system of keeping babies in the ward nursery (to be lifted up for the fathers to view through the nursery window at visiting time) was gradually replaced by extended periods with the mother, up to the present day 'rooming-in' scheme which gives fathers, as well as mothers, freedom to handle the baby as often as they wish. A close psychological and emotional relationship between the baby and its mother in particular has been shown[32-34] to be positively necessary for the baby's complete development and well-being. As not all women can instinctively mother their babies, the midwife has an important part to play in teaching parents before and after birth the fundamental need of babies for love and security, praise and recognition, and new experiences.[35] She can stress the positive value of talking and singing to the baby and of eye-to-eye and skin-to-skin contact.

National Health Reorganisation Act 1973: its Effects on Maternity Services

The National Health Service Reorganisation Act 1973, implemented in 1974, radically changed the management structure of the Health Service. Regional Hospital Boards, Boards of Governors, Hospital Management Committees, Executive Councils and Local Health Authorities were all replaced by Regional and Area Health Authorities, the latter often being subdivided into Districts. Each District, Area and Region was to be managed by teams of officers who displaced, among others, the Medical and Non-medical Supervisors of Midwives: with Reorganisation these terms and posts became obsolete. Following Reorganisation, statutory responsibility for midwives, previously held by Local Government Health Authorities, was transferred to Regional Health Authorities. This supervisory responsibility was then delegated from Region to Area or District Health Authorities, and now rests with the Head of Midwifery Services who is usually also the supervisor of midwives. She is responsible for the training and practice not only of midwives employed in the National Health Service but also of those employed by voluntary and religious organisations, by the Home Office in prisons, and by the Ministry of Defence in the Armed Services, and also of those working for employment agencies and those independent midwives in private practice. No longer were community midwives employed by local government and answerable to a midwife and Medical Officer of Health as their supervisors. Instead they now came under the same employer as the hospital midwives, and the hospital Midwifery Unit Manager (Divisional Nursing Officer, as she was then styled) became responsible for both hospital and community midwifery services. This change of allegiance was psychologically traumatic to some community midwives and also to some managers who found themselves responsible for, as well as being supervisor over, a service unfamiliar to them, which had many commitments and work patterns that differed from those in the hospital service. A large number of the community midwives became 'GP-practice attached', and this demanded of the midwife loyalty and commitment to the practice concerned, as well as to the total midwifery service. The worst blow to many of the community midwives was the loss of their local-authority antenatal clinics because, in many cases, the new attachment to GPs turned out to be nominal rather than actual. Many found themselves completely cut off from any involvement in antenatal care or parentcraft teaching sessions, and so they were simply providing postnatal care to mothers discharged from hospital, many of whom were unknown to them. Even now, in the mid-1980s, there are GP practices that do not have — because they do not wish to have — a midwife attached.

Changes and Innovations

Courses for Midwives and their Supervisors

From 1977 a Research Appreciation element was introduced into Statutory Refresher courses. This 'refreshment' at five-yearly intervals remains exclusive to midwives.

Supervision of Midwives. From 1936 the title 'Inspector of Midwives' has been superseded by 'Supervisor of Midwives' and the qualifications for the holder of the post of non-medical supervisor did not alter until 1977. A new Statutory Instrument (SI 1977, No. 1580) amended the previous regulations regarding qualification of the Supervisor.

> A midwife so appointed will no longer be required to be a State Registered Nurse or to have had a specified period of experience in domiciliary practice, but must be a certified midwife with at least three years' experience as a practising midwife, a year of which must be within the two years immediately preceding her appointment.

This came into operation on 1 November 1977.

Induction Courses for Supervision of Midwives. In 1978, in accordance with the Midwives (Qualifications of Supervisors) Regulations 1977, the Board arranged mandatory induction courses for existing and prospective Supervisors. Supervisors are now required to attend Experienced Supervisors' Courses approved by the English National Board, at intervals of not more than five years.

Courses in Maternity Care and Care of the Newborn. Since 1979 the 'Obstetric Module' known as the Maternity Care and Neonatal Nursing Course has became an integral part of the course leading to State Registration. Its minimum length is 4 weeks and its aim is to introduce student nurses to *normal* pregnancy, labour and puerperium, and to this end it is clinically based.

Men Midwives — 20th-century Style

The British Sex Discrimination and Equal Opportunities Act 1975 exempted midwifery from the list of jobs where there could be no discrimination on the grounds of sex. However, the EEC Directives of 1976 banned discrimination in the midwifery profession on grounds of sex. Subsequently, the DHSS approved two pilot schemes, one in England and one in Scotland, to start in 1977, and a total of 28 male midwives were subsequently trained. This was a very small number for satisfactory evaluation of a scheme which could bring about profound change to a traditionally female profession. The DHSS Report[36] on the two studies, published in 1982, showed that the schemes had not run into any major problems, and that the men student midwives had proved generally acceptable to patients and their families and to professional colleagues. However, certain problems were encountered in the London study where patients from varied ethnic backgrounds had religious and cultural taboos on male involvement with childbirth. In the Edinburgh study, primigravidae expressed a preference for a female midwife, but in both English and Scottish studies it was found that age, marital status and socioeconomic groups did not influence the mothers' acceptance of a male. From September 1983, all Schools of Midwifery have been authorised to accept male student midwives into either the 18-month or the 3-year training.[37] However, the provision of chaperones to protect both the male midwife and the mother has been acknowledged as a potential problem. All Health Authorities have been asked to ensure that every mother will have freedom of choice to be attended by a female midwife, and, when male midwives are employed, the Authorities must make appropriate arrangements for chaperonage as necessary. This could have considerable cost implications, and could also cause difficulties in providing sufficient staff, especially on night duty in small units, in order to allow the mothers to choose between male and female attendants.

One practising male midwife has written of his experiences during training and subsequent practice. He states that he has not encountered hostility from female midwives or mothers. He found that mothers were indifferent to the gender of the care-giver provided kindness and understanding were shown.[38]

The Reaction of Mothers and Midwives to Technology

Formation of Professional and Consumer Pressure Groups. Following the Cranbrook Report and the Peel Report,[39] which recommended almost total hospital confinement, lay pressure groups came into focus and gave expression to their views. Their aims included the right of a woman to freedom of choice as to where and how she gives birth. These organisations included Aims for Improvement in Maternity Services, the National Childbirth Trust, the Society to Support Home Confinements, the Patients' Association, and the Active Birth Movement.

AIMS, the Association for Improvement in the Maternity Services (originally called the Society for the Prevention of Cruelty to Pregnant Women[40]), came into existence in the early 1960s when they mounted a campaign for action on five points. They wanted more government *money* to be allocated to the maternity services and in particular for more beds in new hospitals; more *midwives* and an improvement in their pay, conditions of work and training (there was a critical shortage of midwives at this time); more *home helps* for mothers having their babies at home; '*sitters*' for labouring women, to counteract loneliness in labour, which they recognised could cause unnecessary distress and fear, both of which are counterproductive to progress in labour; they also thought there should be more *research* carried out in obstetrics, particularly into the relief of pain and into the psychological aspects of pregnancy and the postnatal period. This nationally known organisation has grown both in numbers of members and influence. As some of their objectives have been achieved, others have arisen and now the Association's overriding aims are for women to have *choice* as to where and how they give birth, and for sympathetic and sensitive professional attendants.

The National Childbirth Trust, which is an educational charity, was also an early pressure group. Its main aims are to educate women on all aspects of childbearing by means of antenatal classes. The Trust prepares mothers for labour, teaching them psychoprophylaxis and other breathing and relaxation techniques, but its most valuable contribution has been to revive the belief among mothers in the values of breast feeding. Its members discuss the facts, demonstrate techniques, provide practical support and encouragement to women breast feeding, and also loan, for an indefinite period after delivery, any equipment that a mother may need.

The Society to Support Home Confinements was set up by a group of women who had been antagonised by the pressure to conform to the medical view that all confinements should take place in hospital. They felt that in conforming they would be subjected to an inflexible technological doctor-controlled system. The Society's aim is to give advice on how mothers may achieve a home delivery, working on the premiss that home birth must remain an option open to women.

One of the triggers to the rebellion by mothers was the increasingly powerful feminist movement which has swept parts of the Western World

during the last two decades. The increasing mechanisation of birth, allowing women a merely passive role, was a serious affront to the instincts
and deeply felt convictions of women. This state of affairs gave rise to
the comment that 'childbirth is not now something women *do*, but
something *done unto them* by doctors' [our italics].[41]

The unexpressed and submerged dissatisfaction and frustration of
many practising midwives was verbalised by a small group of disillu-
sioned student midwives when they realised that midwives were not
fulfilling the role for which they had been trained. In 1976 they formed
a pressure group through which they could publicise their concern in
articles and letters in the national press and the professional journals.
They were overwhelmed by the response from all grades of midwives,
and what started as a gathering of a handful of determined and articulate
midwives has grown into an influential and structured organisation with
almost a thousand members, and one that is still gathering momentum.

They see midwives as *guardians of normal childbirth*, and their main
aim is to restore the role of the midwife for the benefit of childbearing
women and their offspring. This group eventually called themselves the
Association of Radical Midwives (ARM), using 'radical' to emphasise
the need for the midwife to return to the roots and origins of her profession and to her fundamental skills and role. They established objectives
which they formulated as being:

To re-establish the confidence of the midwife in her own skills.
To share ideas, skills and information.
To encourage midwives in their support of a woman's active participa-
tion in birth.
To reaffirm the need for midwives to provide continuity of care.
To explore alternative patterns of care.
To encourage evaluation of developments in midwifery.

ARM set up local and regional groups, and organised study days and
skill-sharing sessions to ensure individual competence in such procedures
as suturing, venepuncture and intubation. They were anxious to con-
solidate these skills, acknowledging them as part of the total and basic
practice of the midwife. They have also become increasingly outspoken
about the political implications of the present and projected future role
of the midwife. National conferences have been held and have been en-
thusiastically supported. It must be seen as significant that, of the
39 candidates who presented themselves for election to the English National Board for Nursing, Midwifery and Health Visiting, three of

the five elected by the free vote of all practising midwives are 'radical midwives'.

The aims of the lay pressure groups and of the professional group, with their stress on natural rather than interventionist birth, were almost identical. This symbiosis has been mutually beneficial and supportive to both 'consumers' and care-givers.

Private Midwives

The medicalisation of pregnancy and labour, and the subtle takeover even of the normal process by some doctors provoked a reaction on the part of a small number of midwives to opt out of the State system and set up in private practice. Convinced of the value of the traditional supportive role of the midwife, these independent practitioners have met a need among women. They offer total and individualised care, having made themselves experts in every facet of normal midwifery and normal neonatology in order to give positive guidance throughout the pregnancy, birth and recovery period. After a long and searching interview they book mothers who meet the low-risk criteria and they work with General Practitioner-obstetricians willing to give maternity medical care. By performing antenatal examinations in the mother's own home, these midwives are able to establish a relationship with the mother and her family and so provide not only physical care but also psychological and social support. They motivate the mothers towards fitness during pregnancy through diet, exercise, yoga and other relaxation techniques. Independent practice is very demanding physically, mentally and financially on the midwives. These midwives have to provide all their own equipment, their transport is unsubsidised, and their income is somewhat erratic and not necessarily guaranteed. Their reward is in assisting the mother to give birth, having had respect for her wishes and preferences, and in sharing the mother's emotional satisfaction. The ideal would be for two or more independent midwives to work as a team so that at least one is available and 'on call' at all times. This independent practice, where mothers can arrange to have their babies at home with the midwife of their choice, is akin to the type of domiciliary practice that was lost when 100 per cent hospital confinement was advocated.

Differing Perceptions of Need

At the time when pressure groups and the Radical Midwives organisations were gaining strength, a Conference was convened (in 1979) in Glasgow under the title 'Needs and Expectations in Obstetrics'. Its aim was to underline those aspects of obstetric services about which expectant mothers and clinicians had differing perceptions of need. The views of all those involved with childbirth were sought. These included consultant obstetricians, midwives, general practitioners, consumers and the Medical Research Council's Sociology Unit. The views expressed divided the participants into those (mainly doctors) who perceived childbirth as 'pathological and scientific' and those (mainly midwives and lay persons) who perceived it as natural and physiological. All the doctors spoke in favour of birth technology and delivery in a consultant or GP unit. The speaker for the consumers expressed the conviction that 'whatever arguments were put forward to the contrary it was a fact that the experience of pregnancy and childbirth was a biological process set about with many psychological and emotional factors'. The mothers, she said, were asking for selective use of technology and felt that they were 'forgotten' or 'redundant' as persons in the face of medical skill. They felt that they lost their identity and self-esteem and the sense of achievement in giving birth. The representative from the Medical Research Council Sociology Unit, Dr Sally McIntyre, confirmed the adverse effects in women that were brought about by high-powered centralised units. She spoke of depersonalisation and anxiety experienced by many women who were subjected to high technology. She claimed that obstetricians saw women as a homogeneous mass and therefore made statements on their collective behalf such as the following by Professor O'Driscoll of Dublin: 'All primigravidae would be grateful of the reassurance that their labour would not exceed 12 hours'. Such statements, she felt, were based on the fundamental fallacy that all women having babies had identical knowledge, wishes, expectations and psychological needs. This clearly is not so. Ann Thompson, the midwife speaker, highlighted the underuse of midwives' skills in a climate in which 99 per cent of pregnancies and labours were doctor- and machine-managed. She stressed the need for low-risk mothers to be recognised as such and to be allowed to labour naturally in a non-clinical environment which, she claimed, would induce relaxation and thus enhance the physiological process. Such low-risk mothers could be looked after in a midwives unit with midwives giving total care.[42]

The Chelsea Project: Analysis of the Role and Responsibilities of the Midwife

At the end of 1977 the University of London Nursing Education Research Unit at Chelsea College were asked by the Department of Health and Social Security to undertake a research project. Its terms of reference were to analyse the role and responsibilities of the midwife and to develop the curriculum for midwifery training.[43]

The initiative for the project came through the Royal College of Midwives in response to concerns expressed by members of the profession. Many midwives felt confused and uncertain about their role and about the future of their profession in the light of the increasing use of technology in childbirth, the almost total incidence of hospital confinement, and the increasing involvement in and encroachment by other health professionals upon the provision of maternity care. This was to be an in-depth study on precise current clinical midwifery practice and on the views of midwives about this practice. They also wished to elicit what practising midwives thought their role should be. GPs and medical staff concerned with obstetrics were questioned as to their views on the role and responsibilities of the midwife. Age and experience and place of work obviously influenced the role perception.

From a mass of evidence and a welter of detail it emerged clearly that both hospital and community midwives were dissatisfied with their role in antenatal care. There was little uniformity in the clinical responsibility they were allowed to exercise, which was particularly small in teaching hospitals. Some were relegated to acting as scribes and chaperones; others undertook the routine observations and checks although these were often repeated by the doctor. Indeed only a few midwives actually carried out abdominal examinations/palpations, but again these were almost invariably repeated by the doctor.

On the whole, hospital-based midwives seemed slightly less dissatisfied with their role in intra-partum care. The majority of labours were still managed by midwives but many felt they were not as free to use their own clinical judgement as they had been previously. Interference with physiological labour brought about a situation where the doctor had more scope for decision-making and clinical involvement. It was revealed that few labours in hospital were allowed to follow their natural course, and so intra-partum care and delivery undertaken solely by midwives was rare. The scope of the midwife's responsibility was often limited by Unit policy, which could conflict with both her traditional and extended role. Many midwives were using newly permitted and acquired clinical skills, such as topping-up epidural analgesia, perineal infiltration and suturing, application of fetal-scalp electrodes, and intubation of neonates, but others were frustrated because Unit policy did not allow them to learn or practise these permitted techniques. These new skills were increasingly necessary because of the altered nature of labour, but some midwives disliked practising what was termed an 'extended' role at the expense of their traditional one.

The main problem encountered by community midwives was their almost total lack of involvement with intra-partum care. Of the midwives questioned, 44 had had no deliveries in 1978 (at home or in a GP unit), and 25 had had 'only one or two'. Some of the midwives expressed regret at the decline in the number of home confinements, and others, sadly, preferred to have no responsibility for home births.

The current philosophy of individualised *postnatal care* on the basis of demand/need has involved the midwife in a demanding and time-consuming system which applies at home as well as in hospital. This was highlighted by midwives in their response to the Chelsea investigation. They felt unable to give the amount of time required to support each mother and help her establish satisfactory infant feeding. This they felt was one of their most important tasks and they experienced frustration when unable to fulfil this vital function. They felt strongly that although auxiliary staff had a limited role, modern mothers required all the skills and experience of a midwife to provide them with the physical, social and psychological support necessary during their vulnerable post-partum state. They did not experience encroachment on this role by medical staff and most of them accepted the involvement of the Health Visitor in extended postnatal care.[43]

Profound Effects of Prevailing Pattern of Care

Anthropologists, sociologists, medical statisticians and psychologists were becoming alarmed at the trend in obstetrics which they saw as being powerful enough to change the nature of one of life's major events and in so doing to alter irretrievably the basis of British society. The very special and vital role of the midwife in society was being destroyed by modern obstetrics, and people concerned with the quality of childbirth and life expressed their concern at her potential disappearance.

The imposition of nearly 100% hospital delivery has not brought about all the benefits once thought *a priori* likely to follow, and has had disadvantages not foreseen when adequate care was a life and death matter . . . Such a centralising policy might involve booking all women into large units with all technical facilities laid on . . . with induction for the dilatory, anaesthesia for the frightened, early discharge usually on the bottle for the majority of babies, and special care for the rest. This might result in the lowest mortality for the least expenditure but it will not necessarily bring about the greatest happiness and fulfilment for the large body of women who choose motherhood as the best expression of their values and on whose devotion the preservation of our present caring culture depends.[44]

British midwifery is an institution in the process of rapid change, perhaps disintegration. In moving from a home to a hospital work environment the midwife has moved from a culture characterised by personal relations, familiar procedures, active family participation, continuity of care, and a large degree of control over the situation by the mother and her family, to a scientific culture which involves impersonal relations, specialised procedures, a passive role for family members and control by experts.[45]

Eight years later a writer to *The Times* stated 'It does not seem to be appreciated by society as a whole that midwives are a dying species.'[46]

For a while, it therefore seemed that members of the obstetric establishment were inexorably destined to sweep away, in the name of progress, the act of childbirth as a natural phenomenon. Their male preoccupation with science, technology and the purely physical mechanisms of birth seemed to gain dominion over the female characteristics of intuition, emotion and instinct, which have in every culture always been an integral part of childbearing. Midwives had recognised that if the erosion of their role continued, extinction of the midwifery profession as an entity was a distinct probability, and they saw the likelihood of their being replaced by a subservient species of maternity nurse. Many doctors already regarded midwives as 'nurses who assist obstetricians' but who have a little more decision-making delegated to them by doctors than do nurses.[47]

Social anthropologist Sheila Kitzinger also deplored the fact that although the midwife still did most of the work 'she is subservient, has lost professional status, job satisfaction and dignity and mothers have lost her individual caring approach'. She urged mothers and midwives to join forces to reassert the social and psychological importance of childbirth, and resist the growing over-use of technology in normal deliveries. 'Obstetricians', she said, 'with their complex equipment were like little boys playing star wars.' 'All this equipment', she asserted, 'did not help mothers to give birth normally let alone happily.'[48]

Disquiet Expressed by Doctors

The 1970s also saw the beginning of a reaction by some doctors against the drive to control childbirth by technical measures that condemned women to unnatural labours in unnatural positions in intimidating surroundings. Obstetricians, paediatricians, psychologists, radiologists, physiologists and general practitioners began to doubt seriously the obstetrical and statistical justification for the high hospital confinement rate and the mechanisation of labour and birth. They questioned the almost universal use of interventionist procedures by which the mother was tethered to an IVAC machine and to a cardiotocograph machine by leads from an abdominal belt and from a fetal scalp electrode. They were concerned about the psychological effect on the mother, who was reduced to playing a passive part in an event controlled by doctors, in which only the negative aspects of pregnancy were being emphasised. It was also suggested that oxytocics, analgesics and even monitoring itself could be hazardous to the fetus.[49,50] At this time a radiologist, Dr J.G.B. Russell, wrote: 'the mother's pelvic capacity depends on the mother's position at delivery. For maximum outlet dilation the squatting position is best. Perhaps the old-fashioned birth stool is due for reassessment.'[51]

Pioneers of Alternative Philosophy and Practice

Frederick Leboyer was among the first to suggest that the ensuing birth could be not only physically but also psychologically injurious to the baby. In *Birth without Violence*, Leboyer advocated gentle, natural birth in a quiet, non-clinical setting. His view that noise and lack of tranquillity and gentleness could have adverse effects on the baby and on the mother-baby relationship was also held by the psychiatrist, R.D. Laing.

Quite independently, Michel Odent (possibly aware of and sensitive to birth practices in other cultures, for example Russia), working at Pithiviers Hospital near Paris, developed a philosophy of birthing akin to that of primitive peoples.[52] Women are given the opportunity to labour physiologically and to follow their instincts about the positions they wish to adopt during labour and for giving birth. Mothers are given the freedom to walk about, relax in a warm pool, kneel, crouch or squat. The non-clinical environment is conducive to relaxation, which enhances the physiological process. 'Body functions are dependent on ease of mind, and ease of mind is more effective than technology in promoting normal parturition and lactation.'[53] Michel Odent expresses the view that the birth process and care of mother and baby should be left to mothers and midwives.

The Arguments for and against Hospital Confinement

The Cranbrook Report of 1959 recommended a 70 per cent hospital confinement rate 'to meet the needs of all women in whose case the balance of advantage appears to favour confinement in hospital'. It also states: 'the *advantages* of home confinement for the apparently normal case

probably *outweigh* the very slight risk of unforeseen complications . . .'
    However, the Peel Report of 1970 advocated 100 per cent hospital
confinement on the grounds that hospital was the safest place for birth.

> We consider that the greater safety of hospital confinement for mother
> and child justifies the objective of providing sufficient hospital facilities
> for every mother who desires or needs a hospital. (para. 248)

> We consider that the resources of modern technology should be
> available to all mothers and babies and we think that sufficient facilities
> should be provided to allow for 100% hospital delivery. The greater
> safety of hospital confinement for mother and child justifies this ob-
> jective. (para. 277)

The report did not, however, present any statistical evidence to support
this policy. Its assertions were based on yearly statistics which showed
that as the trend to hospital confinement rose so the perinatal mortality
rate fell, and a cause-effect relationship was assumed. Because this
assumption conformed with the predilections of the obstetric establishment, they were quick to accept and build upon it, claiming that their
use of modern technology was a major contributory factor. It seems that
many obstetricians were genuinely convinced that this correlation was
correct. In response to the reaction by the women's movement against
intervention and hospital delivery and towards home confinement, a professor of obstetrics wrote of the 'resentment of the medical profession
to the implication that their attitude is uncaring and who point to the
dramatic fall in maternal and perinatal mortality as *an achievement of
hospital obstetrics*' [our italics].[54]
    The notion that the fall in the perinatal mortality rate was due to an
increase in the hospital confinement rate was 'an obvious fallacy', according to a general practitioner,[55] who reasoned that 'the onus of proof
now seems to lie with those who advocate 100% hospital confinement'.
His very comprehensive paper on the home versus hospital confinement
debate argued that the risk of unpredictable complications occurring at
home does not justify insistence on hospital confinement. He cites other
authors who support his argument.[56-58] Doll, Fryer and Follis point out,
from data available in the United Kingdom, that no simple relationship
exists between perinatal mortality and the place of booking.
    Within the first national Perinatal Mortality Report itself,[59] reference
is made to 'the difficulty in making meaningful comparisons; the danger
in quoting selective figures', and suggests that the reader 'draw his own
conclusions from the original'.

Unfortunately, in 1980 the Social Services Committee (Short Committee) accepted the 'safety of hospital' premiss as undisputed fact and therefore continued to advocate total hospital confinement *and* maximum use of birth technology. They envisaged that with more obstetricians, more paediatricians and more machines the perinatal mortality rate would drop almost to zero. The members of this Committee were unaware of the serious challenge, on statistical grounds, to the belief that birth in hospital was safer. This challenge to the accepted interpretation of the 1958 Perinatal Mortality Survey findings came from Marjorie Tew, a medical research statistician. She found that the correlation between the hospital confinement rate and the perinatal mortality rate was so low as not to be statistically significant, and she was surprised to find no evidence to support the pursuit towards the goal of 100% hospitalisation for birth. By analysing data used for the Perinatal Mortality Report 1958, Tew showed that the number of mothers booked for hospital with high-risk factors relating to parity, social class and pre-eclamptic toxaemia were not sufficiently greater than those booked for GP units or home with identical risk factors to account for the considerably higher overall mortality rate in hospital.[60] Opposite conclusions have been drawn[61] but serious doubts have been cast on them.[62]

Subsequently, by analysing all the available data including the Registrar General's statistics and using sophisticated statistical methods, and taking into account variables such as the fact that the *actual* place of delivery was not necessarily the *intended* place of delivery, Marjorie Tew has been able to conclude that 'there is no causal relationship between hospital birth and lower perinatal mortality rate'.[63] She also explains that the evidence gathered in the 1970 British Births Survey gave no justification whatsoever for intensifying the policy of hospitalisation. 'The statistics support the hypothesis that reductions in mortality are more likely to result from improvements in the general health of the mothers and their fitness to reproduce than from innovations in scientific obstetrics, however sophisticated.'[64] 'Birth in an obstetric hospital is much less safe not only for normal births but also for many births with some kind of abnormality'.[65]

Other doctors pursued the hypothesis that several other interacting factors may contribute to the fall in perinatal mortality.

It may be both misleading and dangerous to attribute improvements in pregnancy outcome to our own professional efforts, and to underestimate the possibility that changes operating within society were at least partly responsible for this change . . . Most of us who

practise obstetrics are prone to make such optimistic statements as
— 'We have managed to get our mortality figures down to 3 per 1000
this year'. However, the uncritical assumptions which underlie these
claims are potentially misleading, and we shall be well advised to in-
sist on the use of randomised controlled trials to provide a more
stringent demonstration of a causal relationship between our interventions and any improvements in outcome.[66]

An obstetrician, analysing the statistics, concluded:

Most of the fall in maternal and perinatal mortality has been attributed
to scientific advance and to the concentration of maternity care in the
hands of specialists. However, the improvements in obstetric performance could equally well be accounted for by social changes such
as more women bearing children at a safer age (i.e. fewer very young
or old women having babies); an overall improvement in standards
of living, especially amongst those least well off; a reduction in the
number of mothers of very large families, a general increase in the
standards of nutrition and stature of women; general improvement
in maternal and child care because more people are better informed;
the more widespread use of contraception and to the Abortion Act
(1967) that has allowed many more women to bear only those children
that they really want.[67]

Such a view is supported by data from the Perinatal Mortality Survey[59]
and from the British Births Survey 1975.
After analysing available data another writer concludes:

Although some doctors tend to over-emphasise their own role in the
greater safety of childbirth today, a few are beginning to recognise
that home confinements — for those who choose them — are safe.
. . . Although there must be some uncertainty about the true situation
. . . two points are beyond doubt: that home confinement under present conditions in Britain is very safe for both mother and child and
that the difference in safety for low-risk cases between home and
hospital confinements is very small.[68]

References

1. Central Midwives Board. *Suggestions and Instructions Regarding the Conduct of
the Course of Training for Pupil Midwives*, 3rd Edn (J. Sherratt & Son, Manchester, 1950).

2. *Central Midwives Board Annual Report, 1952.*
3. *Central Midwives Board Reports, 1950, 1951.*
4. *Central Midwives Board Report, 1954*, containing Memorandum to Guillebaud Committee.
5. Ministry of Health. *Report of the Maternity Services Committee* (Cranbrook) (HMSO, London, 1959, p. 17).
6. Lancashire County Council. *Health Services Handbook, No. 16.*
7. Reference 6, p. 9.
8. Central Midwives Board. Evidence to Cranbrook Committee within *CMB Report, 1957.*
9. *Central Midwives Board Report, 1959.*
10. *Central Midwives Board Report, 1961.*
11. Mason, D. 'Some Aspects of the Work of the Midwife', Research Committee of the Florence Nightingale Memorial Committee (7 Grosvenor Crescent, London, SW1), 1963.
12. HMSO. *A Hospital Plan for England and Wales* (HMSO, London, 1962).
13. *Central Midwives Board Report, 1964* (Discussion Paper).
14. World Health Organisation. 'The Midwife in Maternity Care', Technical Report Series No. 331 (WHO, Geneva, 1966).
15. Doughty, A. 'Epidural Analgesia in Labour', *Journal of Royal Society of Medicine*, December 1978, 879.
16. *Central Midwives Board Report, 1977.*
17. Thompson, M. *The Cry and the Covenant* (Doubleday, New York, 1950).
18. Central Midwives Board. 'Active Management of Labour', *Statement to Training Schools*, 21 January 1974.
19. DHSS *The Future Role of the Midwife in the Maternity Services*, CNO (76)20. (HMSO, London, 1976).
20. *Central Midwives Board Joint Report for Years 1 April 1972 to 31 March 1975.*
21. Central Midwives Board. *Investigation into Education and Training of Midwife Teachers to Meet the Changing Role of the Midwife.* (Conducted at Surrey University, 1970).
22. *Central Midwives Board Report 1972.* Appendix F. Comments on Document *Reorganisation of Group Practice*, 1971.
23. *Central Midwives Board Report, 1978.*
24. *Central Midwives Board Report, 1979.*
25. *Central Midwives Board Joint Report for years 1 April 1972 to 31 March 1975*, Appendix D. Memorandum to the Committee of Inquiry into the Regulation of the Medical Profession (Ref: C/G 26/35).
26. Lynch, M. and Roberts, J. 'Predicting Child Abuse: Signs of Bonding Failure in the Maternity Hospital', *British Medical Journal*, 5 March 1977.
27. Fomon, S.J. *Trends in Feeding by Breast and Bottle* (W.B. Saunders, Philadelphia, 1967).
28. Taitz, L.S. 'Infantile Nutrition among Artificially Fed Infants in the Sheffield Region', *British Medical Journal, 1*, 1971, 315–316.
29. Wallace, A.J. *Syllabus of Lectures on Midwifery* (H. Young & Sons, Liverpool, 1908).
30. Watson, J.B. *Psychological Care of the Infant and Child* (1928).
31. Lindsey (Lincolnshire) County Council. *Advice on the Care and Feeding of Infants* (1929).
32. Bowlby, J. *Child Care and the Growth of Love* (Penguin, 1952).
33. Klaus, H.H. and Kennell, J.H. *Maternal-Infant Bonding: the Impact of Early Separation or Loss on Family Development* (C.V. Mosby, St. Louis, 1976).
34. Macfarlane, A. *The Psychology of Childbirth* (Fontana, London, 1977).
35. Pringle, M.K. *The Needs of Children* (Hutchinson, London, 1975).
36. DHSS *Male Midwives. A Report of Two Studies* (HMSO, London, 1982).

37. DHSS *Male Midwives*, Circular HC(83)15 (HMSO, London, 1983).

38. Lewis. P. 'The Inside Story', *Nursing Mirror*, 2 March 1984.

39. DHSS Welsh Office, Central Health Services Council. *Domiciliary Midwifery and Maternity Bed Needs. Report of the Sub-committee of the Standing Maternity and Midwifery Advisory Committee (Peel Report)* (HMSO, London, 1970).

40. Oakley, A. *The Captured Womb* (Blackwell, London, 1985).

41. Tweedie, J. 'Polished Delivery', *Guardian*, 13 October 1974.

42. Thompson, A. *Needs and Expectations in Obstetrics*. Glasgow Conference, 1979, *Health Bulletin*, May 1980.

43. DHSS *A Study of the Role and Responsibilities of the Midwife*, NERU Department of Nursing Studies, Chelsea College (S. Robinson, J. Golden, S. Bradley) (HMSO, London, 1983).

44. Kitzinger, S. and Davis, J. (eds) Preface to *The Place of Birth* (Oxford University Press, Oxford, 1978).

45. Walker, J. 'The Changing Role of the Midwife', *International Journal of Nursing Studies*, 1972.

46. Anonymous letter to *The Times*, 24 April 1980.

47. Walker, J. 'Midwife or Obstetric Nurse?', *Journal of Advanced Nursing, I*, 1972.

48. Kitzinger, S. 'Midwives Have Lost Status' (Quoted in *Nursing Mirror*, 21 October 1981).

49. Parsons, R.J., Brown, V.A. and Cooke, A.D. 'Second Thoughts on Fetal Monitoring', in *Progress in Obstetrics and Gynaecology* Vol. I. J. Studd (ed.) (Churchill Livingstone, Edinburgh, 1983).

50. Belsey, E.M., Rosenblatt, E.B. *et al.* 'The Influence of Maternal Analgesia on Neonatal Behaviour', *British Journal of Obstetrics and Gynaecology*, No. 188, 398–406, April 1981.

51. Russell, J.G.B. *Radiology in Obstetrics and Ante-natal Paediatrics* (Butterworth, London, 1973).

52. Odent, M. *Birth Reborn* (Souvenir Press, London, 1984).

53. Holt, J. *et al.* 'Lumbar Epidural Analgesia in Labour: Relation to Fetal Malposition and Instrumental Delivery', *British Medical Journal, i*, 14–16, 1977.

54. Beard, R. 'Future Developments in Obstetrics Part I. Hospital v. Home', *Midwife, Health Visitor and Community Nurse*, August 1977.

55. Barry, C.N. 'Home and Hospital Confinement', *Journal of the Royal College of General Practitioners*, February 1980.

56. Doll, R. 'The Effect of Changes in the Environment on the Health of the Community — an Epidemiologist's View', *Journal of the Royal College of General Practitioners, 25*, 326–34, 1975.

57. Fryer, J.G. and Ashford, J.R. 'Trends in Perinatal and Neonatal Mortality in England and Wales', *British Journal of Preventive and Social Medicine, 26*, 1–9, 1972.

58. Follis, P. 'The Safest Place to Have a Baby', *Pulse*, 31 May 1975.

59. Butler, N.R. and Bonham, D.G. *Perinatal Mortality* (E. and S. Livingstone, Edinburgh, 1963).

60. Tew, M. 'Where to Be Born', *New Society*, 20 January 1977.

61. Fedrick, J. and Butler, N.R. 'Intended Place of Delivery and Perinatal Outcome', *Journal of the Royal College of General Practitioners*, 25 March 1978, 763–5.

62. Tew, M. 'The Safest Place of Birth — Further Evidence', *Lancet*, 30 June 1979.

63. Tew, M. 'Intended Place of Delivery and Perinatal Outcome', *Journal of the Royal College of General Practitioners*, 25 March 1978, 1139–46.

64. Tew, M. 'Obstetrics versus Midwifery. The Verdict of the Statistics', *Maternal and Child Health* (May 1982).

65. Tew, M. *Guardian*, 20 June 1981.

66. Kerr, M.G. 'Problems and Perspectives in Reproductive Medicine', University of Edinburgh Inaugural Lecture No. 61 (1975).

67. Huntingford, P. *Obstetric Practice: Past, Present and Future. In Place of Birth* (Oxford University Press, Oxford, 1978).

68. Best & Birke (eds) *The Power of Science over Women's Lives. Alice through the Microscope* (Virago, London, 1980).

10 THE REAPPRAISAL OF CHILDBIRTH PRACTICES AND THE RESTORATION OF THE MIDWIFE

Midwives are now being joined by a growing number of doctors and obstetricians who are expressing their deep unease over the obstetric scene of the 1980s. They are recognising the error of classifying all pregnancies as being at 'risk' or 'high risk', and of subjecting all pregnant women to the indiscriminate barrage of modern technology; indeed they acknowledge that routine inflexible policies and doctor-controlled labours and deliveries have dehumanised the act of birth and at the same time have de-skilled the midwife.

> We have stolen from midwives their role as providers of primary maternity care . . . They must get used to being in charge again as practitioners in their own right in the care of normal women.[1]

> If only we could regain our confidence in the normality of the great majority of women and leave them in the care of midwives and husbands, then there would be ample time to put the remaining 20% under the obstetrical microscope.[2]

It seems extraordinary that the majority of specialist obstetricians, who view an essentially physiological process as a disease, have managed by propaganda and indoctrination to convince their professional colleagues, the politicians and the mothers for so long.

One of the principal protagonists of non-interventionist childbirth is the South American obstetric physiologist Caldeyro-Barcia, who has demonstrated scientifically the physiological benefits of natural labour and birth. In his paper on what he describes as 'The modern and humanised management of normal labour'[3] he shows that women who are mobile during the first stage have contractions which are more effective but less painful than when they are lying down. In consequence the need for analgesia becomes minimal. He also shows that delivery on a birth chair (see Figure 26), which prevents supine hypotensive syndrome and compression in the diaphragm, increases placental perfusion and fetal oxygenation, and that in this position blood gases remain satisfactory even if the second stage lasts 120 minutes, providing organised breath-holding and pushing sessions are avoided. He found that, on the whole, with

Figure 26: Modern Chair in Use at Park Hospital, Manchester

A

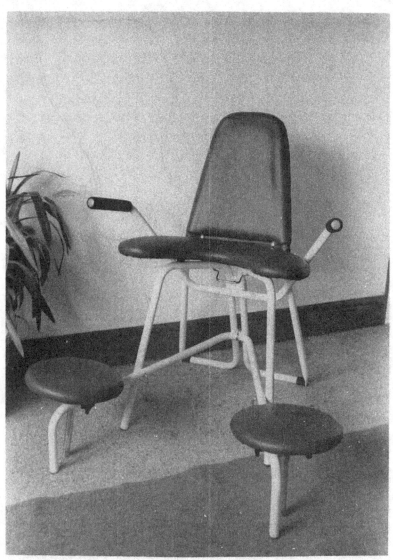

Courtesy of Barry Feldman.

The 'Century' Birth Chair

B

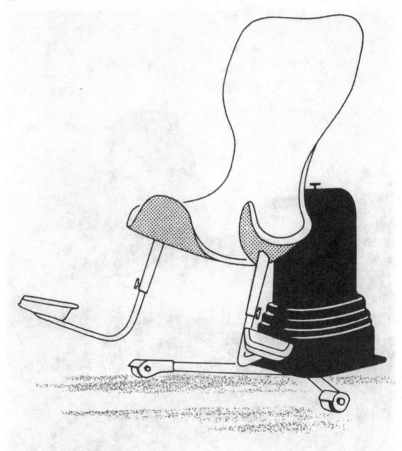

Source: Century Manufacturing Company, Nebraska.

the mother sitting or squatting the delivery phase is shortened both by gravity and the increase in pelvic capacity. The results of other studies concur with his findings.[4-6]

Technology recognises no self-limiting principle — in terms, for instance, of size, of speed or violence. It therefore does not possess the virtues of being self-balancing, self-adjusting and self-cleansing. In the subtle system of nature, technology, and in particular the subtle technology of the modern world, acts like a foreign body, and there are now numerous signs of rejection.[7]

Choice and Responsibility

If mothers are to be free to choose the physiological process for birth, then the following are some of the questions that need to be resolved. When is it appropriate for a woman to take responsibility for decisions about her pregnancy, labour and birth? Or is the appropriate question, when is it *inappropriate* for a woman to make such decisions? Is parental choice consistent with professional judgement and accountability?

Since there appear to be no sound grounds for structuring the maternity services so that almost all deliveries take place in the highly technical-clinical environment of hospital obstetric units, there is no reason why choice as to where mothers have their babies should not be made freely available. They should be given the opportunity of birthing in the non-clinical environment of their own homes, or in a GP/Midwife Unit which allows for other choices to be made in relation to the labour and birth.

Similar recommendations are made in Maternity Care in Action 162 Intra-Partum Care (DHSS Advisory Committee).

Informed Choice

If a mother is to accept responsibility for decisions she makes regarding herself and her unborn baby, her choice must be a well-informed one. It is not enough for her simply to choose between alternatives on intuitive grounds only: her choice must be made in full knowledge of all the pros and cons, facts and facets of the matter; only then can she make a responsible choice. The information she is given must be appropriate to her and sufficiently detailed to enable her to make her choice a real one between real alternatives. The level of information provided must take into account the cultural, social, educational and obstetric background of each mother. Information should not be withheld or biased because of the predisposition of the professionals who give it, and should be realistic and include impartial appraisal of the potential benefits, hazards and implications, as well as probable gains and losses consequential upon the choice.

What is required of the professional is an objective review of the whole gamut of possibilities inherent in each particular obstetric situation.

What is required of the mother is for her to be happy to accept responsibility for her choice, having considered not only the experiential and emotional dimensions of childbirth, but also its physical and obstetric elements.

Although not all women want to make choices, they actually do so (by default) by letting the professional choose for them. However, a growing number of women recognise and resent the denial of choice and are campaigning for patients' rights to be defined in law. They wish to choose where and how to give birth to their children, to receive full information about any drugs, tests and interventions used during pregnancy and birth, and to withdraw consent to routine technological intervention. They believe these to be inalienable human rights.[8]

This rebellion has arisen because the obstetric will has been imposed, albeit on paternalistic grounds. Indeed, a General Practitioner raises the question

> Is it appropriate to allow decision making about obstetric care to remain almost solely in the hands of those who by virtue of making obstetrics their specialty have acquired a perspective that although highly advanced scientifically has restricted their view of the human experience of childbirth?[9]

Some obstetricians choose to withdraw their support from general practitioners (and midwives) who allow their patients to exercise choice as to how and where to give birth. Dr Zander[9] argues that a consultant who does so could be interfering with the right and responsibility of colleagues in general practice to fulfil their functions as personal physicians who are cognisant of the social and psychological as well as the obstetric needs of the woman.

> A review of the official Reports concerned with the development of the maternity services sadly shows how concern for the comfort and wishes of individuals has been sacrificed gradually for the sake of bureaucratic and professional interests and organisations. First the midwife and then the GP have been demoted in obstetric care. Secondly, institutional delivery has replaced home confinement. And thirdly, technology has been allowed to take precedence over the needs of individuals.[10]

Will *normal* midwifery once again fall within the province of the community midwife and general practitioner? If this comes about, it is reasonable to suppose that the primary care-giver should be the midwife, because in the main 'GP obstetrics is in fact Midwife obstetrics with the GP as an appendage'.[11] The writer, after practising GP obstetrics for 20 years in an area with a high GP/community midwifery involvement, came to this conclusion: 'I regard my function as super-fluous, and all ante-natal, intra-partum (including putting up drips and doing episiotomies) and post-natal care could equally well be done by the midwife alone.'[11] This GP could foresee that 70 per cent of all deliveries in his area could be conducted by community midwives, leaving the consultant obstetrician and his team ample time to deal with complicated pregnancies.

Scientific Obstetrics Reviewed

As a result of unparalleled public debate and expressed consumer discontent, official professional bodies (the RCOG, the RCM and the RCGP) were obliged to discuss and review the whole subject of pregnancy and childbirth. Working parties were set up to debate the place and manner of birth and the best use of the skills of the professionals involved — midwives, general practitioners and specialist obstetricians. The Reports containing the deliberations of these Committees were, however, pre-empted by innovatory schemes and alternative patterns of care introduced up and down the country, and often initiated by midwives.

Innovatory Maternity Schemes in the Community

The Sighthill scheme in Edinburgh pioneered *neighbourhood clinics*. Here all mothers attend antenatal clinics at their local health centre where they may be seen by their GP or midwife, or by the Consultant Obstetrician from the city hospital, whose idea the scheme was and who is now in attendance once a month. Mothers with identified low-risk pregnancies attend less frequently than do those whose pregnancies are deemed to be at risk. Midwives can order, on their own initiative, haemoglobin, plasma oestriol, urates and human placental lactogen estimations and also ultrasonic scans and cardiotocograph monitoring. If the Consultant is not available at the clinic, the GP or midwives can contact him or his registrar to discuss any problem cases. Every mother with a raised blood pressure is visited daily by her midwife until it returns to normal level. The perinatal mortality rate has fallen dramatically from 27 per 1000 to 5 per 1000 over a six-year period. However, for Sighthill women not in this scheme the decline in perinatal mortality is in line with the national average of 10 per 1000. The incidences of pre-term labour, low-birth-weight babies and inductions have also fallen. The team at the Health Centre hold a group meeting at the end of each clinic session so that each mother and the plan of her care can be discussed and reviewed if necessary. Although the births take place in hospital, community midwives give continuity of care in the ante- and postnatal periods.[12]

There are other peripheral and neighbourhood clinic schemes in various parts of the country, for example in Huntingdonshire where mothers are seen throughout pregnancy by GPs and midwives, with the obstetrician attending purely in a consultative capacity.

Innovatory Schemes in Hospital

Realising that they were fast succumbing to a doctor-dominated task-oriented antenatal system, midwives in various centres themselves initiated innovatory schemes of antenatal care. These include midwives' clinics held concurrently with consultant clinics, and the reinstatement of separate midwives' clinics. In at least one hospital some mothers are seen by the same midwife, or by one of a small team; this midwife, or one of the team, is called to conduct the labour and delivery. This scheme provides for continuity and personalised care, which includes emotional and social support as well as physical care, and it also aims to respect the mother's wishes as far as possible.[13]

Evaluation of Conventional Current Antenatal Care

The desire on the part of midwives to regain their clinical role coincided with a reappraisal by certain obstetricians of current antenatal care;[14] a recognition that an increasing number of women were presenting with problems of a social rather than an obstetric nature; and a dissatisfaction about the organisation of antenatal care in terms of long waiting times, short contact time with the doctor and/or lack of continuity of care. The question asked was whether routine antenatal care was worth while. Tests (some of which are said to be *sub-judice*[15]) when carried out routinely on all women have been shown to lead to overdiagnosis and conversely to failure of diagnosis,[16] and so the value of such tests for low-risk mothers has been seriously questioned. A study has shown that women who deliver prematurely frequently have high levels of social stress of which the obstetric team were, and remain, unaware.[17] It is now felt that such women would benefit from personalised *midwife* care and support. It is acknowledged that rather than involve women in travelling to a large, impersonal, intimidating hospital clinic it would be in their interest to attend a local or neighbourhood clinic. There the more familiar figures of community midwife and general practitioner would provide the continuity of care that seems to be of great importance and of positive benefit to many women. This care would of course be given in the context of the social, psychological and cultural background of the mother.

Maternity Care in Action — Antenatal Care

Midwives have been encouraged by the document written by the Maternity Services Advisory Committee which was set up by the Government in response to the Social Services Committee Report on perinatal and neonatal mortality (the Short report). The Maternity Services Committee deplored the under-utilisation of the clinical and social skills of midwives in caring for pregnant women and saw 'scope for more midwives' clinics to be established'. The Committee, with consultant obstetricians, consultant paediatricians, senior midwives and general practitioners among its members, reaffirmed the fact that:

> the midwife is qualified to assess both the health of the woman and the growth and development of her unborn child *throughout* the pregnancy. She is able to give comprehensive ante-natal care, including clinical assessment, advice, information and emotional support. This includes the detection of abnormal and potentially abnormal conditions, and referral for appropriate medical advice and care.

Maternity Care: Whose Responsibility?

The question of who should be responsible for maternity care has been raised frequently and over a span of many years. With the advent of obstetricians it was inevitable that they would want to play the largest part, but Sir George Godber, Chief Medical Officer to the Ministry of Health, writing in 1963, felt that the process of specialisation had gone far enough and that 'the first requirement of a specialist obstetric service is that it should deal with that part of the work which *only* the specialist can handle'.[18] He stressed that the midwife and the GP had a significant role to play in the care of every pregnant woman.

> Specialists, as their expertise advances, depend the more on being used, and properly used by others. Even in the specialist work, there is need for the other specialties — paediatricians, physicians . . . anaesthetists . . . pathologists and radiologists; *and constantly and in every case the midwives* [our italics].[18]

Antenatal and Intra-partum Care. Contemporary Obstetricians' Views

In 1979 a Working Party of the Royal College of Obstetricians and Gynaecologists was set up to study antenatal and intra-partum care. Most of the Working Party's discussions have taken place against 'an unparalleled background of public debate about the maternity services'. They admitted in their Report[19] that much of this debate was due to consumer dissatisfaction, particularly relating to interventionist techniques and allegations that 'obstetricians had become over-obsessed with safety in childbirth'. In the discussion on the role of the midwife in antenatal care they acknowledge that her remit is *normal obstetrics*, with the obstetrician concentrating on abnormalities, and in fact they recommend that she should provide antenatal care as part of the team of the obstetrician or general practitioner.

The Working Party did not envisage a striking shift away from the highly technological environment of the conventional labour ward, although they did concede that continuous fetal heart monitoring was an invasive technique which was highly contentious. Although they expressed the view that every woman should have a midwife with her throughout labour, they did not see her as the sole professional taking responsibility for the birth even in normal cases. Implicit in their chapter on intra-partum care was their belief in the dangers surrounding birth and in the necessity for professionals trained to deal with these contingencies to be in the foreground.

Reluctance on the part of the obstetricians to allow the midwife to accept responsibility for care of healthy women in normal labour may be due to fear of litigation against them as they see themselves as ultimately liable for her practice. In 1983 the Royal College of Obstetricians and Gynaecologists, in response to an enquiry, informed the Royal College of Midwives that

> The RCOG *cannot* accept responsibility that within either the Specialist Maternity Units or the GP Units is the midwife responsible for all normal deliveries. The ultimate responsibility must rest with the Consultant (within his Unit) or with the GP under whose care the patient is booked.

In the light of this statement of policy, midwives are placed in an invidious position between what they as professional women know or feel, instinctively and intuitively, another woman's care should be, and what they in their all too often subservient capacity are obliged to do in fulfilling doctor-ordained policies — thus making them appear to be *against* rather than *with* woman.

It is unfortunate that the Central Midwives Board, following the shift from home to hospital confinement in the 1960s, failed to make a definitive statement about the responsibility of the hospital midwife in respect of antenatal, intra-partum and post-partum care for uncomplicated cases. Had they foreseen the implications of the technological takeover, and defined the role of the hospital midwife, then low-risk mothers might well have been allowed non-mechanised birth and the midwife might have been allowed to fulfil her role as a specialist in normal birth. However, the Central Midwives Board, in one of the last documents it produced, did make clear the position of the midwife in a statement entitled 'Limits of the Midwife's Practice'.[20] They affirmed that

> The midwife is a practitioner in her own right in that she takes responsibility for carrying out practices for which she has been trained, either before or after enrolment. She must be aware of the limits within which she is entitled to practise and must take responsibility for maintaining her competence to work within these limits.

This means that the statutory position of the qualified midwife is that she is liable for her *own* practice, thus placing on each midwife the onus of ensuring that every aspect of her practice is of the highest standard. Fortunately the current Midwives' Rules and Code of Practice also make it clear that every midwife is responsible for her own professional practice.

The Place of Birth

From the political viewpoint it would appear that both obstetricians and many general-practitioner obstetricians see hospital as the place for birth, but this does not necessarily mean birth in a consultant unit. They agree that the best alternative for a substantial number of women is a unit adjacent to or within a consultant unit, where care can be given by general-practitioner obstetricians and midwives. Such units can provide a 'sensible and sensitive compromise . . . .'[21] for healthy low-risk normal cases, which constitute the majority of pregnancies. They considered that greater and more active involvement of GPs in obstetrics would ensure that more competent cover was available for home confinements.

An increasing number of GP units and GP-midwife suites are being set up which simulate home conditions and provide an environment conducive to relaxation. Here, labour can be physiological with the mother active rather than passive, having the freedom to walk, sit, kneel or lie and give birth in the position of her choice. The midwife's role is to facilitate the natural process while unobtrusively monitoring the progress and the condition of the mother and fetus. It is disappointing that, despite increasing evidence in support of natural childbirth, and the relentless pursuit of this by both midwives and consumer pressure groups, the Maternity Services Advisory Committee's second document *Care during Childbirth (Maternity Care in Action II) 1983* is ambivalent and conservative in its recommendations. It pays lip-service only to current trends and suggests some flexibility within existing rigid policies. It does, however, recognise that 'for the large majority of women childbirth will be uncomplicated'. It also suggests that women should be allowed to be ambulant in early labour and to state their preferences with regard to fetal monitoring. These are rights rather than concessions, and it is to be hoped that women will exercise these rights.

Innovatory Schemes — Intra-partum Care

Midwives are still the most senior professional person present at over 70 per cent of births but the labours of the majority of mothers delivered in consultant units have until recently been managed according to doctors' policies and dictates. Now, however, in increasing numbers of consultant units, low-risk mothers are being allowed to labour without interference, entirely under the care of midwives; in others, policies are becoming less rigid in that electronic monitoring is no longer continuous but instead is carried out for short periods every hour, which allows mothers to be ambulant in-between if they wish.

Midwives' Units

The concept of *total midwife care*, with the midwife and mother agreeing a plan of care, could also be provided within maternity hospitals. Schemes are in operation, or envisaged, whereby *low-risk* mothers referred initially to the hospital consultant could be identified and referred for midwife-unit care. A team, or teams, of midwives operating from and within a midwives' unit could give complete antenatal, intra-partum and post-partum care, referring any mother with suspected or diagnosed complications, or deviations from the normal, directly to the consultant obstetrician and his team.

The Midwife — Specialist in Normal Childbirth?

What does the future hold for the midwife? Once midwives had won the battle for state recognition at the turn of the century, they assumed that they had secured their future existence and were no longer in danger of extinction — yet once again, in the 1970s, their demise or relegation appears to have been imminent. The attempted total takeover of normal midwifery by obstetricians, with the concomitant discouragement of natural childbirth, created a state of affairs which

deprives the rising generation of midwives, medical students and mothers, of the knowledge that such an event is even possible; and the baseline of *normality* by which we still judge *abnormality*, is in the process of being lost. This medical coup has caused a crisis for the midwives who have suffered loss of identity and reduction in status [author's italics].[22]

Perceiving that medicalised childbirth could become the norm, certain midwives have appealed to their colleagues to recognise what is at stake, to assess the situation and to reclaim their own unique identity.

As the cultural pattern of childbirth becomes increasingly scientific the role of the midwife changes and may disappear completely.[23]

Midwives have recently allowed themselves to wallow in a pool of self-pity, blaming their managers, obstetricians, other health professionals, or even the government for steady and undeniable erosion of their unique role. Midwives must take advantage of the legal framework that affords them the status of independent practitioners and ensure that as individuals they strive to develop the profession rather than be party to its disintegration. If we succeed in developing midwifery and ensure that we undertake the total care of healthy pregnant women, it is obvious that the demand for the obstetrician will be reduced.[24]

We should regain control of the normal process and be seen as clinicians giving ante-partum, intra-partum as well as post-partum care. Revival will only come when each midwife accepts the full professional responsibility implicit in the title midwife.[25]

What is needed is a complete change in the way that midwives have been conditioned to seeing themselves . . . It will take an incredibly strong leadership who have an uncompromising vision of midwives as independent practitioners.[26]

Some lay people appear to have a clear perception of what the role of the midwife in society today should be:

A midwife is unique in the medical world of doctors and nurses. She is neither a nurse nor a doctor — she is a professional trained to work with a large amount of independence and responsibility, calling on the GP or obstetrician when the pregnancy or labour looks as if it is getting into difficulty.[27]

Midwives are legally entitled to act without the presence of a doctor. Midwifery is still a practical craft and its approach, of necessity, empirical. No one birth is exactly the same as another and the midwife's skill lies in adapting her craft to meet each individual woman's labour and requirements . . . Technologised childbirth removes at a stroke the craft skills from midwifery and diminishes the midwives' area of responsibility as practitioners in their own right. It makes childbirth a specialist area.[28]

Obstetricians and Midwives are by definition colleagues not competitors. It is of fundamental importance to maternity services that the midwife is given the deserved recognition and status on which future progress depends.[29]

Holistic Midwifery

For the benefit of future generations midwives should recognise their own potential for giving many-sided help to all pregnant women and total care to healthy women with normal pregnancies; and not allow their status to be further eroded.

It can now be taken for granted that a qualified midwife will possess considerable and tested knowledge, manual and technological dexterity, and practical, social, psychological and interpersonal skills. However, these 'basics' are not enough, because if the midwife is to be of real and special value to a mother she must possess extra but less tangible qualities of empathy, patience and sensitivity to the mother's subjective needs and preferences. With these 'special skills' she has much to offer, particularly to disadvantaged mothers and those with psychosocial stresses. In caring for all mothers she must bring into play her female characteristics of intuition, instinct and emotion in order to enter into the experience 'with woman'. Her virtues of love, tenderness and gentleness should enable the woman to harness her own inner strength and confidence so that her body, mind and emotions work together harmoniously to enable the physiological process to take place unimpeded. An aware, fulfilled mother has a heightened sense of self-esteem and well-being and thus enters motherhood with positive and loving emotions. To womankind the midwife is irreplaceable.

Midwives . . . *Quo Vadis?*

References

1. Anonymous obstetrician in *Sunday Times Health Supplement*, 15 January 1982.
2. Dunn, P. 'Obstetric Delivery Today: for Better or for Worse?', *Lancet*, 10 April 1976.
3. Caldeyro-Barcia, R. *Physiological and Psychological Bases for the Modern and Humanised Management of Normal Labor, 1979*. Scientific Publication No. 858 of the Centro Latino Americano De Perinatologia Y Desarrollo Humano. Casilla de correo 627, Montevideo, Uruguay.
4. Veland, K. and Hansen, J.M. 'Maternal Cardiovascular Dynamics', *American Journal of Obstetrics and Gynaecology*, *103*, 1–18, 1969.
5. Flynn, A.M., Kelly, J., Hollins, F. and Lynch, P.F. 'Ambulation in Labour', *British Medical Journal*, 2, 591–3, 1978.
6. Mendez-Bauer, E. *et al.* 'The Effect of Standing Position on Spontaneous Uterine Contracting and Other Aspects of Labour', *Journal of Perinatal Medicine*, *3*, 89–100, 1975.
7. Schumacher, E. *Small is Beautiful* (Abacus, London, 1975).
8. AIMS. 'Patient's Rights', *AIMS Quarterly Journal*, Summer, 1983.
9. Zander, L. 'The Place of Confinement — a Question of Statistics or Ethics?', *Journal of Medical Ethics*, 7 (1981), 125–7.
10. Huntingford, P. *Obstetric Practice: Past, Present and Future. In Place of Birth* (Oxford University Press, Oxford, 1978).
11. Fogarty, A.J. Letter, 'Home Deliveries and British Obstetrics', *British Medical Journal*, 9 August 1981.
12. Staines, C. 'Moving Forward in Ante-natal Care — the Sighthill Project, Edinburgh', *Midwives Chronicle*, September 1983, 6–8.
13. Flint, C. 'Research Project. Continuity of Care by Midwives. St. George's Hospital, London', *Nursing Mirror*, 16 December 1981.
14. Enkin, M. and Chalmers, I. (eds) *Effectiveness and Satisfaction in Ante-natal Care* (Heinemann, London, 1982).
15. Kerr, M.G. Preface to *Effectiveness and Satisfaction in Ante-Natal Care* (Heinemann, London, 1982).
16. Hall, M. *et al.* 'Is Routine Ante-natal Care Worthwhile?', *Lancet*, 12 July 1980.
17. Newton, R. *et al.* 'Psycho-social Stress in Pregnancy and its Relation to the Onset of Premature Labour', *British Medical Journal*, 18 August 1979.
18. Godber, G. 'Effect of Specialisation on the Maternity Services', *Lancet*, 18 May 1963.

19. Royal College of Obstetricians and Gynaecologists *Report of the RCOG Working Party on Ante-natal and Intra-partum Care*, September 1982.

20. Central Midwives Board Statement, 'Limits of a Midwife's Practice', 2 March 1983.

21. Royal College of Obstetricians and Gynaecologists, and Royal College of General Practitioners. *Report on Training for Obstetrics and Gynaeology for General Practitioners by a Joint Working Party of the RCOG and RCGP*, November 1981.

22. Donnison, J. 'The Role of the Midwife', *Midwife, Health Visitor and Community Nurse*, July 1979.

23. Walker, J. 'The Changing Role of the Midwife', *International Journal of Nursing Studies, 1*, 1972.

24. Newson, K. 'The Future of Midwifery', *Midwife, Health Visitor and Community Nurse*, December 1982.

25. Towler, J. 'A Dying Species? Survival and Revival are up to Us', *Midwives' Chronicle*, 1 September 1982.

26. Royal College of Midwives. Statement by spokesman, 1982. Quoted in 'Larceny of Labour', *Times Health Supplement*, 15 January 1982.

27. Rantzen, E. *The British Way of Birth*, survey by BBC Television 'That's Life' programme 1983.

28. Chamberlain, M. *Old Wives Tales: their History, Remedies and Spells* (Virago Press, London, 1981).

29. Fenney, R.J. Recognition and Regulation of Midwives, *International Journal of Gynaecology and Obstetrics, 17*, 105-7, 1979.

APPENDIX 1: STATUTORY BODIES AND LEGISLATION

A New Governing Body

The Central Midwives Board, the governing body for midwives for 81 years, maintained and consistently expressed its belief that the midwife was the 'expert of the normal'. Its authority for the training and practice of midwives was taken over by the United Kingdom Central Council for Nursing, Midwifery and Health Visiting in 1983, and this new statutory body is now responsible for the rules regulating midwifery practice which will be framed in accordance with the recommendations of its Midwifery Committee. So, in theory, midwives for the first time can control their own practice. The UKCC Midwifery Committee is currently (1985) revising the Rules and Code of Practice and this new legislation will apply to midwives practising in England, Wales, Scotland and Northern Ireland. The UKCC works in collaboration with the other statutory bodies, i.e. the four National Boards, one for each of the countries in the United Kingdom. One of the functions of the National Boards is to implement policies formulated by the UKCC.

Legislation

In addition to amended Midwives' Practice Rules (to be published within a Statutory Instrument in 1986), a revised Code of Practice will be issued at the same time which will give guidance to a midwife in relation to her professional practice.

In future — each midwife as a practitioner of midwifery shall be accountable for her own practice in whatever environment she practises. The standard of practice in the delivery of midwifery care shall be that which is acceptable in the light of current knowledge and clinical developments. In all circumstances the welfare of the woman and/or her baby must be of primary importance.

Midwives are also required to pay due regard to the UKCC *Code of Professional Conduct*. This is distinct from the Code of Practice and is concerned with the responsibility of every Registered Nurse, Midwife and health Visitor to act in a professional manner so as to justify public trust and confidence.

303

The Definition of a Midwife (within Revised Code of Practice 1986)

The definition of a midwife adopted by the International Confederation of Midwives and International Federation of Gynaecologists and Obstetricians, in 1972 and 1973 respectively, following amendment of the definition formulated by the World Health Organisation, is:

A midwife is a person who, having been regularly admitted to a midwifery education programme, duly recognised in the country in which it is located, has successfully completed the prescribed course of studies in midwifery and has acquired the requisite qualifications to be registered and/or legally licensed to practise midwifery.

She must be able to give the necessary supervision, care and advice to women during pregnancy, labour and the post-partum period, to conduct deliveries on her own responsibility and to care for the newborn and the infant. This care includes preventative measures, the detection of abnormal conditions in mother and child, the procurement of medical assistance and the execution of emergency measures in the absence of medical help. She has an important task in health counselling and health education, not only for the patients, but also within the family and the community. The work should involve antenatal education and preparation for parenthood and extends to certain areas of gynaecology, family planning and child care. She may practise in hospitals, clinics, health units, domiciliary conditions or in any other service.

Activities of a Midwife (as Stated within Code of Practice)

The activities of a Midwife are defined in the European Community Midwives Directive 80/155/EEC Article 4 as follows:

Member states shall ensure that midwives are at least entitled to take up and pursue the following activities:

1. to provide sound family planning information and advice;
2. to diagnose pregnancies and monitor normal pregnancies; to carry out examinations necessary for the monitoring of the development of normal pregnancies;
3. to prescribe or advise on the examinations necessary for earliest possible diagnosis of pregnancies at risk;

4. to provide a programme of parenthood preparation and a complete preparation for childbirth including advice on hygiene and nutrition;
5. to care for and assist the mother during labour and to monitor the condition of the fetus *in utero* by the appropriate clinical and technical means;
6. to conduct spontaneous deliveries including where required an episiotomy and in urgent cases a breech delivery;
7. to recognise the warning signs of abnormality in the mother or infant which necessitate referral to a doctor and to assist the latter where appropriate; to take the necessary emergency measures in the doctor's absence, in particular the manual removal of the placenta, possibly followed by manual examination of the uterus;
8. to examine and care for the newborn infant; to take all initiatives which are necessary in case of need and to carry out where necessary immediate resuscitation;
9. to care for and monitor the progress of the mother in the postnatal period and to give all necessary advice to the mother on infant care to enable her to ensure the optimum progress of the newborn infant;
10. to carry out the treatment prescribed by a doctor;
11. to maintain all necessary records.

APPENDIX 2: CENTRAL MIDWIVES BOARD. CHAIRMEN AND DEPUTY CHAIRMEN FROM 1902 TO 1983

Name	Date of appointment	Date of termination of office
Chairmen		
Sir Francis Champneys, Bart., MA, MD, FRCP	December 1902	Died July 1930
John S. Fairbairn, FRCP, FRCS, FRCOG	October 1930	Resigned March 1936
Sir Comyns Berkeley, MC, MD, FRCP, FRCS, FRCOG	April 1936	Died January 1946
Sir Arnold L. Walker, CBE, FRCS, FRCOG	February 1946	Appointment expired March 1967
Sir Alan Moncrieff, CBE, MD, FRCP, FRCOG	April 1967	Resigned March 1968
Humphrey Arthure, CBE, FRCS, FRCOG	April 1968	Appointment expired March 1973
Miss Margaret I. Farrer, OBE, DN (Lond.), SRN, SCM, MTD	April 1973	March 1979
Miss N. Hickey, OBE, SRN, SCM, MTD, DN	April 1979	Until 30 June 1983 (when CMB was dissolved)
Deputy Chairmen		
Sir Arnold L. Walker, CBE, FRCS, FRCOG	April 1944	Elected Chairman February 1946

J. Prescott Hedley, FRCP, FRCS, FRCOG	April 1946	Appointment expired March 1952
Sir Alan Moncrieff, CBE, MD, FRCP, FRCOG	April 1953	Elected Chairman April 1967
Miss Margaret I. Farrer, OBE, DN (Lond.), SRN, SCM, MTD	April 1967	Elected Chairman April 1973
J.S. Tomkinson, FRCS, FRCOG	April 1973	March 1978
F.J.W Miller, MD, FRCP	April 1978	30th June 1983

Members of the Central Midwives Board until June 1983 when its responsibilities were transferred to UKCC and National Boards

Miss N. Hickey OBE, SRN, SCM, MTD, DN *Chairperson* (Appointed by Secretary of State for Social Services)

Miss M. Aynsley SRN, SCM, MTD, B.Ed. (Appointed by Royal College of Midwives, 1980)

Miss V. Crowe SRN, SCM, MTD (Appointed by Royal College of Midwives)

Mrs R. Davies SRN, SCM, MTD (Appointed by Secretary of State for Wales, 1980)

Miss M. Davis SRN, SCM (Appointed by Secretary of State for Social Services)

Miss R.I. Farebrother OBE, SCN, SCM, MTD (Appointed by the Royal College of Midwives)

Mrs J. Greenwood SRN, SCM, MTD (Appointed by Secretary of State for Social Services)

Miss A. King SRN, SCM, MTD (Appointed by Secretary of State for Social Services)

Miss B. Pugh SRN, SCM, MTD (Appointed by Royal College of Midwives, 1980)

Dr A.E. Fyfe FRCOG (Appointed by Royal College of Obstetricians and Gynaecologists)

Mrs E. Halling (Appointed by Secretary of State for Social Services, 1980)

Dr F.J.W. Miller MD, FRCP (Appointed by Royal College of Physicians)

Dr L. McMurdo DPH, MFCM (Appointed by Society of Community Medicine)

Dr A.M. Nelson MB, Ch.B, DPH, FFCM (Appointed by Faculty of Community Medicine)

Dr P. O'Brien OBE, MD, FRCGP (Appointed by Secretary of State for Social Services)

Dr O.M. Reynolds MD, Ch.B. DPH (Appointed by National Association of Health Authorities in England and Wales)

Dr R.E. Robinson FRCS, MRCOG (Appointed by Royal College of Surgeons)

INDEX

Accoucheurs 103, 140, 141, 142, 145, 146, 156, 158, 184
Acts of Parliament
  Adoption, 1976 266
  British Sex Discrimination, 1975 273
  Chronically Sick and Disabled Persons, 1970 266
  Congenital Disabilities (Civil Liabilities), 1976 266
  Emergency Powers (Defence), 1939 232
  Equal Opportunities, 1975 273
  Factory, 1842 136
  Infant Life Protection, 1872 138
  Local Authority Social Services, 1970 266
  Maternal and Child Welfare, 1918 200, 210
  Midwives see Midwives Acts
  National Health Service, 1946 234, 239, 240; reorganisation, 1973 262, 271
  Nurses, Midwives and Health Visitors, 1979 265
  Poor Law, 1601 43, 63
  Poor Law (Amendment), 1834 137
  Public Health, 1848 137
Active Birth Movement 274
Advanced Diploma in Midwifery (A.D.M) 264
Aeginetta 17, 18
Aetites (Eagle-stones) 31, 85, 95
Agnodike 13
Aims for Improvements in Maternity Services (Aims) 274
Andro-Boethygynist 71, 106
Anglo-Saxon
  Chronicle 22
  People 22, 23
Ante-natal
  Advice 53, 68, 69, 142, 155, 184
  Care 68, 155, 200, 216, 219, 233, 234, 237, 252, 259, 271, 276, 294, 295, 296; midwives in 219, 224, 240, 294; shared 259

Classes 274
Clinics 200, 205, 219, 236, 238, 239; hospital 218, 236, 259, 294; local authority 218, 219, 225, 226, 236, 240, 252, 262, 271; midwives 294, 295; neighbourhood 293, 294
  Investigations 206
  Visits 216
Apothecaries 27, 55, 101, 102, 130, 131, 140, 145, 217
  Worshipful Society of 102, 141, 142, 161, 177, 188, 248
Aristotle 12, 84, 85
  Masterpiece of 84-5
Association for Promoting Compulsory Registration 168
Association for Radical Midwives (A.R.M.) 275-6
Aveling, J.H. 18, 123, 159, 163
Avicenna 18

Babies
  Care of 50, 82, 84, 106, 121, 126, 217, 228, 257, 267, 268-70
  Rearing of 68
  Resuscitation of 73, 122, 126, 256, 278
Baptism 37, 38, 53, 59, 60, 144, 153
  By Midwives 30, 53-5, 57
Barber-surgeons 28, 29, 44, 77, 101
  Company of 101, 102
Biblical Era
  Peoples of 6
Birth 1, 3, 8, 16, 23, 30, 247
  Attendants 3, 4, 16, 22, 70, 75, 85, 88, 114, 126, 135, 160, 192, 203, 207, 208, 248, 267, 274
  Chair 9, 66, 101, 120, 121, 288
  Chamber 19, 75
  Manner of: interventionist 276; mechanisation of 261, 275, 281; natural 49, 74, 75, 76, 92, 103, 112, 121, 146, 156, 170, 261, 276, 277, 280, 281,

Printed in the United States
by Baker & Taylor Publisher Services